TECHNICAL PROBLEMS IN PATIENTS ON HEMODIALYSIS

Edited by **Maria Goretti Penido**

Technical Problems in Patients on Hemodialysis
Edited by Maria Goretti Penido

Published by InTech
Janeza Trdine 9, 51000 Rijeka, Croatia

Publishing Process Manager Masa Vidovic

Technical Editor Teodora Smiljanic

Cover Designer InTech Design Team

Additional hard copies can be obtained from orders@intechopen.com

Technical Problems in Patients on Hemodialysis, Edited by Maria Goretti Penido
p. cm.
ISBN 978-953-307-403-0

For EU product safety concerns:
IN TECH d.o.o., Prolaz Marije Krucifikse Kozulić 3, 51000 Rijeka, Croatia,
info@intechopen.com or visit our website at intechopen.com.

Meet the editor

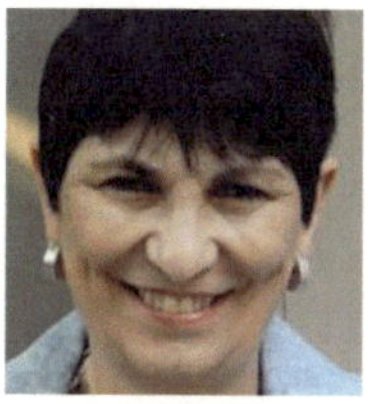

Maria Goretti Moreira Guimarães Penido, MD, PhD is Associate Professor of Pediatrics and Pediatric Nephrology at the Federal University of Minas Gerais, School of Medicine, Department of Pediatrics and Pediatric Nephrology Unit. She graduated medicine in 1980 at the Federal University of Minas Gerais, and obtained her Master Degree in Pediatric Nephrology in 1995 at the same institution, as well as a PhD in Pediatric Nephrology in 2000. She was a Postdoctoral Fellow in the Bone and Mineral Disorders Clinic and Research Laboratory, Section of Pediatric Nephrology, The Children's Mercy Hospitals and Clinics, University of Missouri, Kansas City School of Medicine, US. She is member of the Unity of Pediatric Nephrology, Clinics Hospital, School of Medicine, Federal University of Minas Gerais, Belo Horizonte, Brazil.

Contents

Preface

This book provides an overview of technical aspects in treatment of hemodialysis patients. Authors have contributed their most interesting findings in dealing with hemodialysis from the aspect of the tools and techniques used.

Each chapter has been thoroughly revised and updated so the readers are acquainted with the latest data and observations in the area, where several aspects are to be considered. The book is comprehensive and not limited to a partial discussion of hemodialysis. To accomplish this we are pleased to have been able to summarize state of the art knowledge in each chapter of the book.

This book provides practical and accessible information. It is quite comprehensive as it covers various established as well as emerging techniques and equipment. We wish to thank each author for taking considerable time and effort to ensure their chapter provides state of the art information. We hope that readers achieve the same level of acquisition of new knowledge as we have attained by editing this book.

Dr. Maria Goretti Penido
Department of Pediatrics
School of Medicine
Federal University of Minas Gerais
Minas Gerais
Brasil

1

Bedside Linear Regression Equations to Estimate Equilibrated Blood Urea

Elmer A. Fernández[1,2], Mónica Balzarini[2,3] and Rodolfo Valtuille[4]
[1]*Faculty of Engineering, Catholic University of Córdoba*
[2]*National Council of Scientific and Technological Research (CONICET)*
[3]*Biometry Department, National University of Córdoba*
[4]*Fresenius Medical Care*
Argentina

1. Introduction

Three decades ago Sargent and Gotch established the clinical applicability of Kt/V, a dimensionless ratio which includes clearance of dialyzer (K),duration of treatment(t) and volume of total water of the patient (V), as an index of Hemodialysis (HD) adequacy (Gotch & Keen, 2005). This parameter, derived from single-pool(sp) urea(U) kinetic modelling, has become the gold standard for HD dose monitoring and it is widely used as a predictor of outcome in HD populations (Locatelli et al., 1999; Eknoyan et al., 2002; Locatelli, 2003). However, this spKt/V overestimates the HD dose because it does not take into account the concept of U rebound (UR). UR begins immediately at the end of HD session and it is completed 30-60 minutes after. UR is related to disequilibriums in blood/cell compartments as well as the flow between organs desequilibriums, both produced during HD treatment.

Therefore, equilibrated (Eq) Kt/V is the true HD dose and it requires the measurement of a true eqU when UR is completed. A blood sample to obtain an eqU concentration has several drawbacks that make this option impractical (Gotch and Keen,2005). For this reason in the last decade several formulas were developed to predict the eqU and also (Eq) Kt/V eliminating the need of waiting for a equilibrated urea mesurement. For instance, the "rate formula" (Daurgidas et al., 1995) is the most popular and validated equation. It is based in the prediction of (Eq)Kt/V as a linear function of (sp)Kt/V and the rate of dialysis(K/V). Another approach has been proposed by Tattersall, a robust formula based on double-pool analysis (Smye et al.1999). However, spite this eqU prediction approach is conceptually rigorous, it is not accurate (Gotch, 1990; Guh et al., 1999; Fernandez et al., 2001). Consequently, the availability of a model to predict subject-specific equilibrated concentration will be very helpful.

Although the behaviour of urea is non-linear since its extraction from blood follows some exponential family model as a function of time, we found that prediction of its equilibrated concentration after the end of the treatment session by means of linear models is accurate. In this study, we have shown how to build linear models to predict equilibrated urea based on two statistical procedures and a machine learning method that can be implemented in hemodialysis centres. The fitted model can be used for daily treatment monitoring and is easily implemented in common available spreadsheets. A linear model is based on linear combinations of unknown parameters which must be estimated from data. The first step in looking for an appropriate model relies on prior knowledge or basic assumptions about the problem at hand that should be expressed in a hypothesized mathematical structure. The model can be expressed as $E(Y)=f(\mathbf{X},\beta)$, where $E(\mathbf{Y})$ is the expected value of the output vector, "f " is a linear function, i.e. $E(y_i)=f(\mathbf{x}_i,\boldsymbol{\beta})=\beta_0+x_{i1}\beta_1+x_{i2}\beta_2+.....+x_{ip}\beta_p$, $\mathbf{X}$ is a matrix of input variables and $\boldsymbol{\beta}$ is a vector of parameters that needs to be estimated. In this way a set of potential mappings has been defined. The second step implies the estimation of the components of the vector $\boldsymbol{\beta}$. This step includes the selection of a specific mapping (a 'proper' $\boldsymbol{\beta}$) from the set of possible ones, choosing the parameter vector $\boldsymbol{\beta}$ that performs best according to some optimization criteria. There are several techniques to find a proper $\hat{\boldsymbol{\beta}}$ when using a linear model, being $\hat{\boldsymbol{\beta}}$ an estimation of $\boldsymbol{\beta}$ vector. Each of them has its own assumptions and requirements. Here we explore three different approaches for the estimation of the parameters of the $\boldsymbol{\beta}$ vector. They are: the Ordinary Least Square (OLS) procedure, based on the minimization of the sum of squared residuals $\sum_{i=1}^{N}\left(y_i-f\left(\mathbf{x}_i,\hat{\boldsymbol{\beta}}\right)\right)$ which assume independence on the $\mathbf{X}$ matrix columns. The Partial Least Square (PLS) method based on decomposition schema maximizing the estimated covariance between the input and its outputs, and which is able to handle co-linearity or lack of independence among the $\mathbf{X}$ matrix columns. Finally, we use the Support Vector Machine algorithm (SVM) which is based on the minimization of the empirical risk over ε-sensitive loss functions. In this study, the three regression procedures were used to estimate the $\boldsymbol{\beta}$ coefficients in order to predict the equilibrated urea concentration at the end of the dialysis session. The input variables were the intradialysis urea concentrations (U_0, U_{120}, U_{240}), the predialysis body weight and ultrafiltration patient data. Data analysis and modeling requires performing several tasks. In this work we use the Knowledge Discovery in Data Base (KDD) strategy as an ordered analysis framework. In this sense several steps involving different KDD stages such as problem/data understanding, collection, cleaning, pre-processing, analysis-modeling and results interpretation were implemented.

2. Material and methods

2.1 Data collection

2.1.1 Patients

One hundred and nine stable patients were selected from two dialysis units as follows: sixty one from Unit1 (mean age 56±3.5 years and mean time on dialysis (MTD) 32±12.3 months) and 48 from Unit2 (mean age 58±18.0 and MTD of 42±23.5). All patients were from Buenos Aires, Argentina, and were subjected to chronic HD treatment for at least 3 months. The selection criteria to include patients in the study were: (1) patients without infection or hospitalization in the previous 30 days; (2) patients with an A-V fistula (70% autologous fistula and 30% prosthetic fistula) with a blood flow rate (QB) of $\geq$ 300 ml/min, and (3) patients having consented to participate in the study. The study protocol complied with the Helsinki Declaration and was approved by the Ethical Committee of the Catholic University of Córdoba. All patients received HD three times a week with current hemodialysis machines using variable bicarbonate and sodium. Hollow-fiber polysulfone and cellulose diacetate dialyzers were used (see Fernandez et al, 2001 for more details). For the purpose of this study, all patients were dialyzed over 240 min and the flows of blood (QB) and dialysate (QD) were fixed at 300 and 500 ml/min, respectively. It is known that hemodialysis dose is influenced by several factors including dialysis time, hemodialysis schedule and blood and dialysate flow (Daugirdas et al. 1997). In order to decrease the complexity, such variables were handled externally, fixing their values to control their effects on the equilibrated urea prediction model.

2.1.2 The input and output variables

Blood samples were obtained at the mid-week HD session. They were taken from the arterial line at different times to obtain urea determinations: 1) predialysis urea (U_0), at the beginning of the procedure; 2) intradialysis urea (U_{120}), in the middle of the HD session (at 120 min from the beginning); 3) postdialysis urea (U_{240}), at the end of the HD session.
For the intradialysis urea (U_{120}) and postdialysis urea (U_{240}), QB was slowed to 50 ml/min and blood was sampled 15 seconds later. At this point, access recirculation ceased and the dialyzer inlet blood reflected the arterial urea concentration. Regarding the protocols for intradialysis samples, it is worth noting that originally Smye et al. 1997 proposed taking them within 60 min from the beginning of the session and at 20 min before its finalization. We, however, decided to take the intradialysis sample 120 min after the beginning of the HD session (U_{120}), which allowed us to compare our results with those reported by Guh et al. 1999.
Urea (U) determinations were performed in triplicate on each blood sample using autoanalyzers (see Fernandez et al, 2001 for more details). The urea averages were calculated and recorded with an accuracy of 1% for both machines. For information about the pre- and post-treatment status of the patient, we used the pre- and post-dialysis body weights (BW_0, BW_{240}). Both variables are commonly used in clinical practice to decide the treatment schedule as well as to calculate the treatment dose. These variables were recorded in the same dialysis session when the blood samples were taken.
The output variable was the equilibrated urea. For the purpose of this study, the patients were retained one hour in the dialysis center and the equilibrated urea levels (U_{eq}) were extracted 60 min after the end of HD. The summary statistics for the input and output variables are shown in Table 1

	U_0	U_{120}	U_{240}	Bw	UF	U_{eq}
Min	59	31	21	45.3	0.0	23
1st Quantile	127	64	40	59.4	2.0	50
Median	149	77	49	71.0	2.7	59
Mean	149	80	53	72.0	2.7	62
3rd Quantile	169	96	62	83.8	3.3	76
Max	221	144	98	119.0	5.5	112

Table 1. Summary statistics of the patient data distribution.

2.2 Ordinary least squares

The Ordinary Least Square approach estimates the β coefficient vector by minimizing the sum of squared residuals from the data

$$L(\boldsymbol{\beta}) = \sum_{i=1}^{N} \left(y_i - f(\tilde{x}_i, \boldsymbol{\beta}) \right)^2 \tag{1}$$

where $\tilde{x}_i = (1, x_i)$ with x_i the "*i-th*" row of the input matrix **X**. The algorithm looks for the $\boldsymbol{\beta}$ that minimize (1). This is achieved taking derivatives of equation 1 and setting them to zero, yielding the following closed solution:

$$\hat{\boldsymbol{\beta}}_{OLS} = \left(\tilde{\mathbf{X}}^t \cdot \tilde{\mathbf{X}} \right)^{-1} \cdot \tilde{\mathbf{X}}^t \cdot \mathbf{Y} \tag{2}$$

where "*t*" means "transpose" and $\left(\tilde{\mathbf{X}}^t \cdot \tilde{\mathbf{X}} \right)$ is a singular matrix with $\tilde{\mathbf{X}}$ the extended input matrix holding $\tilde{x}_i = (1, x_i)$ in each row.

2.3 Partial least squares

Partial Least Squares not only generalizes but also combines features from regression and Principal Component Analysis, to deal with correlated explanatory variables in linear models (abdi, 2003, Shawe-Taylor & Cristianini, 2005). It is particularly useful when one or several dependent variables (outputs) must be predicted from a large and potentially highly correlated set of independent variables (inputs). In the PLS algorithm (Wood et al., 2001), **X** and **Y** are expressed as:

$$\mathbf{X}^{N \times p} = \mathbf{T}^{N \times A} \left(\mathbf{P}^{p \times A} \right)^t + \mathbf{H}^{N \times p} \tag{3}$$

$$\mathbf{Y}^{N \times p} = \mathbf{U}^{N \times A} \left(\mathbf{C}^{1 \times A} \right)^t + \mathbf{R}^{N \times p} \tag{4}$$

where A is the number of PLS factors ($A \leq p$) and **H** and **R** are error matrices. The columns of **T** and **U** ("score" matrices) provide a new representation of the **X** and **Y** variables in an orthogonal space. The matrices **P** and **C** are the projections ("loadings") of the **X** and **Y** columns into the new set of variables in **T** and **U**. The **T** matrix is calculated as $\mathbf{T}=\mathbf{X} \cdot \mathbf{W}$ where $\mathbf{W}=\mathbf{U}(\mathbf{P}'\mathbf{U})^{-1}$. In the PLS algorithm, **U** and **P** are built iteratively (Wood et al.,2001) by means of matrix products between consecutive deflations of the original matrices **X** and **Y**. Thus, the **T** matrix is also a good estimator of **Y**, so

$$\mathbf{Y}^{N \times p} = \mathbf{T}^{N \times A} \left(\mathbf{C}^{1 \times A} \right)^t + \mathbf{E}^{N \times p} \tag{5}$$

where $\mathbf{C}^{1\times A}$ is the "loadings" matrix of **Y** that projects it over the new space represented by **T**. The error term in **E** represents the deviations between the observed and predicted responses. Replacing **T** in the above equation yields:

$$\mathbf{Y} = \mathbf{X} \cdot \mathbf{W} \cdot \mathbf{C}^t + \mathbf{E} = \hat{\boldsymbol{\beta}}_{PLS} \cdot \mathbf{X} + \mathbf{E} = \hat{\mathbf{Y}} + \mathbf{E} \tag{6}$$

where $\hat{\mathbf{Y}}$ is the predicted output.

The number of factors chosen impacts the estimation of the regression coefficients. In a model with "A" factors, the $\boldsymbol{\beta}$ coefficients are calculated as follows:

$$\hat{\boldsymbol{\beta}}_{PLS}^{p\times 1} = \mathbf{W}^{p\times A}\left[\mathbf{C}^{1\times A}\right]^{t} \tag{7}$$

In the PLS algorithm the input and output data are centered prior to calculate the different matrices. In addition the input training matrix **X** could be scaled dividing each column by its standard deviation. Thus, regression coefficients estimated by means of equation (7) lives in the scaled **X** domain. The values of the **β** coefficients in the raw data domain are calculated as follows:

$$\hat{\mathbf{Y}} = \mathbf{V}^{-1}\hat{\boldsymbol{\beta}}_{PLS}\mathbf{X}_{raw} + \mathbf{V}^{-1}\hat{\boldsymbol{\beta}}_{PLS}\overline{\mathbf{X}}_{raw} + \overline{Y} = \hat{\beta}_0 + \hat{\boldsymbol{\beta}}_{raw}\mathbf{X}_{raw} \tag{8}$$

where $\hat{\mathbf{Y}}$ is the estimated Ueq, $\mathbf{V}$ is a diagonal matrix of standard deviations for each column of **X** and $\overline{\mathbf{X}}$ is the vector of columns means from **X**. $\overline{Y}$ is the mean of the response variable from the training data set, and $\hat{\beta}_0 = \mathbf{V}^{-1}\hat{\boldsymbol{\beta}}_{PLS}\overline{\mathbf{X}}_{raw} + \overline{Y}$ is the intercept.

2.4 Support vector machine

In previous cases, the sum of squared deviation of the data can be viewed as a loss function measuring the amount of loss associated with the particular estimation of **β**. In the Support Vector Machine framework (Vapnik, 2000), the loss function only provides information on those data points from which the loss is beyond a threshold ε yielding to

$$L_{\varepsilon}^{p}\left(\mathbf{x},y,f\right) = \left|y - f\left(\mathbf{x}\right)\right|_{\varepsilon}^{p} = \max\left(0,\left|y - f\left(\mathbf{x}\right)\right|^{p} - \varepsilon\right) \tag{9}$$

with *p=1* or 2. Then the algorithm try to minimize an empirical risk defined as

$$R_{emp}\left(\boldsymbol{\beta}\right) = \frac{1}{N}\sum_{i=1}^{N}\left(\left|y_i - f\left(x_i,\boldsymbol{\beta}\right)\right|_{\varepsilon}^{p}\right) \tag{10}$$

constrained to $\left\|\boldsymbol{\beta}\right\|^2 \le C$ where C is a user defined constant, playing a role of regularization constant, a trade-off between complexity and losses.
The optimization problem, in primal form, can be defined as follows

$$\text{minimize } \left\|\boldsymbol{\beta}\right\|^2 + C\sum_{i=1}^{N}\left(\xi_i^p + \xi'^p_i\right)$$

$$\text{subject to} \begin{cases} \left(\left\langle\boldsymbol{\beta}\cdot x_i\right\rangle + \beta_0\right) - y_i \le \varepsilon + \xi_i \;; i = 1 \ldots N \\ y_i - \left(\left\langle\boldsymbol{\beta}\cdot x_i\right\rangle + \beta_0\right) \le \varepsilon + \xi'_i \;; i = 1 \ldots N \\ \xi_i, \xi'_i \ge 0 \;; i = 1 \ldots N \end{cases} \tag{11}$$

The ξ and ξ' symbols represent slack variables for those points above or below the target in more than ε and $\xi_i\xi'_i = 0$. This minimization problem can be rewritten in terms of Lagrange multipliers (dual form) as

$$\text{Maximize} \sum_{i=1}^{N} y_i(\alpha'_i - \alpha_i) - \varepsilon \sum_{i=1}^{N} (\alpha'_i - \alpha_i) - \frac{1}{2} \sum_{i,j=1}^{N} (\alpha'_i - \alpha_i)(\alpha'_i - \alpha_i)\left(\langle x_i \cdot x_j \rangle + \frac{\delta_{ij}}{C}\right)$$

$$\text{subject to} \begin{cases} \sum_{i=1}^{N} (\alpha'_i - \alpha_i) = 0 \\ \alpha'_i ; \alpha_i \geq 0, i = 1..N \end{cases} \quad (12)$$

where α, α' are Lagrangean multipliers satisfying $\alpha_i \alpha'_i = 0$ and $\frac{\delta_{ij}}{C} = 0$ for *p=1*. The following Karush-Kuhn-Tucker conditions should also be satisfied

$$\alpha_i\left(\langle \boldsymbol{\beta} \cdot x_i \rangle + \beta_0 - y_i - \varepsilon - \xi_i\right) = 0, i = 1...N$$
$$\alpha_i\left(y_i - \langle \boldsymbol{\beta} \cdot x_i \rangle - \beta_0 - \varepsilon - \xi'_i\right) = 0, i = 1...N$$

Then the link between the dual and primal representation is given by

$$\hat{\boldsymbol{\beta}}_{SVM} = \sum_{i=1}^{N} (\alpha_i - \alpha'_i) x_i$$

where $\alpha_i, \alpha'_i \geq 0$ (Cristianini and Shawe-Taylor,2000).

In our application, for the SVM case, both input and output training data where centered and scaled to have zero means and unity standard deviation. The values of the $\boldsymbol{\beta}$ coefficients in the raw data domain were calculated as follows:

$$\hat{\mathbf{Y}} = sd_{\mathbf{y}} \mathbf{V}^{-1} \hat{\boldsymbol{\beta}}_{SVM} \mathbf{X}_{raw} + sd_{\mathbf{y}} \mathbf{V}^{-1} \hat{\boldsymbol{\beta}}_{SVM} \overline{\mathbf{X}}_{raw} + \overline{Y} = \hat{\beta}_0 + \hat{\boldsymbol{\beta}}_{SVM} \mathbf{X}_{raw} \quad (13)$$

where $\hat{\mathbf{Y}}$ is the estimated Ueq, $\mathbf{V}$ is a diagonal matrix of standard deviations for each column of $\mathbf{X}$ and $\overline{\mathbf{X}}$ is the vector of columns means from **X.** The mean and standard deviation of Ueq from training data set are $\overline{Y}$ and $sd_{\mathbf{y}}$, respectively. The intercept is expressed as $\beta_0 = sd_{\mathbf{y}} \mathbf{V}^{-1} \hat{\boldsymbol{\beta}}_{SVM} \overline{\mathbf{X}}_{raw} + \overline{Y}$.

2.5 Statistical modeling of equilibrated urea

The three estimation procedures (OLS, PLS, and SVM) to obtain the regression coefficients $\boldsymbol{\beta}$ of a linear model where applied to build bed side equations to estimate equilibrated urea from intradialysis urea samples and anthropometric data in 109 hemodialyzed patients. Estimation, selection and validation of the model were implemented in R language (www.r-project.org) (see appendix).Prior to fit a model, the appropriate number of factors (A) ,the best cost (C) and epsilon (ε) pairs values were chosen for PLS and SVM, respectively. For this purpose, a 15 fold cross validation strategy was applied over 70% randomly chosen patients from the data set. In the PLS case, models including 1 to *A* factors with *A=1, 2, 3, 4* and *5* were tested. For each model the cross validation root mean prediction error (RMPE) was calculated. Then the expected value of the RMPE over all partitions was obtained. The model achieving the smaller RMPE mean was chosen. For the linear SVM case, a Cxε 10x10 grid searches was performed. The ranges were from *4* to *6* for *C* and from *0.001* to *2* for ε. A linear SVM model was built for each (C,ε) pairs and the cross validation RMPE was calculated and compared. The smaller RMPE mean was used as selection criteria. The predictive ability of the fitted models was evaluated using a 20 fold cross-validation strategy over the whole data set. The data set was split in 20 consecutive sets of equal size and 19 were alternatively used for **β** estimation and one for prediction from the estimated model.

3. Results

In table 2, cross validation statistics for PLS models with different number of factors is shown. Table 2 summarizes mean and standard deviation of Mean Prediction Error (RMPE) and mean and standard deviation of correlations between estimated and measured Ueq (*R*). It is possible to see that a PLS model with 3 or 4 components are very competitive. We chose a linear fit with 3 Factors because it yields the lowest RMPE with a parsimonious model

# Factors	$\overline{\text{RMPE}}$
1	27.03
1,2	20.69
1,2,3	19.28
1,2,3,4	19.69
1,2,3,4,5	19.82

Table 2. Expected prediction error for PLS model with different number of factors.

In Fig.1 the achieved RMPE of the SVM models are shown for each C×ε grid point. The chosen C×ε pair was *C= 4.2222* and *ε= 0.2223* (filled circle in Fig.1)

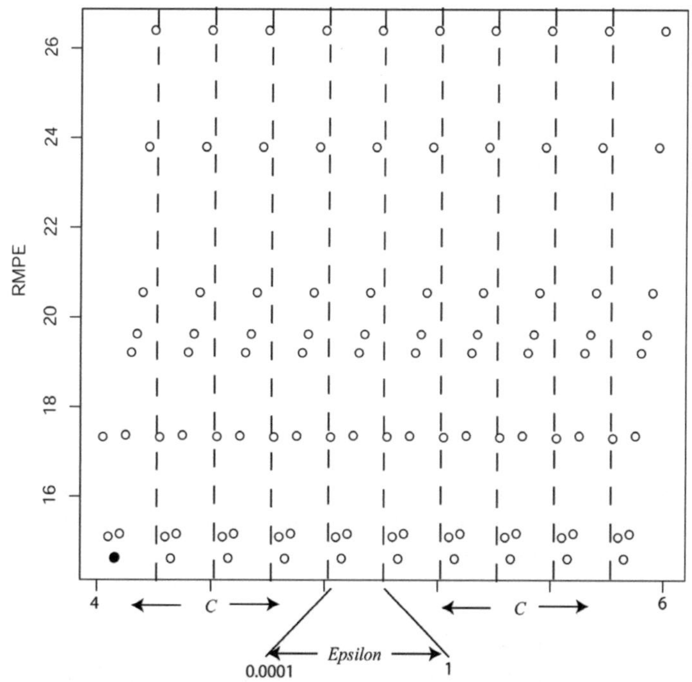

Fig. 1. Cross-validation MSE for each C×ε combination in the SVMR algorithm. The best C×ε combination pair is indicated with a filled circle

Once the PLS and SVM models where selected, *i.e.* a 3 PLS factor model and a SVM trained with *C= 4.2222* and *ε= 0.2223,* the 3 methods (OLS, $PLS_{A=3}$ and $SVM_{C=4.222,\varepsilon=0.2223}$) where evaluated over the whole data set with a 20-fold cross-validation strategy. In Fig. 2 the relative prediction error (%PE) vs. true equilibrated Urea and its corresponding smooth trend are shown for the three estimation strategies. In open circles the OLS (dashed smooth trend) approach, in * PLS errors (dot-dashed smooth trend) and in "+" symbol the SVM errors (dotted smooth trend). It is possible to see that OLS and PLS performs almost equal with a small tendency to increased over estimation for PLS in high Ueq values (the PLS smooth trend curve shows greater %PE than in the other cases). On the contrary, SVM performs better for low Ueq (dotted smooth trend closer to zero %PE). In the midrange of Ueq the three methods performs similar. All the methods tend to overestimate small Ueq values and under estimate high Ueq values.

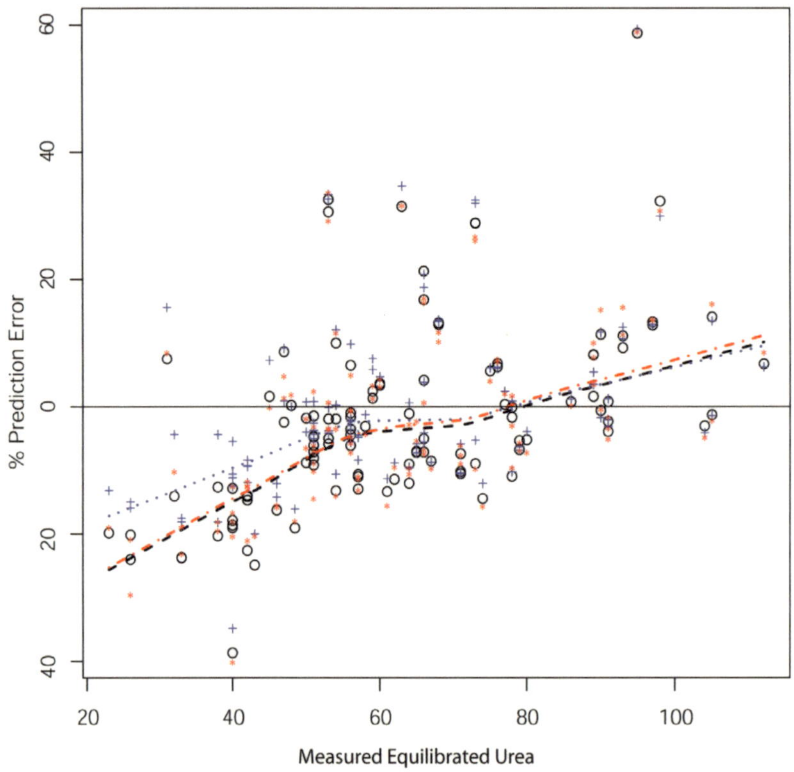

Fig. 2. 20-Fold cross-validation % prediction errors (%PE) for each tested model. Open circles for OLS model, "*" for PLS and "+" for SVMR. The smooth trend curve for each model is also presented (see text for references)

In Table 3, summary statistics for PE and the number of data points which have a %PE in the ±10 and ±20 ranges is shown. The PLS model achieves the lowest %PE and SVM the highest but with lesser standard deviation across runs. In terms of median we can see that all the methods tend to overestimate the response, however SVM presents the lower median of %PE suggesting robustness to outliers.

	Prediction Error			Percentage of data points with %PE in the range	
	Mean	SD	Median	-10≤%PE≤10	-20≤%PE≤20
OLS	0.08	9.59	-2.44	55.05%	85.32%
PLS	0.06	9.60	-.255	55.96%	87.16%
SVM	1.08	9.26	-1.72	63.30%	90.83%

Table 3. Summary statistics for prediction errors and number of data points laying in the ±10 and ±20 %PE interval

In Fig. 3 the distribution for the $\hat{\boldsymbol{\beta}}$ coefficients that weights each input variable ($\beta_1$for U0, $\beta_2$for U_{120}, $\beta_3$for U_{240}, β_4 for Bw_0, and β_5 for Uf) in the input scale (equation 8 for PLS and 13 for SVM) are shown. It is possible to see that coefficient β_5 (associated to Uf) is very variable. This coefficient is mainly estimated as positive by OLS, negative by PLS case and both by SVM. In the first two cases, β_5 was statistically different from zero ("t test" p<0.01). SVM estimation of $\boldsymbol{\beta}$ seems to be more robust than the other cases. In particular, the β coefficient related to Uf (β_5) shows significant less dispersion than in the other models. In the OLS and PLS cases, all except Uf coefficient, show similar behaviour. The Uf coefficient for PLS is the most variant among the rest.

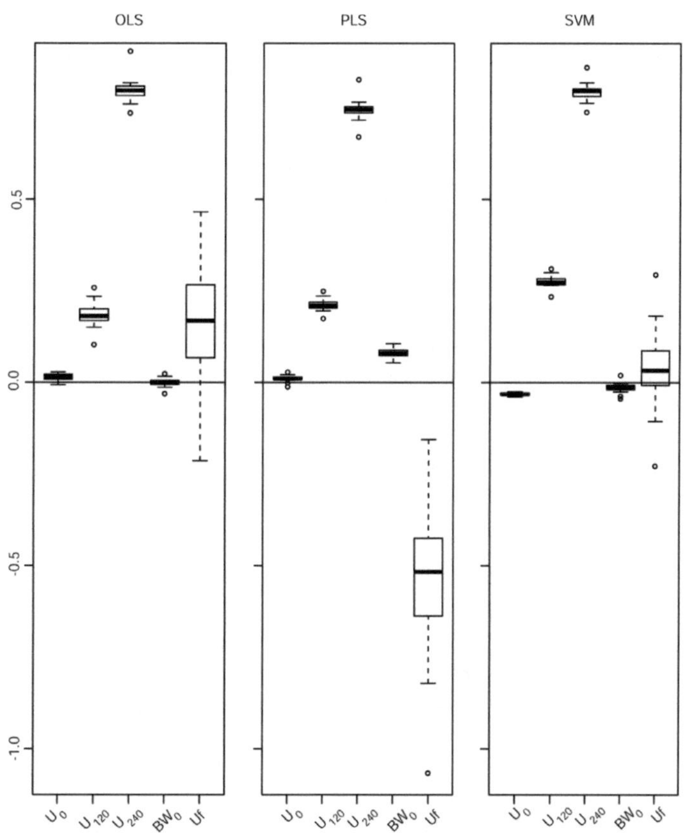

Fig. 3. Distribution of the $\hat{\boldsymbol{\beta}}$ coefficients for each input variable from the 20-Fold cross-validation.

3.1 Bed side equations for equilibrated urea prediction

Final models were built using the whole patients and using the parameters found in the previous section (for PLS and SVM). We found that the coefficients estimated using the full data set (equations 14 to 15) where similar to the mean of the cross validation coefficients for OLS and SVM. On the contrary, coefficients estimated by PLS where different when using the whole data set compared to those estimated in the cross validation evaluation.
In the OLS case the final bed side equation was the following:

$$\hat{Y} = 3.02449 + 0.01381 \cdot U_0 + 0.18576 \cdot U_{120} + 0.79713 \cdot U_{240} - 0.00028 \cdot BW_0 + 0.16252 \cdot Uf \quad (14)$$

In the PLS case and accounting only the first three PLS factors the achieved model is

$$\hat{Y} = 0.84616 + 0.00810 \cdot U_0 + 0.20652 \cdot U_{120} + 0.75386 \cdot U_{240} + 0.06862 \cdot BW_0 - 0.26812 \cdot Uf \quad (15)$$

For the SVM we get

$$\hat{Y} = 4.27754 - 0.03362 \cdot U_0 + 0.27904 \cdot U_{120} + 0.78921 \cdot U_{240} - 0.01210 \cdot BW_0 + 0.02323 \cdot Uf \quad (16)$$

The SVM identify 77 support vectors. This means that the $\hat{\boldsymbol{\beta}}$ coefficients were estimated using only %70 of the data base. On the contrary, the other two methods require the full data set to build the solution.

4. Discussion

In this work we show how to build linear models from three different linear regression estimation procedures relying on different optimization algorithms. Ordinary Least squares is based on the minimization of the sum of squared residuals while Partial Least Squares uses maximization of co-variance information by means of repetitive deflation of the input and output matrices based on correlation. Finally, the Support Vector Machine Regression is based on the empirical risk minimization of non-linear loss function. Theoretically, none of the method requires any specific assumption; however, it is known that if the observed variable (the equilibrated urea in this case) follows a normal distribution, the statistical significance of the $\boldsymbol{\beta}$ coefficients estimated by OLS and PLS can be proved.
Even though all the models predict similarly well, they show different estimates not only in value but also in sign for U_0, body weight and ultrafiltration. Analyzing the "raw" data relationships between these variables (see Fig. 4) and urea rebound $\left(U_{eq} - U_{240}\right)/U_{eq}$ it is possible to see the known [Gotch & Kleen, 2005] slightly inverse relationship (see smooth trend curves) between BW and Uf with urea rebound. This behaviour seems to be capture for Uf by PLS (negative β_5). The β_5 estimated by OLS method seems to follow the positive linear relationship mostly found in the Uf vs Ueq pairs plot. The SVM finds a solution in between, estimating much smaller values for β_5 than the others two. For the case of body weight coefficient (β_4), estimations by OLS and SVM are smaller than for PLS, however, SVM method captures the known small tendency between BW and urea rebound. In this sense, PLS is able to capture known biological relationships while still providing broad ranges for the estimation of the Uf coefficient. On the opposite OLS does not reflect the biological effect of Uf. The SVM method provides an in-between solution providing small estimates of the Uf coefficient. Thus, those methods that account for co-linearity (PLS and in some extent SVM) provide better solutions than OLS which do not account for it.

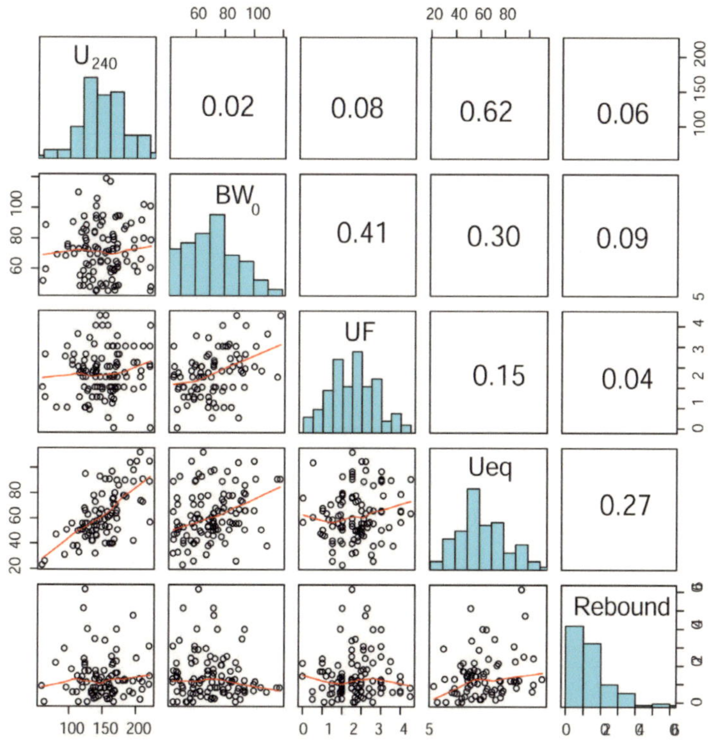

Fig. 4. Pairs plots and correlation coefficients between U_{240}, BW_0 Uf, Ueq and urea rebound.

We showed that by means of linear models we were able to build bedside equations that can be easily implemented in any calculator or electronic spreadsheet such as Excel®.
All the presented methods performed better than traditional methods (Smye et al, 1999) over the same data (Fernández et al, 2001) suggesting the appropriateness of the simple linear approaches. In addition, each hemodialysis centre can build its own predictor based on its own patient population by following the described process or implementing the accompanying source code (see appendix).
In this work we show that the use of an intradialysis sample (U_{120}) provided valuable information to predict the equilibrated urea. Smye et al. (1999) were the first to use an intradialysis sample to model Ueq. In clinical practice the extraction of an additional blood urea sample could be very problematic. In a recent publication (Fernandez et al, 2008) we showed that a linear model built without this urea sample can also provide accurate Ueq estimation. Future challenges for Ueq prediction by linear models are emerging with the implementation of different HD schedule proposals based on the variation of session time and/or weekly frequency.

5. Appendix: R source code for OLS, PLS and SVM linear models for estimate equilibrated urea

In order to apply the R (www.r-project.org) algorithm to build the linear models presented in this work, we assume that the patient data base is stored in a comma separated values (CSV) file as follows (any electronic spreadsheet program allows to save CSV files).

PatientID	U_0	U_{120}	U_{240}	BW_0	Uf	Ueq
1	121	63	47	94.5	2.9	51
2	166	87	68	59.4	1.4	71
3	196	68	40	61.6	1.9	42
4	167	73	43	45.7	2.6	43
5	128	64	46	54.8	1.1	46
6	127	77	50	72.6	1.8	56
7	139	49	28	45.3	2.5	32
…	…	…	…	…	…	…
…	…	…	…	…	…	…

Table 4. Data base in comma separated file format. The R code assumes this file for processing (PP: Body weight)

```
#set path to data directory
path=paste(base.path,"C:/....../UreaData/",sep="")
#we assume that the data base is a comma separated file
datafile="naneofpatientdatabase.csv"
#read file
udata=read.csv(paste(path,datafile,sep=""),h=T)
#load required libraries
library(pls)
library(e1071)
### SVM auxiliary functions ###############
coef.svm<-function(model){
# return the beta coefficients in the possibly standardized space
  w=t(model$coefs)%*%model$SV
  w=c(-model$rho,w)
  names(w)=c("(Intercept)",attr(model$terms,"term.labels"))
  return(w)
}

getScaledCoef.svm=function(obj){
# return the beta coefficients in the raw scale
  if(obj$kernel!=0) stop("getScaledCoef: only for linear svm")
  ym=unlist(obj$y.scale["scaled:center"])
  sdy=unlist(obj$y.scale["scaled:scale"])
  xm=unlist(obj$x.scale["scaled:center"])
  sdx=diag(1/unlist(obj$x.scale["scaled:scale"]))
  beta=coef(obj)
  b0=beta["(Intercept)"]

  sdbeta=sdx%*%beta[-1]

  Intercept=b0-sdy*(xm%*%sdbeta)+ym
  betanew=sdy*sdbeta
  ret=c(Intercept,t(betanew))
  names(ret)=names(beta)
 return(ret)
}
```

```
###########################################
## PLS auxiliary functions ############
getScaledCoef.pls=function(obj,comps=1:obj$ncomp){
  if(missing(comps) || is.null(comps))
    comps =1:model$ncomp
  beta = rowSums(coef(obj,comps=comps,cumulative=F),2)
  ym=obj$Ymeans
  xm=obj$Xmeans
  if(is.null(obj$scale)==TRUE){
   sdx=1
  }else sdx=diag(1/unlist(obj$scale))

  sdbeta=sdx%*%beta

  Intercept= ym-(xm%*%beta)
  betanew=sdbeta
  ret=c(Intercept,betanew)
  names(ret)=c("(Intercept)",attr(mpls$terms,"term.labels"))
 return(ret)
}
########################################

####  Data set for model selection ###
samp=sample(nrow(udata),round(0.7*nrow(udata),0))
seldata=udata[samp,]
kfold=cvsegments(length(samp),15)#15 fold CV

####  SVM parameters selection ##########
scalar=TRUE
RESsvm=NULL
RESMsvm=NULL # cross validation result matrix
#set grid CxEps ranges
C.range=seq(4,6,length.out=10)
epsilon.range=seq(.0001,1,length.out=10)
for(cc in C.range){
  for(ep in epsilon.range){
   RESsvm=NULL
    for(cv in 1:length(kfold)){
        bestmod=svm(Ueq~Upre+U120+Upos+PP+UF,data=seldata[-
kfold[[cv]],],cost=cc,epsilon=ep,kernel="lin",scale=scalar)
        pp=predict(bestmod,seldata[kfold[[cv]],])
        #save squared errors, and correlation
        RESsvm=rbind(RESsvm,
c(sqrt(sum((pp-seldata[kfold[[cv]],"Ueq"])^2)),
```

```
 for(cv in 1:length(kfold)){
        bestmod=plsr(Ueq~Upre+U120+Upos+PP+UF,data=pdata[-
kfold[[cv]],],comps=nc)
        pp=predict(bestmod,newdata=pdata[kfold[[cv]],],
type="response",cumulative=F,comps=1:nc)
        RESpls=rbind(RESpls,
c(sqrt(sum((pp-
pdata[kfold[[cv]],"Ueq"])^2)),cor(pp,pdata[kfold[[cv]],"Ueq"])))

    }
   RESMpls=rbind(RESMpls,c(nc,mean(RESpls[,1]),
sd(RESpls[,1]),mean(RESpls[,2]),sd(RESpls[,2])))
  }

b=which.min(RESMpls[,2])
RESMpls[b,] #print the best parameters
###########################################
##....................................###
#### Testing the final models ############
cv.sets=cvsegments(nrow(udata),20)#20 cross validation partition

model=formula("Ueq~Upre+U120+Upos+PP+UF")

### OLS method ####
coefslmnc=NULL
predlmnc=NULL
Ylmnc=NULL
i=2
for(i in 1:20){
  mlmnc=lm(Ueq~Upre+U120+Upos+PP+UF,data=pdata[-cv.sets[[i]],])

predlmnc=c(predlmnc,predict(mlmnc,pdata[cv.sets[[i]],]))#prediction
  Ylmnc=c(Ylmnc,pdata[cv.sets[[i]],"Ueq"])#real data

  coefslmnc=rbind(coefslmnc,coef(mlmnc))
}
errlm=Ylmnc-predlmnc#prediction error
errrellm=100*errlm/Ylmnc #relative error
#ploting and smooth trend lines
plot(y=predlmnc-Ylmnc,x=Ylmnc,ylim=c(-65,60))
lines(stats::lowess(x=Ylmnc, y=predlmnc-Ylmnc),col="black",lty=2)

###  SVM method ###
coefssvm=NULL
```

```
errsvm=Ysvm-predsvm #prediction error
errrelsvm=100*errsvm/Ysvm #relative prediction errors
points(y=predsvm-Ysvm,x=Ysvm,col="blue",pch="+")
lines(stats::lowess(x=Ysvm, y=predsvm-Ysvm),col="blue",lty=3)
abline(h=0)
### PLS method ###
coefspls=NULL
predpls=NULL
Ypls=NULL
sccpls=NULL
for(i in 1:20){

  mpls=plsr(Ueq~Upre+U120+Upos+PP+UF,data=pdata[-
cv.sets[[i]],],scale=T)
  predpls=c(predpls,predict(mpls,newdata=pdata[cv.sets[[i]],],
type="response",cumulative=F,comps=1:RESMpls[b,1]))
  Ypls=c(Ypls,na.omit(pdata[cv.sets[[i]],"Ueq"]))
  coefspls=rbind(coefspls,coef(mpls))
  sccpls=rbind(sccpls,getScaledCoef.pls(mpls,1:3) )
}
#boxplot(coefspls)
errpls=Ypls-predpls
errrelpls=100*errpls/Ypls

points(y=predpls-Ypls,x=Ypls,col="red",pch="*")
lines(stats::lowess(x=Ypls, y=predpls-Ypls),col="red",lty=4)
abline(h=0)

#### FULL model (final beta) #####

coef(lm(model,data=udata))
getScaledCoef(svm(model,data=udata,scale=T,kernel="lin",type="eps-
reg",cost=RESMsvm[b,1],epsilon=RESMsvm[b,2]))
getScaledCoef.pls(plsr(Ueq~Upre+U120+Upos+PP+UF,data=udata,scale=T)
,1:3)
```

6. References

Abdi H. (2003) Partial Least Squares (PLS) Regression. In: Lewis-Beck M, Bryman A, Futting T (Eds). *Encyclopedia of Social Sciences Research Methods*. Thousand Oaks, CA.

Cristianini, N., Shawe-Taylor, J.,(2000) *An Introduction to Support Vector Machines*, Cambridge University Press,.

Daugirdas J. (1995) Simplified equations for monitoring kt/v, pcrn, ekt/v and epcrn. *Adv. in Renal Replacement Therapy*. 2(4) 295-304,

Depner, T.A. (1999) History of dialysis quantification. *Sem. Dial*. 12:S1:14-19

Eknoyan, G.; Beck, G.J.; Cheung, A.K. et al (2002). Effect of dialysis dose and membrane flux in maintenance hemodialysis. *New Engl J Med* 347: 2010–2019

Fernández EA, Valtuille R, Willshaw P, Perazzo CA.(2001) Using Artificial Intelligence to predict the Equilibrated Blood Urea Concentration. *Blood Purification*. 19(3) 271-285

Fernández EA, Valtuille R, Willshaw P, Balzarini M. (2008) Partial Least Squares Regression: A Valueble Method for Modeling Molecular Behaviour in Hemodialysis. *Annals of Biomedical Engineering*. DOI: 10.1007/s10439-008-9492-1,

Ghu J, Yang J, Chen IU lai Y. (1998) Prediction of equlibrated BUN by an artificial neural network in high efficient hemodialysis. *Am. J. Kid. Dis.* 3: 638-646.

Gotch, F.A. (1990) *Kinetic modeling in hemodialysis*. W: Nissenson A.R., Fine R.N., Gentile D.: Clinical dialysis, 2nd ed., Appleton and Lange, Norwalk, CT

Gotch,FA, Keen, M. (2005) *Kinetic modeling in Hemodialysis in: Clinical Dialysis*,fourth edition,Nissenson,a and Fine,R,editors.

Locatelli, F.; Hannedouche, T.; Jacobson, S. et al (1999). The effect of membrane permeability on ESRD: design of a prospective randomized multicentre trial. *J. of Nephrol.* 12: 85-88.

Locatelli, F. (2003) Dose of dialysis, convection and hemodialysis patients outcome- what the HEMO study doesn't tell us: the European viewpoint. *Nephrol. Dail. Transp.* 18:1061-1065

Roa LM, Prado M. (2004) The role of urea kinetic modeling in assessing the adequacy of dialysis. Crit. Rev. Biomed. Eng. 32 (5-6): 461-539,

Tattersal J, Detakats D, Chamney P, Greenwood R, Farrington K. (1996) The post dialysis rebound: Predicting and quantifying its effect on Kt/V. *Kidney Int.* 50(6) 2094-2102,

Shawe-Taylor J and Cristianini N. Kernel. (2005) *Methods for pattern analysis*. Cambridge UP. Cambridge

Smye S.W,. Will E.J, Lindley E.J. (2002) Postdialysis and Equilibrium Urea Concentrations. *Blood Purification*. 20: 189-189,

Smye S, Tattersal J, Will E. (1999) Modeling the post-dialysis rebound: The reconciliation of current formulas. *ASAIO*. 45(6) 562-569

Wold S, Sjöström M, Eriksson L. (2001) PLS-regression: a basic tool of chemometrics. *Chem. Int. Lab. Sys.* 58: 109-130

Vapnik. VN.(2000) *The Nature of Statistical Learning*. 2d ED. Springer

2

Hemodialysis Access: The Fistula

Mary Hammes
University of Chicago
United States

1. Introduction

The primary aim of this chapter is to understand the importance of placement and maintenance of arteriovenous fistula (AVF) in the patients with advanced renal failure prior to the need for dialysis. Vascular access complications contribute significantly to the morbidity and mortality associated with end-stage renal disease patients on hemodialysis. The major concern this publication will address is that with the recommendation for an increased number of AV fistulas, we are faced with the fact that many fistulas fail, with limited data to understand complications of AVF specifically stenosis and thrombosis. Attempts to understand underlying mechanisms of stenosis and thrombosis will aide in access design, treatment options, and hence improve morbidity and mortality.

The care and outcome of the patient with end-stage renal failure (ESRD) on chronic hemodialysis is dependent on their access. Although a variety of techniques have been developed for providing hemodialysis access, there have been no major advances in the past three decades. This contributes to the fact that hemodialysis access dysfunction is one of the most important causes of morbidity and mortality in the hemodialysis population. In addition, the expense of providing ESRD care in the US is a significant portion of the Medicare budget, totaling $23.9 billion in 2007, of which a significant portion is spent on placement and maintenance of vascular access (USRDS, 2009).

The fistula provides the best outcome and can be placed with the least expense and complication rate when compared to a catheter or graft. Therefore, regional and network indicators promote the placement of AVF. Several recent initiatives have focused on vascular access and ways to improve outcomes. The National Foundation for Kidney-Dialysis Outcomes Quality Initiative (K-DQOL), End Stage Renal Disease Clinical Performance Measures (CPM) and Fistula First Initiative (FFI) have provided guidelines that mandate fistula access in patients on hemodialysis (Vasquez, 2009). FFI, developed to promote fistula placement, had an initial goal of 40% of prevalent patients with fistula access. This goal was achieved in 2005, with a goal of 66% set for 2009. Nationwide, however, there are only 54.4% of prevalent hemodialysis patients with fistula access as of November, 2009, with the number of fistula access placements falling for the first time in 2007 (USRDS, 2009).

New insights into the care and maintenance of fistula access will help to ensure duration of long term access patency. With national initiatives to place more fistulas, the number of fistulas has and will continue to increase. There are gaps in knowledge as to surveillance, maturation, cannulation techniques and mechanism and treatment of stenosis and thrombosis. The following chapter on fistula access for hemodialysis will help to fill these voids.

2. Types of vascular access

Permanent vascular access in the patient with ESRD on hemodialysis is provided through a central venous catheter (CVC), arteriovenous graft (AVG), or AVF. The central venous access is provided by a cuffed catheter placed subcutaneously in the internal jugular vein. The most frequent complications of CVC with significant clinical consequences include infection and thrombosis; therefore this access is not a recommended option for permanent vascular access. An AVG is placed if the venous or arterial supply is inadequate. It is created by insertion of a synthetic conduit usually polytetrafluororthylene between an artery and vein. AV grafts have a high rate of thrombosis and infection with an average survival of only 2-3 years (KDQOL, 2006). An AV fistula is created by a surgical anastomosis between and artery and vein. When a fistula is created the vein and artery may be in their normal positions, or the distal end of the vein is moved to a position that is better located for cannulation (vein transposition). A translocation is done when the entire vein is moved from one anatomic location to another requiring an arterial and venous anastomosis.

The fistula with the best outcome is the lower arm radiocephalic (RCF); however this access often fails to mature in the elderly patient with underlying vascular disease, particularly in diabetics (Miller,1999; Rodriquez, 2000). The second recommended fistula is the upper arm brachiocephalic fistula (BCF). This type of fistula is being placed with increased frequency because of the high failure rate of RCF. The third recommended fistula is the brachiobasilic fistula (BBF), which usually involves a two step surgical procedure and may be difficult to cannulate given the medial location of the basilic vein.

2.1 Radial-cephalic fistula

The RCF was the first fistula designed in 1966 by Brescia (Brescia, 1966). The RCF is created by an anastomosis between a radial artery and a cephalic vein usually with a transverse

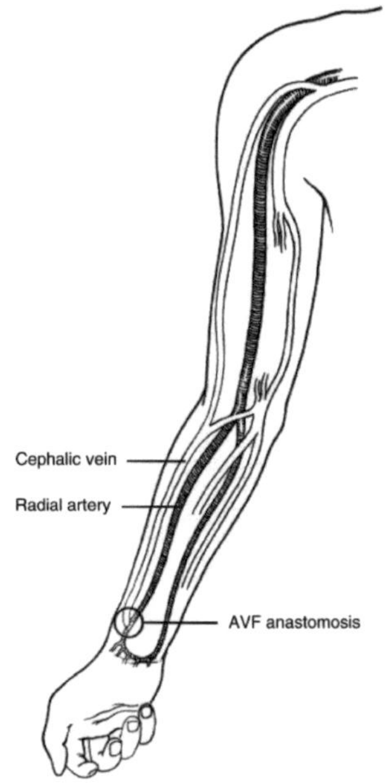

Fig. 1. Radial-cephalic fistula. Figure reprinted by permission from Macmillan Publishers Ltd: Kidney International, 62, 2002

incision at the wrist (Fig 1). This access is easy to place and once mature and used for dialysis has a low complication rate. The classic Cimino fistula is constructed with a side-to side anastomosis but this design may lead to venous hypertension. Therefore an end-to-side anastomosis is commonly used. The most frequent clinical problem is that this access has a higher primary failure rate when compared to BCF or BBF (Miller, 1999). However, if a RCF matures, the 5 to 10 year cumulative patency rate is 53 and 45 percent respectively (Bonalumi, 1982, Rodriguez, 2000). Placement of a lower arm fistula is desirable as it preserves the upper arm for future use.

2.2 Brachial-cephalic fistula

The BCF is a suitable second choice for access (Reubens, 1993). The cephalic vein in the upper arm is larger with increased flow as compared to the lower arm. The anastomosis for a BCF is usually in the antecubital fossa between the brachial artery and cephalic vein (Fig 2). The location of the BCF enables ease of cannulation with the benefit of a large surface area. The major complication with a BCF is the steal syndrome (see complications) as compared to RCF or BBF. In a retrospective review of 2,422 patients with vascular access, the BBF had a superior patency rate in diabetic pateints when compared to diabetic pateints who had a RCF (Papanikolaou, 2009). The authors even went so far as to argue that the BCF may be the best access option for the older diabetic patient on hemodialysis.

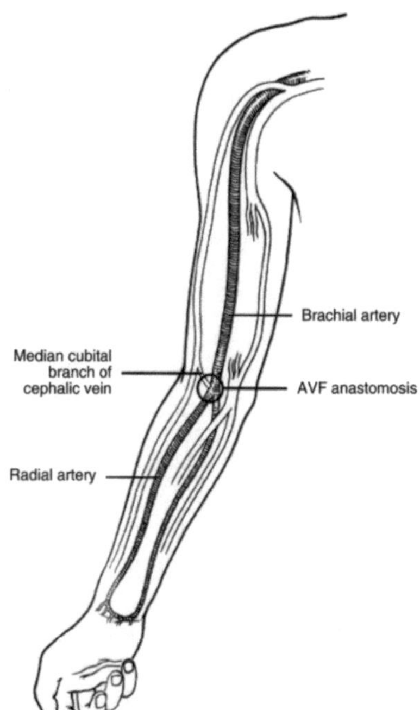

Fig. 2. Brachial-cephalic fistula. Figure reprinted by permission from Macmillan Publishers Ltd: Kidney International, 62, 2002

2.3 Brachial-basilic fistula

The BBF is the third choice for fistula placement (Dagher, 1976). Because the basilic vein is less accessible to venipuncture it tends to be better preserved and less involved with traumatic post-phlebitic changes when compared to the cephalic vein. When the BBF is placed more surgical skill is required with an initial anastomosis deep between the brachial artery and basilic vein (Fig 3). The BBF is left to mature for two months and then a second surgical procedure is preformed to "lift" the vein to allow ease of cannulation. The anatomic location of this fistula is often located in a position which is difficult to cannulate. Overall, the failure rate of the BBF is worse than BCF or RCF (Taghizadeh, 2003).

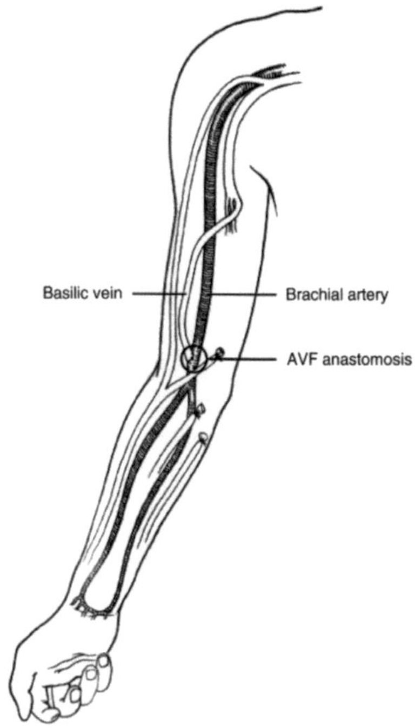

Fig. 3. Brachial-basilic fistula. Figure reprinted by permission from Macmillan Publishers Ltd: Kidney International, 62, 2002

3. Complications of fistula access

Even though complications of fistula access are far less than a graft or a catheter, they do occur and need to be addressed. Complications occur in approximately one-third of fistulas and include: aneurysms, infection, stenosis, thrombosis, steal syndrome and heart failure. These complications have historically been classified as early and late failure. The etiology of both early and late are somewhat similar because if the cause is not diagnosed early on it may progress and lead to late access failure. Fistula failure may also be classified as primary defined as a fistula which fails prior to cannulation or secondary defined as failure after a radiologic intervention such as angioplasty or stent or surgical revision.

3.1 Early failure/complications

Early failure of an AVF is defined as a fistula which never matures or is unable to be used by three months of time. It is well known from several studies that there is a significant primary failure rate for all AV fistulas that are placed (Schild,2004; Biuckians,2008; Dember 2008). Causes of early fistula failure are due to inflow problems from inadequate arterial supply, anastamotic stenosis which may result from trauma during creation, or outflow problems of the venous segment. Outflow problems may occur because of underlying fibrosis of the vein. Other factors which contribute to the primary failure of fistulas include demographic factors such as age, obesity, non-white ethic group, female sex , history of diabetes or peripheral vascular disease (Lok, 2006; Huijbregts, 2008) The size of the underlying vein may also influence the ability of a fistula to mature. A cephalic vein diameter of less than 2.0 mm on ultrasound in the forearm and less venous distensibility increases the risk of primary failure (Silva, 1998).

A cause of poor maturation is the development of collateral circulation. Often times a fistula is placed and when developing, collateral vessels may form which decrease the amount of flow through the designated vein to be used for cannulation. The physical exam may often help diagnosis this problem as you may palpate extra accessory vessels with an apparent augmentation in the vein when it is occluded. Small assessory vessels less than one-forth the diameter of the main AVF are likely to be insignificant. If a fistula is not maturing by 6 weeks, many algorithms suggest a vengram by 6 weeks. If collateral vessels are identified they may be coiled by interventional radiology techniques or ligated by surgical techniques (Rodriguez, 2000).

Prevention of early fistula thrombosis with pharmacologic intervention has been the subject of several recent trials, which have shown only minimal effect. The Dialysis Outcomes -Practice Patterns Study (DOPPS) noted a lower risk of failure of established fistulas in patients who used aspirin consistently over a year (Hassegawa, 2008). The Dialysis Access Consortium Fistula Trial (DAC) was a multi-center trial which compared the effects of the anti-platlet agent Clopidrogrel with placebo on early fistula failure. The proposed sample size was 1284, but the study was terminated after enrollment of 877 patients as interim data analysis showed that Clopridrogel reduced the risk of fistula thrombosis by 37% (Dember, 2008). In the DAC study 61% of newly created fistulas failed. These findings and others have shown a primary failure rate of 31-61% (Schild,2004; Biuckians,2008; December 2008). This suggests that failure of the fistula to mature is the main obstacle to successful fistula use.

3.2 Late failure/complications

Late failure of the fistula is defined as occurring greater than three months after creation and is often due to outflow stenosis. Venous stenosis occurs less frequently in AVF when compared to AVG, but nonetheless it is a common cause of AVF failure. Venous stenosis is usually detected clinically by symptoms of swelling of the extremity, prolonged bleeding post dialysis, difficulty cannulation or poor clearance. When these symptoms develop, the patient may be sent for an ultrasound for diagnosis or more commonly an interventional venogram. The venogram is desirable as a patient may have the venogram/angioplasty as a treatment option during the same procedure.

The most common anatomic location for an outflow stenosis in a RCF is 3 cm from the arteriovenous anastomaosis (Rajan, 2004). Outflow stenosis in RCF may be treated successfully by angioplasty with favorable primary and secondary patency rates (Rajan, 2004). Inflow lesions from inadequate arterial flow are often detected by a negative arterial pressure during hemodialysis and by physical examination using pulse augmentation. An arterial lesion may be present in 15-30% of fistulas (Leon, 2008). This type of lesion also is successfully treated by angioplasty or surgical revision (Turmel-Rodrigues, 2000).

One of the leading causes of failure of BCF is due to stenosis in the cephalic arch, which is the final bend in the cephalic vein prior to entry into the axillary vein (Fig 4). Cephalic arch stenosis (CAS) is found to occur in up to 77% of patients with BCF compared to 30% of patients with RCF with an average clinical significance at 2 years necessitating a venogram with intervention. The risk of development of CAS is less in diabetics for unclear reasons (Hammes, 2008). The BCF has been shown to be a superior access in older diabetic patients (Papanikolaou, 2009). Once CAS occurs it leads to head and neck swelling, high venous pressures and resultant thrombosis with complex treatment options. The arch is elastic, resistant to repeated angioplasty and often requires stent placement resulting in further stenosis (Hammes, 2008).

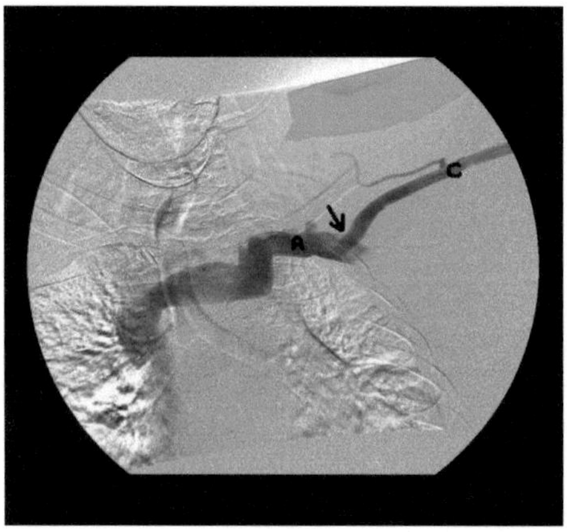

Fig. 4. Radiograph of Cephalic arch represented by arrow; C is the cephalic vein;A is the axillary vein

3.2.1 Aneurysms

The incidence of aneurysm formation in fistulas varies in studies from 5-7% (Lo, 2007). A traditional definition of an aneurysm is that it is considered true if it involves all layers of a venous wall or false if the wall is lined by thrombus or fibrous tissue. Aneurisms form for many reasons which include repeated cannulation at repetitive sites or altered turbulent blood flow from stenosis. As aneurysms are both a physiologic and cosmetic complication that may lead to the need for surgical revision and subsequent failure an approach to address aneurysms should be developed. Moreover, if a thrombosis occurs and significant aneurysm is present, the clot burden may be large and the thrombectomy procedure may be difficult. Aneurysms may also lead to an increased infection risk and prolonged bleeding post dialysis.

The treatment of aneurysms is prevention and if they form surgical correction. Preventative measures start with careful cannulation techniques (see cannulation techniques). Surgical options for correction include longitudinal stapling to reduce the lumen, open placation, excision with primary anastomosis, excision with interposition of prosthetic graft, and ligation (Pierce, 2007; Lo, 2007; Georgiadis, 2008). All of these techniques have been used with success and a decision for surgical treatment should be made on a case-by-case basis.

3.2.2 Steal syndrome

Steal syndrome is defined as distal hypoperfusion of the extremity in patients with severe peripheral vascular disease due to shunting of arterial blood flow into the fistula (Leon 2007). Reverse flow occurs if the diameter of the fistula opening is greater than the diameter of the feeding artery. Symptomatic steal occurs when there is a failure of adequate collateral flow and/or excessive blood flow. This problem complicates approximately 3-5% of fistulas and grafts. It is likely to occur more frequently with BCF (6%) verses RCF. Hand ischemia from steal syndrome may require distal revascularization with interval ligation (DRIL) procedure or complete ligation in severe cases. The DRIL procedure was first proposed by Harry Schanzer in 1988 (Schanzer, 1988). A short distal bypass is created and the artery just distal to the AV anastomosis is ligated. The DRIL procedure has been used successfully to relieve the ischemic symptoms in a significant number of patients with steal syndrome (Waltz, 2007).

3.2.3 Infection

The incidence of infection of an AVF is relatively low given that the native vein is used as a conduit. Predisposing factors to infection include: inadequate skin disinfection prior to cannulation, pseudo aneurisms, perifistular hematomas (often due to inappropriate cannulation), puritis with skin excoriation over needle sites, or the use of the fistula for IV drug use. Infection occurring in native fistulas can usually be treated with intravenous antibiotics and, if necessary surgical drainage.

3.2.4 Cardiac failure

AVF creation causes an increased blood flow and resultant cardiac output, Creation of a fistula is associated with a 15% increase in cardiac output and 4% increase in left ventricular end-diastolic diameter There is also an observed increase in ANP and BNP (Iwashima, 2002). These changes often go unnoticed, however high output failure from fistula access occurs in less than 1% of cases. The decision for permanent access placement in patients with category III or IV heart failure is challenging. Patients with ESRD in this subset should be considered for peritoneal dialysis. If this is not possible a lower arm fistula could be considered (decreased blood flow when compared to an upper arm fistula) with close monitor for worsened heart failure.

3.2.5 Venous hypertension

Venous hypertension in an extremity occurs because of incompetent venous valves or central venous stenosis. This problem may cause severe swelling in an extremity with associated complications of skin discoloration and thickening predisposing to infection. Doppler exam is used for diagnosis to demonstrate reversal of blood flow. Diagnosis and treatment with a venogram by an interventional radiologist may also be preformed. Treatment is aimed at correcting the underlying problem if present. Careful clinical practice includes obtaining a central venograms prior to fistula placement if there are clinical clues of venous hypertension such as, a history of ipsilateral catheter placement or dialated chest wall veins.

3.2.6 Median nerve injury

A very difficult problem with AVF access is median nerve injury. It may occur from ischemic injury from steal, compression of the nerve if there is extravasation of blood or local amyloid deposition in long term dialysis patients. The treatment is first to rule out vascular compromise and confirm diagnosis with an EMG. If traditional therapy to treat neuropathy does not resolve the pain, the fistula may need to be ligated.

4. Physiology of a fistula access

The creation of a fistula results in blood flow from an artery to a vein that is inherently non-physiologic in many ways. The initial flow rate in the radial artery of 20-30 mL/min increases to 200-300 mL/min immediately after creation of an AV fistula, reaching flow rates of 600-1200 mL/min after maturation (Wedgewood, 1984). In addition, the blood flow in the vein is not pulsatile prior to fistula insertion, whereas it is after the fistula is created. High fistula blood flow, a prerequisite for venous dilation and a requirement for easy cannulation and adequate dialysis, is accompanied by high arterial pressure being transmitted to the vein. This intense increase in flow rate and pressure has a profound effect on the hemodynamics in the downstream vein (Albayrak, 2006). The dramatically increased arterial blood flow at the time of fistula creation ultimately leads to an overall increase in shear stress, early on an observed low shear stress is evident which is thought to contribute to intimal hyperplasia and resultant venous stenosis and ultimate thrombosis.

5. Mechanism of stenosis and thrombosis

The mechanism responsible for the development of intimal hyperplasia and resultant venous stenosis is poorly understood. Stenosis, leading to thrombosis may require repeated procedures to maintain access patency and is the number one contributor to access failure. Several factors contributing to the development of intimal hyperplasia include: endothelial cell (EC) dysfunction from high blood flow and resultant shear stress; underlying histology of the vein; geometry of the anastomosis and angles of bends in vein; vascular remodeling; oxidative stress and inflammatory mediators that result from the hemodialysis procedure itself, and rheological factors such as viscosity (Table 1). Future studies that look at these factors will guide treatment trials to improve outcomes.

Shear Stress
Histology
Geometry
Vascular Remodeling
Oxidative Stress
Rheology

Table 1. Factors influencing Intimal Hyperplasia

5.1 Shear stress

When a fistula is created a vein is subjected to intense arterial pressure and flow. A vein is asked to behave as an artery perhaps without the anatomic make-up to undergo remodeling. The anatomy and physiology in a native artery is a constructive model to understand the mechanism of stenosis as it applies to venous stenosis in an AVF. A blood vessel is made of endothelial cells (EC) which form the lining of the vessel. These cells are normally aligned longitudinally. Vascular smooth muscle (VSM) cells align around the EC circumferentially. An arteriole has a thicken VSM layer when compared to a vein. Blood flow exerts pressure on the EC in a perpendicular direction. Shear stress is the frictional force per unit area from flowing blood which acts parallel to the EC that line the vessel. In straight regions of vessels, blood flow is in the same direction (laminar) and EC are quiescent with high laminar shear stress and resultant low oxidative stress, cell turnover and permeability. When a fistula is created blood vessels divide or curve and complex flow patterns may develop. When this happens EC are subjected to disturbed shear stress with higher levels of oxidative stress and inflammation which may result in vascular remodeling (Hahn, 2009).

The anastomosis of the fistula is also important to the development of intimal hyperplasia. The primary mode of failure of a fistula access relates to outflow stenosis caused by anastomotic intimal hyperplasia. When an anastomosis is created, the trauma causes activation of chemotactic factors which result in smooth muscle migration from the media to the intima. The resultant EC dysfunction with abnormal NO production may cause dysregulation of vascular tone. Smooth muscle cells continue to migrate and proliferate with resultant intimal hyperplasia. The end result may be decreased anastomotic compliance (Lin 2005).

This schematic of this process eventually leading to fistula failure is depicted in Figure 5. When a fistula is placed there is a bend or curve created at the anastomosis. This causes a turbulent blood flow, injury to EC, decreased WSS and resultant intimal hyperplasia. There is flow restriction that results and eventual worsened intimal hyperplasia that leads to further flow restriction with the end result of stenosis. The stenotic surface leads to heamostasis and further thrombus formation. Ultimately the fistula fails as a consequence of the stenosis.

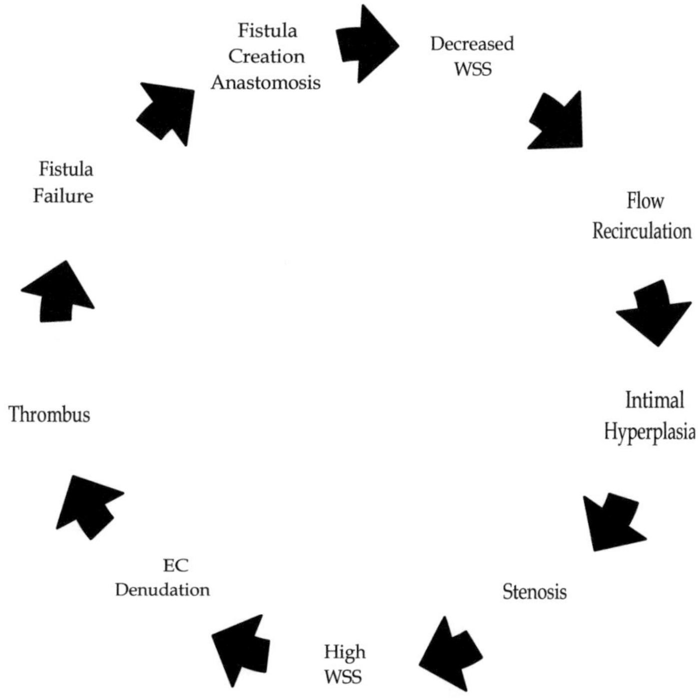

Fig. 5. Proposed cycle of fistula creation which eventually leads to intimal hyperplasia and fistula failure

5.2 Histology of the vein

Arterial and venous dialation is critical for fistula maturation. There is no exact definition of fistula maturation, but it is considered mature when it can routinely be cannulated with 2 needles and deliver a minimum blood flow (typically 350 to 450 mL/min) for a total duration of dialysis (usually 3-5 hours). Impaired dialation may be due to both structural and or functional factors. Pathologic analysis of the muscular artery and cephalic vein from patients with ESRD have demonstrated neo-intimal thickening (Wall, 2006). Other findings include increase radial artery intimal-media thickness which is correlated with decreased fistula maturation (Dixon, 2009). Many of these pathologic findings are present in the vein at the time of fistula placement and influence the outcome of the fistula.

5.3 Geometry

A fistula is created by an anastomosis creating a curve or bend to the vessel. The anastomosis is usually by and end-to-side design but occasionally by a side-to-side design. This creates a change from laminar flow to turbulent flow and as described above, the result is increased shear stress on EC with resultant intimal hyperplasia. This process may also be occurring in native conditions such as occurs in the cephalic arch. Hammes reviewed 45 venograms from BCF access and made measurements of the cephalic arch angle (global) and minimum radius of curvature and cephalic vein diameter (local measurements). Both global and local measurements showed evidence of having two distinct arch angles. Diabetics more commonly had a wider angle and less evidence of cephalic arch stenosis whereas non-diabetics had a wider angle and increased incidence of stenosis. (Hammes, 2009). These findings suggest that geometry influences hemodynamics and resultant stenosis.

5.4 Vascular remodeling

Vascular remodeling, first described by Glagov in 1987, refers to the ability of a vessel to change dimensions by vasoconstriction or vasodilatation, adjusting to flow changes to prevent stenosis. He reported that atherosclerotic arterial lumen narrowing was not simply the result of enlargement of the plaque lesion, but rather the vascular failure of the vessel to remodel to maintain a diameter so as not to inhibit blood flow (Korshunov, 2007). In a fistula, the vein and artery must remodel to a certain degree so as not to develop intimal hyperplasia or fibrosis.

In experimental models, when a fistula is first created, the cross-sectional area of the arterial wall increases with increased elastin, collagen and possibly smooth muscle cells(Driss, 1997). In human studies, this does not occur, but after a year, the artery appears to thicken circumferentially which may lead to defective remodeling (Dammers, 2005). Venous dialation occurs rapidly after the anastomosis due to increased areterial pressure and continues to dilate over several weeks attaining blood flow by 4-6 weeks (Dixon, 2006). Over time, venous thickening occurs and is characterized by intimal hyperplasia, smooth muscle cell proliferation and increased extracellular matrix production (Nath, 2003). If intimal hyperplasia develops and leads to clinically significant stenosis a venogram with angioplasty is usually preformed to dialate the venous stenosis. Early on the lesion may be responsive to angioplasty. At this point, there is no doubt remodeling taking place that is maintaining the diameter of the lumen. Over time with repeated use of the fistula, trauma and resultant inflammation may develop with repeated interventional angiography ultimately leading to fibrosis of the vein and eventual access failure.

5.5 Oxidative stress and inflammation

When a fistula is placed, matures and is cannulated for hemodialysis an inflammatory environment is created which leads to changes in vascular biology that may contribute to the development of intimal hyperplasia. EC dysfunction from altered shear stress as described above leads to release of nitric oxide and arterial dialation in response to increase flow rates (Dixon, 2009). It has been observed that when arterial dialation occurs, there is continued increase in shear stress that does not always normalize, suggesting that arterial adaptation to fistula creation may be incomplete. (Damers, 2005)

With evidence of histologic inflammation, there is upregulation of numerous cytokine and genes the cause smooth muscle proliferation and collagen deposition. Histologic injury to the vein is mediated by easly upregulation of mRNA for MCP-1, PAI-1, and endothelin -1 and later upregulation of mRNA for fibrogenic cytokine, transforming growth factor-B. (Dixon 2009). These studies demonstrate that the vein responds to pressure and shear stress by upregulating genes that lead to NIH. Future attempts to decrease these inflammatory mediators with pharmacologic therapy may prove effective to avert the inevitable intimal hyperplasia and fibrosis that may develop.

5.6 Rheology

Another significant factor which affects blood flow through a fistula is rheology, the characteristics of blood cells. The size, shape, deformeability, aggregation and whole blood viscosity (WBV) of blood have been shown to affect circulatory hemodynamics (Cho, 2008). Increased WBV may be detrimental causing increased peripheral resistance and sludging in post capillary venules (Pop, 2002). Patients with a history of peripheral vascular disease and diabetes, which are common in patients with ESRD, are associated with increased WBV. Over half of patients with ESRD have underlying diabetes and hypertension and it is predicted that these patients have elevated WBV.

Given that elevated WBV causes impaired circulation, it is likely that rheology, specifically WBV, contributes to the development of fistula stenosis and thrombosis. This area is the subject of future investigation.

6. Cannulation techniques for AVF

When a patient begins hemodialysis the start of hemodialysis is accompanied with anxiety regarding the surgical placement of the access along with needle cannulation. Excessive dilation of the fistula may be of major concern for patients. These issues should be addressed through education and not prevent patients from receiving the benefits of a well functioning access. The education and timing of the access placement to coincide with the initiation of hemodialysis is of paramount importance. It is imperative that attention to the placement of dialysis access is discussed when it is determined that a patient will need chronic hemodialysis.

Once an AVF is surgically placed, it usually takes two months for the vein to mature to allow for cannulation. Although some fistulas mature within weeks, others may require up to 6 months before they provide reliable hemodialysis access so catheters may be removed. The timing of when to cannulate is determined by clinical examination. The vein should be palpable, visualized and long enough to accommodate two needles. The fistula should be within 1 cm of the skin surface in order for reliable cannulation. If the venous segment is too deep, a transposition may be preformed. There is consensus that fistulas should be l eft to mature for at least 30 days. In general cannulation before 2 weeks should be avoided.

Accurate cannulation of the fistula by experienced personal is mandatory for successful outcomes. Trauma including laceration and infiltration of the vein may cause local damage making future cannulation difficult. It has been estimated that one infiltration may delay catheter removal by 3 months. Techniques for cannulation include rotation of sites or the buttonhole technique. The buttonhole cannulation method is gaining increased acceptance among patients as there is less pain with the needle stick and decreased long term risk of aneurism formation.

6.1 Rope-ladder technique

The rope and ladder technique is the traditional method for access cannulation. This was developed so as not to weaken the integrity of the vein with repeated cannulation. The fistula is thought of as a rope or ladder and the needles are placed one to two inches apart, similar to rungs on a ladder or knots in a rope. The site is left to heal prior to the subsequent cannulation. This technique is useful to prevent aneurysms and prolong the life of the fistula. Complications may arise if the same site is cannulated which may be the case if sites are limited and one site becomes easier to cannulate.

6.2 Buttonhole technique

The buttonhole technique was introduced in Poland over 25 years ago when dialysis supplies including AVF needles were limited (Twardowski, 1979). AVF needles were reused for multiple cannulations and become dull with repeated use. The "dull" needle would enter smoothly if the exact same cannulation site and angle was used. The buttonhole technique was used to successfully solve the dull needle problem, with this method, the needles are inserted at exactly the same spot at consecutive dialysis sessions, establishing a channel in the AVF. The procedure of the buttonhole cannulation involves: identifying an optimal site such as a long venous segment without previous trauma, removal of the scab from previous puncture site using an aseptic technique and cannulation of the fistula at exactly same angle (approximately 25°). Initially sharp needles are used but once the track is developed which usually takes 2 weeks a blunt needle is used. This method has gained wide acceptance among patients as there is less pain associated with the cannulation and a decreased incidence of aneurysms. The buttonhole technique is gaining widespread acceptance in patients who practice self-cannulation (Verhallen, 2007). It is a technique that promotes independent self-care.

The main risk associated with buttonhole cannulation is infection. There may also be problems with "one-site-itis" which occurs if the same site is stuck technique include those with heavily scarred fibrous or a large amount of subcutaneous tissue in the upper arm. multiple times, the skin can become heavily scarred. Both infection or development of a fibrous track require placement of a new buttonhole.

6.3 Self cannulation

Patients who are able to use self cannulation have excellent outcomes, establishing independence, confidence and less pain. The technique of self cannulation allows the patient to feel where to place the needles and with experience there is a lower risk of infiltrations. This is an excellent cannulation option for home hemodialysis.

7. Routine surveillance

While fistula access is recommended for all patients with ESRD on hemodialysis, complications such as stenosis and resultant thrombosis lead to access failure. Therefore, surveillance of hemodialysis access is mandated by regulatory agencies (NKF: K/DOQI, 2006). Prior research attempts to substantiate a surveillance protocol for AV grafts have failed, showing no improvement in the outcome of thrombosis. There is a paucity of data on the benefit of surveillance for fistulas (Allon 2009). Once the factors that cause venous stenosis in fistulas are known, early detection provides the necessary framework to develop protocols to mitigate the onset of intimal hyperplasia. Treatment trials in future studies could then be initiated to change factors that contribute to venous stenosis.

Although there is a lack of adequate surveillance methods to detect fistula stenosis prior to thrombosis, there are some clues in the physical exam that may prove helpful in clinical practice. The physical examination may be the best test as to fistula adequacy for dialysis. Pre-procedure physical examination has been shown to accurately detect significant venous stenosis. The pre-dialysis physical exam of the fistula to detect significant stenosis may include: inspection, palpation from the anastomosis all the way to the chest wall, and auscultation. The characteristics of the pulse such as pulsatile, normal or weak, and if the thrill or bruit is continuous or discontinuous should be noted. Pulse augmentation and arm elevation tests may also be preformed to detect inflow or outflow stenosis. These elements of the physical exam have been reproduced and substantiated to correlate with venous stenosis (Asif, 2007).

8. Conclusions

This chapter has reviewed important aspects of AVF access for patient with ESRD on hemodialysis. The current enigma is that with increased need for placement the failure rate is high. Multiple factors cause fistula failure including: underlying demographic variables, stress of the dialysis treatment itself, along with flow changes and characteristics as illustrated in Fig. 6. Careful research to identify a comprehensive understanding of these factors will enhance fistula maturation thereby improving the outcomes for patients with ESRD on hemodialysis.

The AVF is by far the best access with the least risk of complications for patients with ESRD. If a patient starts hemodialysis with a mature fistula, their transition to renal replacement therapy occurs with less risk of morbidity and mortality. As more fistulas are being placed, there is an increased awareness of complications including venous stenosis. We need to review and improve the surgical techniques of fistula placement and maintenance while optimizing novel therapies that promote fistula maturation. The etiology of venous stenosis in an AVF is the subject of future investigation with treatment trials to follow.

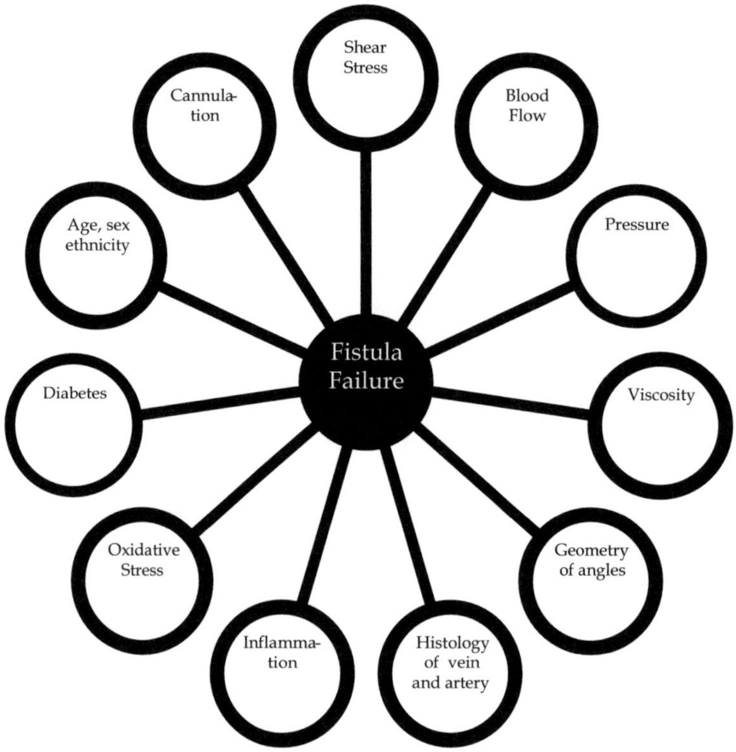

Fig. 6. Factors contributing to fistula failure

9. References

Albayrak R, Yuksel S, Colbay M, s B, Acarturk G, Haktanir A & Karaman O. (2006). Hemodynamic changes in the cephalic vein of patients with hemodialysis arteriovenous fistula. *J Clinical Ultrasound,* Vol.35, No.3, pp.133-137, (April, 2006), PMID 17274035

Allon M. (2007). Current management of vascular access. *Clin J Am Soc Nephrol* Vol.2 , No.4, (July, 2007), pp. 786-800, PMID 17699495, ISSN 1555-9041/204-0786

Asf A, Leon C, Oroco-Vargas CO, Krishnamurthy G, Choi KL, Mercado C, Merrill D, Thomas I, Salmon L, Artikov S & Bourgoignie JJ. (2007). Accuracy of physical examination in the detection of arteriovenous fistula stenosis. *Clin J Am Soc Nephrol,* Vol.2, No.6, (November, 2007), pp. 1191-1194, PMID 17928468, ISSN 1555-9041/206-1191

Bonalumi U, Civalleri D, Rovida S, Adami GF, Gianetta E, & Griffanti-Bartoli F. (1982). Nine years experience with end-to-end arteriovenous fistula at the "anatomical snuffbox" for maintenance haemodialysis. *Br J Surg,* Vol.69, No.8, (August 1982), pp. 486-488 PMID 7104641

Biuckians A. Scott EC, Meier GH, Panneton JM, & Glickman MH. (2008). The natural history of autologous fistulas as first-time dialysis access in the K-DOQI era. *J Vasc Surg,* Vol.47, No.2, (Feburary, 2008), pp.415-421, PMID 18241764

Brescia MJ, Cimino JE, Appel K& Hurwich BJ.(1966). Chronic hemodialysis using venipucture and a surgically creat arteriovenous fistula. *N Engl J Med,* Vol. 275, No. 20, (November, 1966), pp.1089-1092, PMID 5923023

Cho YI, Mooney MP& Cho DJ. (2008). Hemorheological Disorders in Diabetes Mellitus. *J of Diabetes Sci Technol,* Vol.2, No.6, (November, 2008), pp. 1130-1138 PMID 19885302

Dagher F, Gelber R, Ramos E& Sadler J. (1976) The use of basilic vein and brachial artery as an A-V fistula for long term hemodialysis. *J Surg Res,* Vol.20, No.4, (April, 1976), pp.373-376, PMID 933493

Damers R,Tordoir JH, Kooman JP, Welton RJ, Hameleers IM, Kitslaar PJ, Hoeks AP (2005). The effect of flow changes on the arterial system proximal to the arteriovenous fistula for hemodialysis. *Ultrasound Med Biol,* Vol.3, No.10, (October, 2005) pp. 1327-1333, ISSN 16223635

Dember LM, Beck GJ, Alton M, Delmez JA, Dixon BS, Greenberg A, Himmelfarb J, Vasquez MA, Gassman JJ, Greene T, Radeva MK, Braden GL, Ikizler T, Rocco MV, Davidson IJ, Kaufman JS, Meyers LM, Kusek JW, & Feldman HI, Dialysis Access Consortium Study Group (2008). Effect of clopidrogigrel on early failure of arteriovenous fistulas for hemodialysis: a randomized controlled trial. *JAMA,* Vol. 299, No.18, (May, 2008), pp.2164-2171, PMID 18477783

Dixon BS. (2006) Why don't fistulas mature? *Kidney Int,* Vol.70, No.8, (October, 2006), pp. 1413-1422, PMID 16883317

Driss BA, Benessiano J, Poitevan P, Poitevn P, Levy BI,& Michel JB (1997), Arterial expansive remodeling induced by high blood flows. *Am J Physiol,* Vol.272, No.2 Pt 2, (October, 2005) pp.H851-H858, PMID 9124448 Georgiadis GS, Lazzarides MK, Panagoutsos SA, Kantartzi KM, Lambidis CD, Staramos

DN, Vargemezis. (2008) Surgical revision of complicated false and true vascular access-related aneurysms. J Vasc Surg, Vol.47, No.6, (June, 2008) pp.1284-91, PMID 18514844

Hahn C, Schwartz MA. (2009) Mechanotransduction in vascular physiology and atherogenosis. *Nature Reviews Molecular Cell Biology,* 10, (January, 2009) pp.3-62, PMID 1917332

Hammes MS, Boghosian ME, Cassel KW, Funaki B, Coe FL. (2009). Characteristic differences in cephalic arch geometry for diabetic and non-diabetic ESRD patients. *Nephrol Dial Transplant,* Vol.24, No.7, (July, 2009) pp. 2190-2194, PMID 19244227

Hammes M, Funaki B, Coe FL. (2008). Cephalic arch stenosis in patients with fistula access for hemodialysis: relationship to diabetes and thrombosis. *Hemodialysis International,* Vol.12, No.1, (January, 2008), pp.85-89, PMID 18271847

Hasegawa T, Elder SJ, Bragg-Gresham JL, Pisom RL, Yamazakis S, Akizawa J, Tadou IM, Port FK, & Fukuham S (2008). Consistent aspirin use associated with improved arteriovenous fiatula survival among incident hemodialysis patients in the dialysis outcomes and practice patterns study. *Clin J Am Soc Nephrol* Vol. 3, No.5, (September, 2008) pp.1373-8, PMID 18596119

Huijbrets HJ, Bots ML, Wittens CH, Schrama YC, Moll FL, Blankenstien J, Cimino Study Group (2008). Hemodialysis arteriovenous fistula patency revisited: results of a prospective, multicenter initiative. *Clin J Am Soc Nephrol*, Vol.3, No.3, (May, 2008) pp.714-721, PMID 18256379

Iwashima Y, Horio T, Takami Y, Inenega T, Nishikimi T, Takishitas, Kawano Y, (2002). Effects of the creation of arteriovenous fistula for hemodialysis on cardiac function and natriurectic peptide levels in CRF. *Am J Kidney Dis,* Vol. 40, No.5, (November, 2002), pp. 974-982, PMID 12407642

K-DOQI. (2006). Clinical practice guidelines for vascular access. *Am J Kidney Dis,* Vol.48, No. S1, (July, 2006) pp.S176-S247, PMID 16813991

Korshunov VA, Schwartz SM & Berk BC. (2007). Vascular remodeling: hemodynamic and biochemical mechanisms underlying Glagov's phenomenon. *Arterioscler Thromb Vasc Biol,* Vol. 27, No.8, (July, 2007) pp.1722-1728, PMID 17541029

Leon C, Asif A. (2007) Arteriovenous access and hand pain: the distal hypoperfusion ischemic syndrome. *Clin J Am Soc Nephrol* , Vol. 2, No.1, (Januray, 2007) pp.175-183, ISSN 17699402

Lin PH, Bush RL, Nguyen L, Guerrero MA, Chen C & Lumsden AB. (2005) Anastomotic strategies to improve hemodialysis access patency - a review. *Vasc Endovasc Surg,* Vol. 39, No.2, (March-April, 2005) pp. 135-142, PMID 15806274

Lo HY, Tan SG. (2007) Ateriovenous fistula aneurysm - plicate, not ligate. *Ann Acad Med Singapore,* Vol. 36, No.10, (October, 2007), pp.851-853, PMID 17987237

Lok CE, Allon M, Moist L, Oliver MJ, Shah H, & Zimmerman D. (2006) Risk equation determining unsuccessful cannulation events and failure to maturation in arteriovenous fistulas (REDUCE FTM 1). *J Am Soc Nephrol,* Vol.17, No.11, (November, 2006), pp.3204-12, PMID 16988062

Miller PE, Tolwani A, Luscy CP, Deierhoi MH, Bailey R, Redden DT & Allon M (1999) Predictors of adequacy of arteriovenous fistulas in hemodialysis patients. *Kidney Inter,* Vol.57, No. 1 (July, 1999, pp.347-8 PMID 10411703

Papanikolaou V, Papagiannis A, Vrochides D, Imvrios G, Gakis D, Fouzas I, Antoniadis N, Takoudas D.(2009) The natural history of vascular access for hemodialysis: A single center study of 2,422 patients. *Surgery* Vol. 145, No.3, (February, 2009), pp.272-9, PMID 19231579

Pasklinsky G, Meisner RJ, Labropoulos N, Leon L, Gasparis AP, Landao D, Tassiopoulos AK & Pappas PJ. (2011).Management of true aneurysms of hemodialysis access fistulas. *J Vasc Surg* (January, 2011), doi:10.1016/j.jvs.2010.11.100,PMID 21276676

Pierce GE, Thomas JH, Fenton JR. (2007) Novel repair of venous aneurisms secondary to arteriovenous dialysis fistula, *Vasc Endovascular Surg,* 41(1), (Feburay-March, 2007), pp. 55-60, PMID 17277244

Pop GAM, Duncker DJ, Gardien P, Vranckx P, Versluis S, Hasan D & Slager CJ. The clinical significance of whole blood viscosity in (cardio)vascular medicine. *Netherlands Heart Journal,* Vol. 10, No. 12, (December, 2002), pp. 512-516

Port FK, Pisoni RL, Bommer J, Locatelli F, Jadoul M, Eknoyan G, Kurokawa K, Canaud BJ, Finley M &Young EW. (2006) Improving outcomes for dialysis patients in the International Dialysis Outcomes and Practice Patterns Study. *Clin J Am Soc Nephrol,* Vol. 1, No.2, (March, 2006) pp.246-255, PMID 17699213

Rajan DJ, Bunston S, Misra S, Pinto R & Lok CE. (2004) Dysfunctional autogenous hemodialysis fistulas: outcomes after angioplasty-are there clinical predictors of patency? *Radiology*, Vol. 232, No.2, (August, 2004), pp. 508-515, PMID 15286321

Rodriguez JA, Armandans L, Ferrer E, Olmos A, Cordina S, Bartolome J, Borrelas J, Piers L. (2000) The function of permanent access. *Nephrol Dial Transplant*, Vol.15, No.3, (March, 2000), pp. 402-408, PMID10692528

Roy-Chaudury P, Sukhatme VP, Cheung AK.(2008). Hemodialysisvacular access dysfunction: a cellular and molecular viewpoint. *J Am Soc Nephrol*, Vol. 17, No.4, (April, 2008). pp. 1112-1127 ISSN 1046-6673/1704-1112 PMID 16565259

Ruebens F, Wellington JL. (1993) Brachiocephalic fistula: a useful alternative for vascular access in chronic hemodialysis. *Cardiovasc Surg* Vol.1, No.2, (April, 1993), pp. 128-30, PMID 8076013

Schanzer H, Schwartz M, Harrington E, Haimov M (1988). "Treatment of ischemia due to "steal" by arteriovenous fistula with distal artery ligation and revascularization.". J Vasc Surg Vol. 7, No.6,(June, 1988), pp. 770–773. PMID 3373618

Schilid AF, Prieto J, Glenn M, Livingstone J, Alfieri K, & Raines J. (2004). Maturation and fistula rates in a large series of arteriovenous dialysis access fistulas. *Vasc Endovasc Surg*, Vol. 38, No. 5, (October, 2004),pp. 449-453. PMID 15490043

Silva MB, Hobson RW, Pappas PJ, Jamil Z, Anaki CT, Goldberg MC, Gwertzman G, Padberg FJ (1998), A strategy for increasing use of autogenous hemodialysis access procedures: impact of preoperative noninvasive evaluation. *J Vasc Surg*, Vol. 27, No.2, (Febuary, 1998), pp.302, PMID 9510284

Taghizadah A, Dasgupta P, Khan MS, Taylor J, Koffman G.(2003) Long-term outcomes of brachiobasilic transposition fistulas for haemodialysis. *Eur J Vasc Endovasc Surg*, Vol. 26, No.6, (December, 2003), pp. 670-672, PMID 14603429

Tessitore N, Mansueto G, Bedogna V, Lipari G, Poli A, Gammaro L, Baggio E, Morana G, Loschiavo C, Laudon A, Oldrizzi L, Maschio G (2003): A prospective controlled trial on effect of percutaneous transluminal angioplasty on functioning arteriovenous hemo. *J Am Soc Nephrol*, Vol.14, No.6, (June, 2003), pp. 1623-1627, PMID 12761264

Turmel-Rodrigues L, Pengloan J & Rodrigue H, Pengloan J, Rodigue H, Brillet G, Lataste A, Pierre D, Jourdan JL & Blansard D (2000), Treatment of failed native arteriovenous fistulae for hemodialysis by interventional radiology. *Kidney Int*, 57(3), (March, 2000), pp. 1124–1140, PMID 10720965

Twardowski ZJ, Kubara H. (1979) Different sites vs. constant sites of needle insertion into arteriovenous fsitulas for treatment by repeated dialysis. *Dial Transplant*, Vol.8, pp. 978-980

Verhallen AM, Kooistra MP, Jaarsveld BC. (2007) Cannulating in heaemodialysis: rope-ladder or buttonhole technique? *Nephrol Dial Transplant*, Vol.22, No.9, (September, 2007) pp. 2601-2604, PMID 1755776

Vazquez MA. (2009) Vascular access for dialysis: recent lessons and new insights. *Current Opinions in Nephrology and Hypertension*, 18 (2), (March, 2009), pp. 116-121, PMID 19434049

Waltz P, Ladowski JS, Hines A. (2007) Distal Revascularization and interval ligation (DRIL) procedure for the treatment of ischemic steal syndrome after arm arteriovenous fistula. *Annals of Vasc Surgery* Vol. 21, No.4, (July, 2007), pp. 468-473, PMID 17419003

Wedgewood KR, Wiggins PA, Guillou PJ. (1984) A prospective study of end-to-side verses side-to side arteriovenous fistulas for hemodialysis *Br J Surg* Vol.71, No.8, (August, 1984) pp. 640-642, PMID 6743990

Wali MA, Eid RA, Dewan M, Al-Homrany MA. (2006) Pre-existing histopathological Changes in the cephalic vein of renal failure patients before arterio-venous fistula (AVF) construction *AnnThorac Cardiovasc Surg* 2006, Vol.12, No.5, (October, 2006), pp.341-348, PMID 17095976

US Renal Data System, USRDS (2009) Annual Data Report: Atlas of chronic kidney disease and end-stage renal disease in the United States. National Institute of Health, National Institute of Diabetes and Digestive and Kidney Disease: Bethesda Maryland, http://www.usrds.org

The Brachio-Brachial Arteriovenous Fistula

Lucian Florin Dorobanţu, Ovidiu Ştiru, Cristian Bulescu, Şerban Bubenek and Vlad Anton Iliescu
UMF "Carol Davila" Bucureşti
Romania

1. Introduction

The autogenous arteriovenous fistula (AVF) is the preferred access for chronic hemodialysis in patients with end-stage kidney disease. Careful examination of the upper extremity is essential for the creation of a successful fistula. The quality of the arterial and venous circulation should be well established prior to surgery. However, there are cases when the superficial venous system of the upper extremity is unsuitable for the creation of an autogenous AVF. This problem has two solutions: the use of a prosthetic graft or the creation of a brachio-brachial AVF. Prosthetic grafts have a 1-year patency rate of 65-75%(Haimov, 1978), mostly due to the frequent and varying complications that they may sustain, especially ischemia, thrombosis, infection, and aneurysms. The brachio-brachial AVF, a relatively new type of angioaccess, is shown to have similar patency rates to the prosthetic grafts, but without their number of complications and is a very good alternative for patients with an unsatisfactory superficial venous system (Dorobanţu et al., 2006, 2010).

2. Anatomy of the brachial artery and the venous system of the upper arm

The brachial artery is the continuation of the axillary artery beyond the inferior margin of the teres major muscle. It continues down the anterior aspect of the arm to the cubital fossa, being accompanied by two venae comitantes and the brachial nerve. Proximally, the nerve is lateral to the artery but it crosses the medial side of the artery distally, lying anterior to the elbow joint. The brachial artery divides into its terminal branches, the radial and the ulnar, 2 cm below the elbow bend (Gabella, 1995).

The venous system of the upper extremity comprises the superficial and the deep veins. Both groups have valves. The superficial veins (figure 1) are the the cephalic, the basilic and the median vein of the forearm; they are subcutaneous in the superficial fascia. The cephalic vein forms over the "anatomical snuffbox" and ascends along the forearm's radial side and then in front of the elbow, in a groove between the brachioradialis and the biceps. It then crosses anteriorly the lateral cutaneous nerve and continues along the lateral border of the biceps, up to the delto-pectoral groove. It pierces the clavipectoral fascia and joins the axillary vein below the clavicular level.

The basilic vein begins medially in the hand's dorsal venous network and continues on the medial side of the forearm and then anterior to the elbow. Just distally to the elbow, it is joined by the median vein of the forearm. It ascends superficially between the biceps and the pronator teres, between filaments of the medial cutaneous nerve. It perforates the deep fascia midway in the arm, continuing medial to the brachial artery to the lower border of the teres major, where it becomes the axillary vein.

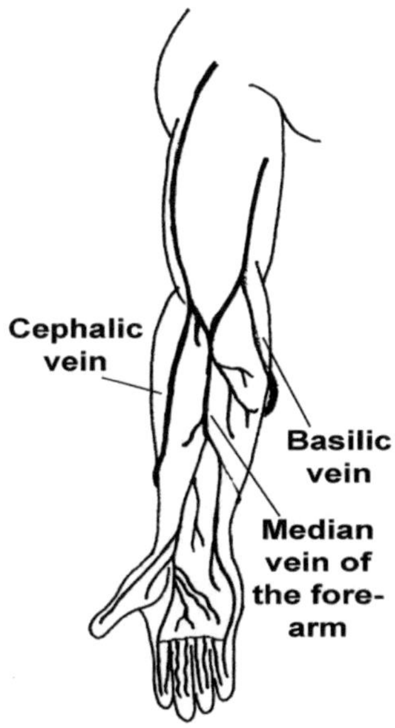

Fig. 1. The superficial veins of the upper limb

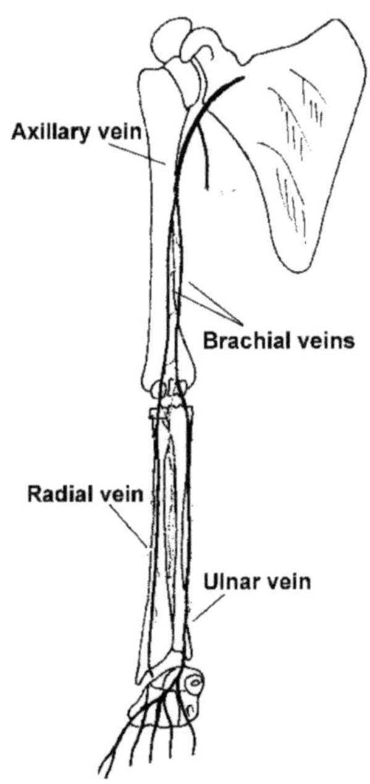

Fig. 2. The deep veins of the upper limb

The brachial veins (figure 2) share their path with the brachial artery. They begin at the junction between the radial and the ulnar veins and end at the inferior margin of the teres major muscle, where they are joined by the basilic vein, forming the axillary vein. There are many collaterals between the two veins and small tributaries that drain the muscles of the upper arm (Lupu et al., 2010).

3. Hemodynamics of an arteriovenous fistula

The arteriovenous fistula is an abnormal connection between a donor artery and a receiving vein. The permeability of the fistula depends on several factors. One of them is the resistance of the outflow vascular bed, which in this case is venous, and thus has a low pressure and a low resistance. As the vein's diameter increases through the maturation process, the venous resistance decreases. This process occurs during the first 4-8 weeks after the creation of the AVF and comprises a thickening of the venous wall, an increase in diameter for the vein, its distal branches, and for the arterial segment proximal to the anastomosis. As the vein is connected to a high-pressure, high-velocity artery, the blood flow through the vein induces an increased wall shear stress. Experiments have shown that acute increases in wall shear stress results in endothelial release of nitric oxide, which in turn increases the lumen radius. This is available for both acute and chronic wall shear alterations (Zarins et al., 2004). Experimentally produced arteriovenous fistulas produce an immediate 10-fold increase in blood flow and a three-fold increase in wall shear stress. Within 24 hours, vessel enlargement begins, and at the end of 4 weeks lumen radius enlarges twofold and wall shear stress returns to normal (Masuda & Bassiouny, 1989).

The flow through the AVF is insignificant as long as the vein's diameter doesn't exceed that of the artery by at least 20%; however, a palpable thrill means that the AVF is functional. When the diameter of the vein exceeds that of the artery by 75%, the venous resistance is virtually null, and the flow through the fistula is limited only by the arterial flow. Between 20 and 75%, the flow through the AVF increases on an exponential basis and it depends mainly on the venous resistance (Hobson et al., 1973).

It is noteworthy that the portion of the artery distal to the AVF does not suffer any modifications, thereby maintaining its high resistance relative to the outflow of the fistula. This can lead to a reversal of flow in this segment, the so-called "steal syndrome", which can result in ischemic complications. This is especially true in proximal fistulas.

The body's adaptation to the presence of an AVF includes global decreased vascular resistance and an increase in cardiac output, which can lead to a hyperdynamic syndrome or even to congestive heart failure. This is easily explained when the flow through a fistula ranges from 650 ml/min (for a radio-cephalic fistula) to 1000-1100 ml/min (for a brachio-cephalic, brachio-brachial or prosthetic fistula) (Schanzer, 2004; Ştiru, 2006). Any cardiovascular comorbidity can alter these patients' long-term prognosis.

4. Advantages of an autogenous arteriovenous fistula

A great number of studies have proven higher patency rates and lower complication rates for autogenous AVF when compared to synthetic bridge AVF (Palder et al., 1985; Enzler et al., 1996; Matsuura et al., 1998; Kherlakian et al., 2006; Kappos et al., 2007). Taking this into account, the National Kidney Foundation Dialysis Outcomes Quality Initiative (NKF-DOQI) guidelines for vascular access emphasize the use of the former over the latter (NKF-DOQI,

2001). Prosthetic and autologous AVF have similar patency rates for the first 4 postoperative weeks. After this period of time, synthetic bridge grafts require further interventions for angioplasty. Even with newer types of grafts, such as the Vectra Vascular Access grafts, the primary assisted rate of the prosthetic AVF is lower that of the autogenous AVF at 18 months of follow-up (58% vs 78%, respectively) (Kappos, 2007). The same study shows an overall access thrombosis rate of 17% for autogenous AVF and 34% for the Vectra graft. This rate is higher for other materials, such as ePTFE (Segal et al., 2003; Choi et al., 2003).
Most complications can be treated conservatively, without compromising the fistula (Matsuura et al., 1998). Severe hand ischemia, necessitating surgical treatment, occurs in 1% of patients with AVF and 2.7-4.3% of patients with graft AVF (Porter et al., 1985). Also, steal syndrome occurs in 73% of autogenous AVF and in 91% of graft AVF, as demonstrated by hemodynamic studies. Therapeutic options for hand ischemia always involve surgical interventions and include banding of the AVF (which is sometimes impractical, especially with prosthetic AVFs) and complex revascularization procedures.
Infection is a rare complication of the autogenous AVF; because there is no foreign body, it responds well to drainage and antibiotics. On the other hand, an infected prosthetic graft is a potentially lethal complication. The presence of foreign material makes this complication very difficult to treat. Prophylactic antibiotics are given before constructing the prosthetic AVF. Treatment requires removal of the whole prosthetic segment, debridement and systemic antibiotics.
Perigraft seroma is a very rare complication of the autogenous AVF (Blumenberg et al., 1985). It is more common with prosthetic grafts, because of changes in the structure of the ePTFE and of certain biological alterations in the host (Sladen & Mandl, 1985; Ahn & Machleder, 1986). Minimally invasive treatment is often unsuccesful, so more aggressive measures must be taken, leading even to replacement of the graft.
There is also a decreased risk of intimal hyperplasia because the anastomosis is much smaller compared to the one used with a prosthetic graft (Lumsden & Chen, 1997). In the rare case of fistula failure, the surgeon still has the backup possibility of creating a synthetic bridge fistula, an option that he would lose should he employ a prosthetic fistula in the first place.

5. Surgical technique

We use the two-stage approach in creating a functional brachio-brachial fistula. Although a single-stage approach has been described by Bazan and Schanzer (Bazan & Schanzer, 2004), we found the two-stage procedure to be safer as mobilization of the arterialized vein is easier than the thin-walled initial vein (Dorobanţu et al., 2010).
The first stage involves anastomosing the brachial vein to the brachial artery. The upper extremity is circumferentially prepared up to the axilla and is placed in extension and abduction, with the hand in supination. Local anesthesia is used, infiltrating 1% Lidocaine in the cutaneous and subcutaneous tissue. A 4-5 cm longitudinal incision is made in the antecubital fossa, following the medial border of the biceps muscle. The muscle is retracted slightly laterally in order to allow access to the thin aponeurotic sheath which contains the neuro-vascular bundle. The sheath is opened and the artery is dissected clear of the median nerve, passing a loop tape underneath it. With the arteries are two venae comitantes, connected by fragile transverse and oblique branches. The vein with the greater diameter is chosen for the AVF. All of its branches are ligated and a longitudinal venotomy is performed. Flushing the vein with a heparinated saline solution (2500 units in 250 ml of

saline) verifies the vein's permeability. The entire length of the catheter is inserted into the vein. Now the brachial artery is cross-clamped proximally and distally to the proposed site of anastomosis and a longitudinal arteriotomy is performed. An end-to-side anastomosis is performed using a running nonabsorbable 7-0 polypropilene suture. The posterior wall is performed first and the brachial vein is divided distally before completing the anastomosis. Before tying the suture, the permeability of the fistula, as well as of the brachial artery should be evaluated. The vein should be inspected for a thrill; its absence indicates poor outflow and the surgeon must look for a potential problem and correct it (figure 3). All bleeding sources should be controlled and the skin is closed using interrupted simple sutures, without drainage (Ştiru, 2006; Iliescu, 2007).

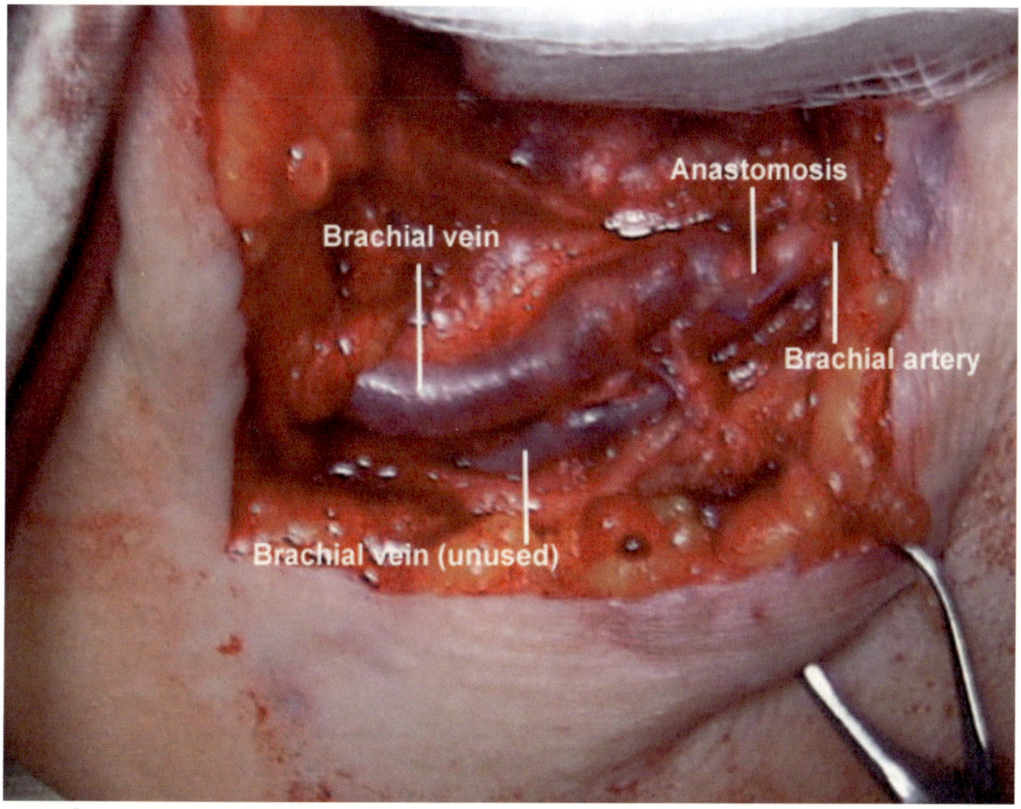

Fig. 3. The brachio-brachial fistula - intraoperative view

After 4 weeks, the vein is evaluated using Duplex scanning and, if its diameter is greater than 4 mm, it is transposed in a superficial plane in order to ease access for punctures. A longitudinal incision is performed on the antero-medial side of the arm, from the antecubital fossa to the axillary region. The neuro-vascular bundle is exposed, with the vein on the lateral side, the artery in the middle and the median nerve on the medial side. All of the venous collaterals are ligated, thus mobilizing the vein so that the aponeurosis can be closed underneath the vein with interrupted sutures (figure 4). A drainage tube is inserted and kept in place for 24 hours. The skin is closed with interrupted sutures, making sure that there is a 1.5 cm layer of tissue between the vein and the skin's surface to allow healing between needle punctures. The fistula can be used for hemodialysis after 3 weeks (Schanzer, 2004; Ştiru, 2006).

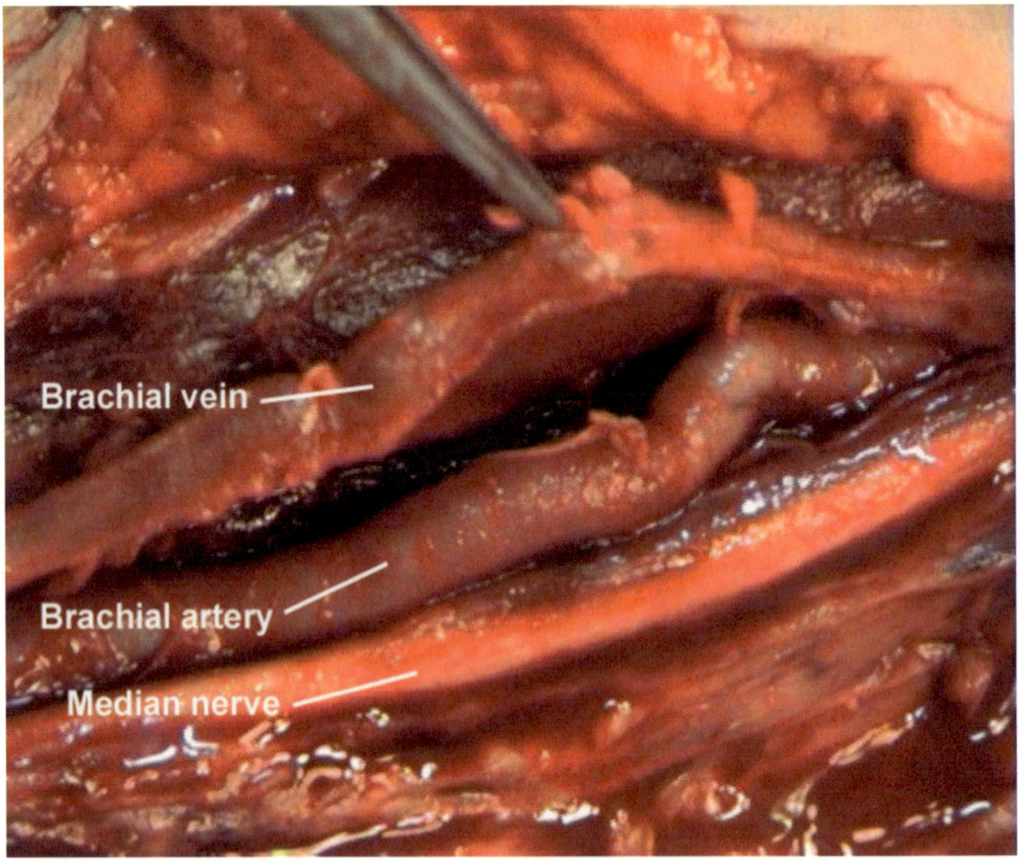

Fig. 4. Mobilization of the brachial vein

6. Results

Between 2004 and 2007 our team has operated on 49 patients with an upper arm venous system unsuitable for long term hemodialysis access, creating 49 brachio-brachial fistulas (Dorobantu et al., 2010). To date, this is the largest reported cohort of patients with a brachio-brachial AVF. Other groups have reported 17 (Casey et al., 2008), 20 (Angle et al., 2005) and 21 patients (Elwakeel et al. 2007). Thirty-nine patients (79,6%) had a functional fistula at the time of brachial vein transposition, after 4 weeks. The follow-up study was performed only in patients with a native functional brachio-brachial fistula after the two-step procedure. Mean follow-up period was 18.0 ± 11.1 months (range 3-37 months), longer than that of other published works, which ranged from 8 to 15.85 months. The overall patency rate at 37 months was 82.1%, compared to 75.89% at 1 year and 55.39% at 2 years reported by Elwakeel and 40% at 1 year reported by Casey. During this period, only seven patients presented with fistula occlusion 6, 6.4, 7.1, 9.4, 12.3, 23.5 and 35.0 months, respectively after superficialization.

No major complications have occurred with the patients. In 17 cases (43.6%) we noted discrete edema of the forearm, which disappeared after the first post-operative month; in only two cases has the edema extended to the entire arm. This was probably related to the greater pressure at the level of the remaining brachial vein, due to arterial pressure at the level of the brachio-brachial fistula, and numerous collaterals between the two brachial veins. In nearly all the patients we noted the presence of a collateral superficial venous network, as an adaptive reaction to the greater pressure in the deep venous system. After the superficialization and the ligation of the collaterals between the two brachial veins, this edema disappeared. We noted only one important edema of the arm, which regressed after the transposition in the subcutaneous tissue of the arterialized brachial vein. We believe that the absence of other complications like persistent forearm edema, ischemic lesions, etc, was related to the presence of two satellite brachial veins; therefore, the remaining brachial vein sustains the deep venous drainage. Other groups have reported a higher number of complications, including hematomas, wound infections (Casey, 2008) and steal syndrome which required reintervention and revascularization of the upper extremity.

	Casey	**Angle**	**Elwakeel**	**Dorobanțu**
No. of patients	17	20	21	49
Mean follow-up (months)	8	14 ± 4	15.85 ± 9	18 ± 11.1
Maturation rate at 4 weeks	47%	100%	66.6%	79.6%
Patency rate				
At 12 months	40%		75.89%	
At 24 months			55.39%	
At 37 months				82.1%
Major complications				
• Hematoma	• 2		• 1	0
• Infection	• 2		• 1	
• Steal sdr.	• 3		• 0	
• Aneurysm	• 0		• 2	

Table 1. Comparison between several groups of patients with brachio-brachial fistulas

There were two cases of technical difficulties in mobilization of the brachial vein that had not been reported before: in one case we managed to maintain the native AVF (due to successful reconstruction of the arterialized vein in front of the median nerve) (figures 5 & 6), while in the other case where the arterialized vein remained too small, we were forced to make a prosthetic fistula. That was a rare event and we believe that it does not diminish the good results achieved with this technique.

No operative deaths occurred, but three patients died (after 2, 8 and 10 months) due to non-related causes and another three patients were lost at follow-up.

We consider that pre-operative ultrasound deep vein evaluation for the first step of the procedure is useless because the brachial vein is always a good native conduit with a variable diameter which does not influence the future of the AVF. Although there are authors that used only brachial veins with a diameter superior to 3 mm, they did not resolve the non-maturation problem (Pisoni et al., 2002).

When compared to the more traditional brachio-cephalic and brachio-basilic AVF, the brachio-brachial fistula shows similar patency and complications rates. A study published by Woo et al. in 2007, analyzing 190 patients with brachio-cephalic and brachio-basilic AVFs shows a patency rate of 56% for the brachio-cephalic and 71% for the brachio-basilic at 1 year. At 5 years, the patency rate was 40% for the brachio-cephalic and 56% for the brachio-basilic. Complications rates were low, including 6 cases of steal syndrome (3.15%), 7 cases of bleeding (3.68%), 3 cases of infection (1.57%) and 1 case of early thrombosis (0.52%), but greater than in the brachio-brachial AVF.

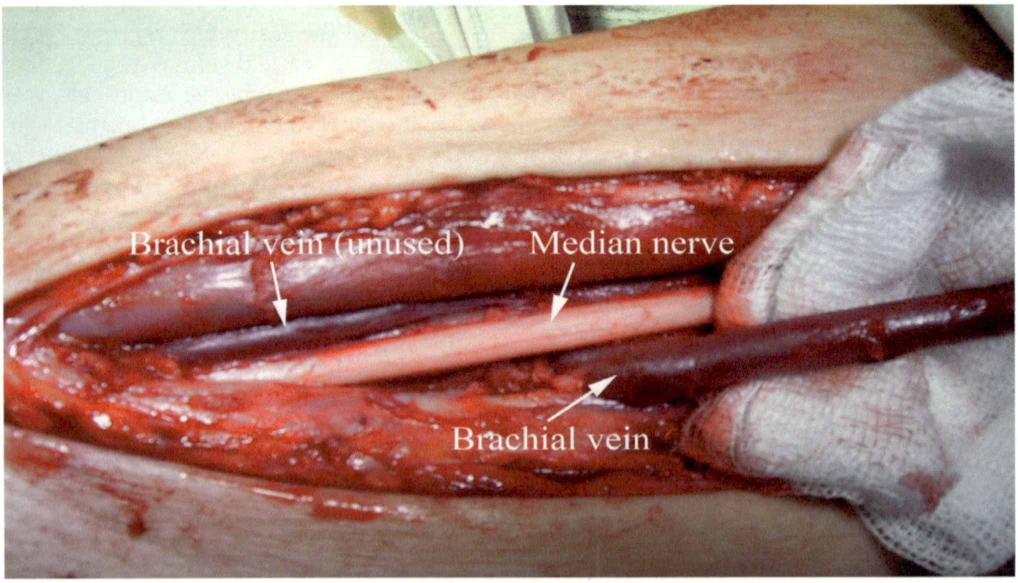

Fig. 5. The arterialized brachial vein runs under the median nerve

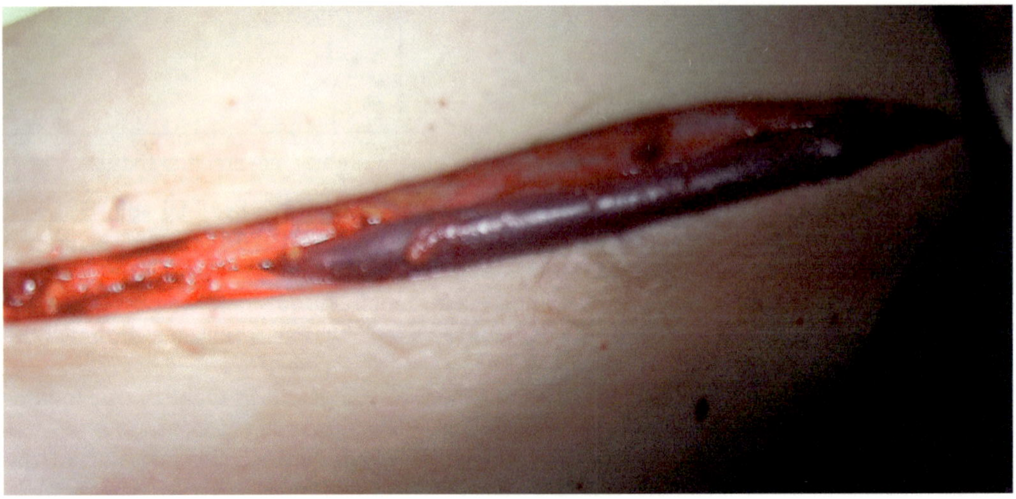

Fig. 6. Final result, after the vein has been divided and reconnected using an end-to-end anastomosis

7. Conclusions

The brachio-brachial arteriovenous fistula is a viable solution for patients with an unsuitable superficial venous system. It can also be used in patients who already have malfunctioning arteriovenous fistulas using the superficial veins of the upper extremity. Studies have shown that it has good patency and low complication rates, therefore its construction can postpone the use of a prosthetic bridge graft or a long-life hemodialysis catheter by several years. The surgical technique includes the same principles of other venous transpositions, so it should be incorporated into the arsenal of techniques that are routinely used by vascular access surgeons.

8. References

Ahn, S.; Machleder, H., et al. (1986). Pathogenesis of perigraft seroma: evidence of a humoral fibroblast inhibitor. *Surg Forum*, No.37 (1986), pp. 460–461, ISSN 1522-666

Angle, N.; Chandra, A. (2005). The two-stage brachial artery- brachial vein autogenous fistula for hemodialysis: An alternative autogenous option for hemodialysis access. *J Vasc Surg*, No.42 (2005), pp. 806-810, ISSN 0741-5214

Bazan, H.A.; Schanzer, H. (2004). Transposition of the brachial vein: a new source for autologous arteriovenous fistulas. *J Vasc Surg*, No.40 (2004), pp. 184-186, ISSN 0741-5214

Blumenberg, R.M.; Gelfand, M.; Dale,W. (1985). Perigraft seromas complicating arterial grafts. *Surgery*, No.97 (1985), pp. 192–203, ISSN 0039-6060

Casey, K.; Tonnessen, B.K.; Mannava, K.; Noll, R.; Money, S.R. & Sternbergh W.C.III (2008). Brachial versus basilic vein dialysis fistulas: A comparison of maturation and patency rates. *J Vasc Surg*, No.47 (2008), pp. 202-206, ISSN 0741-5214

Choi, H.M.; Lal, B.K.; Cerveira, J.J.; Padberg, F.T.; Silva, M.B.; Hobson, R.W. & Pappas, P.J. (2003). Durability and cumulative patency functional patency of transposed and non-transposed arteriovenous fistulas. *J Vasc Surg*, No.38 (2003), pp. 1206-1212, ISSN 0741-5214

Dorobantu, L.F.; Stiru, O.; Iliescu, V.A.; Novelli, E. (2006). The brachiobrachial fistula: a new method in patients without a superficial venous system in the upper limb. *J Vasc Access*, No. 7 (2006), pp. 87-89, ISSN 1129-7298

Dorobantu, L.F.; Stiru, O.; Iliescu, V.A.; Bubenek, S.; Novelli E. (2010). The brachio-brachial arteriovenous fistula: mid-term results. *J Vasc Access*, No.11 (2010), pp.23-25, ISSN 1129-7298

Elwakeel, H.A.; Saad, E.M.; Elkiran, Y.M. & Awad, I. (2007). Unusual vascular access for hemodialysis: transposed venae comitante of the brachial artery. *Ann Vasc Surg* Vol.21, No.5 (2007), pp. 560-563, ISSN 0890-5096

Enzler, M.A.; Rajmon, T.; Lachet, M.; Lagrader, F. (1996). Long-term function of vascular access for hemodialysis. *Clin Transplant*, Vol.10, No.5 (1996), pp. 511-515, ISSN 0890-9016

Gabella, G. (1995). Arterial system, In Williams, P.L. (Ed.), *Gray's Anatomy*, 38th ed, pp. 1538-1539, Churchill Livingstone, ISBN 0-443-05717-6, Edinburgh, UK

Haimov M. (1978). Clinical experience with the expanded polytetrafluoroethylene vascular prosthesis. *Angiology*, Vol.29, No.1 (1978)

Hobson, R., Croom, R., Swan, K. (1973). Hemodynamics of the distal arteriovenous fistula in venous reconstruction. *J Surg Res*, No.14 (1973), pp. 438, ISBN 0022-4804

Huber, T.S.; Carter, J.W.; Carter, R.L.; Seeker, J.M. (2003). Patency of autogenous and polytetrafluoroethylene upper extremity arteriovenous hemodialysis accesses: a systematic review. *J Vasc Surg*, No.38 (2003), pp. 1005-1011, ISSN 0741-5214

Iliescu, V.A.; Stiru, O. & Dorobantu, L.F. (2007). *Fistula arteriovenoasa protetica*, Editura Academiei Romane, ISBN 978-973-27-1542-0, Bucharest, Romania

Kakkos, K.S.; Andrzejewski, T.; Haddad, J.A.; Haddad, G.K.; Reddy, D.J.; Nypaver, T.J.; Scully, M.M.;RN & Schmid, D.L. (2008). Equivalent secondary patency rates of upper extremity Vectra Vascular Access Grafts and transposed brachial-basilic fistulas with aggressive access surveillance and endovascular treatment. *J Vasc Surg*, No.47 (2008), pp. 407-414, ISSN 0741-5214

Kherlakian, G.M.; Roedersheimer, L.R.; Arbaugh, J.J., et al, (1986). Comparison of autogenous fistula versus expanded polytetrafluoroethylene graft fistula for angioaccess in hemodialysis. *Am J Surg*, No.152 (1986), pp. 238-243, ISSN 0002-9610

Lumsden, B.M.; Chen, C. (1997). Accelerated neointimal hyperplasia in haemodialysis access grafts, In: Henry ML, Ferguson RM, (Ed.), *Vascular access for haemodialysis*, 5th ed., pp. 43-50, WL Gore and Precept Press, ISBN 0-944496-50-4, Chicago, Illinois, USA

Lupu, G.; Terteliu, F.; Bulescu, I. (2009). Vascularizatia membrului superior, In Lupu, G. (Ed.), *Anatomie - Membrele*, pp. 47, Editura Universitara "Carol Davila", ISBN 978-973-708-428-6, Bucharest, Romania

Masuda, H.; Bassiouny, H., et al. (1989). Artery wall restructuring in response to increased flow. *Surg Forum*, No.40 (1989), pp. 285–286, ISSN 1522-666

Matsuura, J.H. ; Rosenthal, D. ; Clark, M., et al. (1998). Transposed basilic vein versus polytetrafluoroethylene for brachial-axillary anteriovenous fistulas. *Am J Surg*, No.176 (1998), pp. 219-221, ISSN 0002-9610

Palder, S.B.; Kirkman, R.L.; Whittemore, A.D., et al. (1985). Vascular access for hemodialysis: Patency rates and results of revision. *Ann Surg*, No.202 (1985), pp. 235-239, ISSN 0003-4932

Pisoni, R.; Young, E.W.; Dykstra, D., et al. (2002). Vascular access use in Europe and the United States: results from the DOPPS. *Kidney Int*, No.61 (2002), pp. 305-316, ISSN 1523-1755

Porter, J.A.; Sharp, W.V.; Walsh, E.J. (1985). Complications of vascular access in a dialysis population. *Curr Surg*, No.42 (1985), pp. 298-300, ISSN 0149-7944

Schanzer, H.; Schanzer, A. (2004). Vascular access for dialysis, In Ascher, E. (Ed.), *Haimovici's Vascular Surgery*, 5th ed., pp.1015-1030, Blackwell Science, ISBN 978-0-632-04458-0, Malden, Massachusetts, USA

Segal, J.H.; Kayler, L.K.; Henke, P.; Merion, R.M.; Leavey, S.; Campbell, D.A. Jr. (2003). Vascular access outcomes using the transposed basilic vein arteriovenous fistula. *Am J Kidney Dis*, No.42 (2003), pp. 151-157, ISSN 0272-6386

Sladen. J; Mandl. M., et al. (1985) Fibroblast inhibition: a new and treatable cause of prosthetic graft failure. *Am J Surg*, No.149 (1985), pp. 588–590, ISSN 0002-9610

Stiru, O.; Iliescu V.A. & Dorobantu, L.F. (2006). *Tehnici de fistule arteriovenoase native la nivelul membrului superior*, Editura Universitara "Carol Davila", ISBN 973-708-126-9, Bucharest, Romania

The National Kidney Foundation Kidney Disease Outcomes Quality Initiative (2001). Clinical practice guidelines for vascular access: update. *Am J Kidney Dis*, No.37 (2001), pp. 137-181, ISSN 0272-6386

Woo, K.; Farber, A.; Doros, G.; Killeen, K. & Kokanzadeh, S. (2007). Evaluation of the efficacy of the transposed upper arm arteriovenous fistula: A single institutional review of 190 basilic and cephalic vein transposition procedures. *J Vasc Surg*, No.46 (2007), pp. 94-101, ISSN 0741-5214

Zarins, C.K.; Xu, C. ; Bassiouny, H.S.; Glagov, S. (2004). Intimal hyperplasia, In Ascher, E. (Ed.), *Haimovici's Vascular Surgery*, 5th ed., pp. 165-167, Blackwell Science, ISBN 978-0-632-04458-0, Malden, Massachusetts, USA

4

Vascular Access for Hemodialysis

Konstantinos Pantelias and Eirini Grapsa
University of Athens
Greece

1. Introduction

A progressive rise in the number of patients accepted for renal replacement therapy has been reported world wide [1]. Permanent vascular access (VA) is the life-line for the majority of these patients, when hemodialysis is the treatment of choice. Thus, the successful creation of permanent vascular access and the appropriate management to decrease the complications is mandatory. A well functional access is also vital in order to deliver adequate hemodialysis therapy in end-stage renal disease (ESRD) patients. Unfortunately, despite the advances in hemodialysis technology, the introduction of the polytetrafluoroethylene (PTFE) graft and the cuffed double lumen silicone catheter were the only changes in the field of vascular access in the last years. However the cost of vascular access related care was found to be more than fivefold higher for patients with arteriovenous graft (AVG) compared with patients with a functional arteriovenous fistula (AVF) [2]. It seems that the native arteriovenous fistula that Brescia and Cimino described in 1966, still remains the first choice VA [3]. Thereafter, vascular access still remains the "Achilles' heel" of the procedure [4] and hemodialysis vascular access dysfunction is one of the most important causes of morbidity in this population [5]. It has been estimated that vascular access dysfunction is responsible for 20% of all hospitalizations; the annual cost of placing and looking after dialysis vascular access in the United States exceeds 1 billion dollars per year [6, 7]. Nowadays, three types of permanent vascular access are used: arteriovenous fistula (AVF), arteriovenous grafts (AVG) and cuffed central venous catheters. They all have to be able to provide enough blood flow in order to deliver adequate hemodialysis, have a long use-life and low rate of complications. The native forearm arteriovenous fistulas (AVF) have the longest survival and require the fewest interventions. For this reason the forearm AV is the first choice, followed by the upper-arm AVF, the arteriovenous graft (AVG) and the cuffed central venous catheter as a final step [8-10].

2. History of vascular access

Vascular access for hemodialysis is closely associated with the history of dialysis. Glass needles were employed as vascular access when hemodialysis came into view in 1924. The first haemodialysis treatment in humans was carried out by Haas G. who used glass cannulae to acquire blood from the radial artery and reverting it to the cubital vein [11]. Venipuncture needles were used as means for blood acquisition from the femoral artery and its reinfusion to the patient by vein puncture, in 1943 by Kolff W. [12, 13]. Regular hemodialysis treatments were possible in 1950s through the use of a medical apparatus (Kolff 's twin-coil kidney [14]), thus projecting the problem of a reliable, capable of repeated use vascular access. Nowadays, the artery-side-to-vein-end-anastomosis has become a standard procedure [15]. In 1952, Aubaniac had described the puncture of the subclavian vein [16].

In the 60s, by using Alwall's experience, Quinton, Dillard and Scribner developed arteriovenous Teflon shunt [17]. This procedure involved two thin-walled Teflon cannulas with tapered ends inserted one into the radial artery and the other into the adjacent cephalic vein. The external ends were connected by a curved Teflon bypass tube. Later, the Teflon tube was replaced by flexible silicon rubber tubing. After the advancement of permanent vascular access, the possibility of maintenance hemodialysis was a fact and therefore a groundbreaking procedure.

In the subsequent years, many variants of the AV shunt were used, with the majority of them concerning temporary vascular access from the onset of chronic dialysis treatment, compensating for the time of AV fistula's absence or maturity. In 1961, Shaldon performed hemodialysis procedures by inserting catheters into femoral artery and vein, using the Seldinger-technique [18, 19]. Over time, vessels in different sites were used, including the subclavian, jugular and femoral vein.

In 1962 Brescia MJ described a 'simple venipuncture for hemodialysis' [20]. In 1963 Fogarty TJ et al invented an intravascular catheter with an inflatable balloon at its distal tip, designed for embolectomy and thrombectomy [21]. The first surgically created fistula was placed in 1965, followed by further 14 operations in 1966 [22]. In 1966 Brescia, Cimino, Appel and Hurwich published their paper about arteriovenous fistula. Appell had performed a side-to-side-anastomosis between the radial artery and the cephalic antebrachial vein. One year later, in 1967, Sperling M. et al reported the successful creation of an end-to-end-anastomosis between the radial artery and the cephalic antebrachial vein in the forearm of 15 patients using a stapler [23]. In the next few years this type of AV anastomosis received widespread acceptance. However this procedure was cast aside as first choice AV, due to the increasing numbers of elderly, hypertensive and diabetic patients with demanding vessels and high risk of steal syndrome. End-to-end-anastomoses are still a common place technique in revision procedures but it seems that they correlate with higher mortality risk due to infection [24].

In 1968 Röhl L. et al published thirty radial-artery-side-to-vein-end anastomoses [25]. After anastomosis was performed, the radial artery was ligated distal to the anastomosis, thus resulting in a functional end-to end-anastomosis. Today, the artery-side-to-vein-end-anastomosis has become a standard procedure [15]. In 1970, Girardet R. [26] and Brittinger W.D. [27] described their experience with the femoral vein and artery for chronic hemodialysis. Experimental trials have been done by several authors in order to establish a permanent vascular access using subcutaneous tunnel. Brittinger W. was the first to implant a plastic valve as a vascular access in an animal model but unfortunately his efforts did not proceed to a human one [28]. Moreover, during the early 70s, Buselmeier T.J. developed a U-shaped silastic prosthetic AV shunt with either one or two Teflon plugged outlets which communicated to the outside of the body. The U-shaped portion could be totally or partially implanted subcutaneously [29]. Subsequently pediatric hemodialysis patients were extremely favored by this procedure. New materials for AV grafts were presented in 1972, one biologic and two synthetic. In 1976, Baker L.D. Jr. presented the first results with expanded PTFE grafts in 72 haemodialysis patients [30]. In the years to come, several publications indicated the benefits and the shortcomings of the prosthetic material in question, remaining the primary choice of graft for hemodialysis VA to date. The same year, two authors, Mindich B. and

Dardik H., had worked with a new graft material: the human umbilical cord vein [31, 32]. Regrettably so, this material did not succeed in becoming a revolutionary graft material, due to its inadequate resistance against the trauma of repeated cannulation and its complications (aneurysm and infection). After the subclavian route for haemodialysis access was firstly introduced by Shaldon S et al in 1961, it was further processed in 1969 by Erben J et al, using the intraclavicular route [33]. In the next 20 years or so, the subclavian vein was the preferred access for temporary vascular access by central venous catheterization. Today, due to phlebographic studies revealing a 50% stenosis or occlusion rate at the cannulation site, subclavian route has been discarded. Subclavian stenosis and occlusion predispose to oedema of the arm, especially after creation of an AV fistula [34].

The first angioplasty described by Dotter CT et al who introduced a type of balloon, was immensely conducive to the resolution of one of the most significant predicaments in vascular surgery and vascular access surgery [35].

In 1977, Gracz KC et al created the "proximal forearm fistula for maintenance hemodialysis", a variant of an AV anastomosis [36]. An adjustment of this AVF became quite significant in the old, hypertensive and diabetic patients on the grounds that it allows a proximal anastomosis with a low risk of hypercirculation [37]. In 1979 Golding A.L. et al developed a "carbon transcutaneous hemodialysis access device" (CATD), commonly known as "button", by which, blood access does not require needle puncture [38]. As a procedure of third choice, these devices were expensive and never gained widespread acceptance. Shapiro F.L. described another type of "button", a device similar to that developed by Golding [39].

3. Angioaccess classification

Years after the initial efforts to create the appropriate vascular access in order to perform a safe hemodialysis, modern Nephrologists have now the possibility to select the appropriate access for their patients. Thus, the first distinction is made between temporary and permanent VA [40]. Temporary VA with expected half-life less than 90 days, peripheral arteriovenous shunts and non cuffed double lumen catheters are included. Mid-term VA with expected half-life from 3 months to 3 years include veno-venous accesses (tunneled cuffed catheters and port catheter devices) and arteriovenous internal shunts, requiring vascular graft synthetic (PTFE) or biologic (saphenous vein, Procol, etc.) material ,or external shunt. Long-term VA with an expected half-life more than 3 years includes virtually the native arteriovenous fistulas [4] and the new generation of PTFE grafts .

3.1 Acute hemodialysis vascular access

When an urgent hemodialysis has to be performed, the need for an appropriate vascular access becomes immediate. This type of access must have some specific features such as ease of insertion and availability for immediate use. Two types of such accesses are currently available: non-tunnelled dialysis catheters and cuffed, tunnelled dialysis catheters (Figure 1-5).

Double-lumen, non-cuffed, non-tunnelled hemodialysis catheters are the preferred method for immediate hemodialysis when a long-term access is not available. They are made of polymers which are rigid at room temperature to facilitate insertion but soften at body temperature to minimize vessel injury and blood vessel laceration. In order to minimize recirculation, the distance between the proximal and distal lumens should be at least 2cm [41].

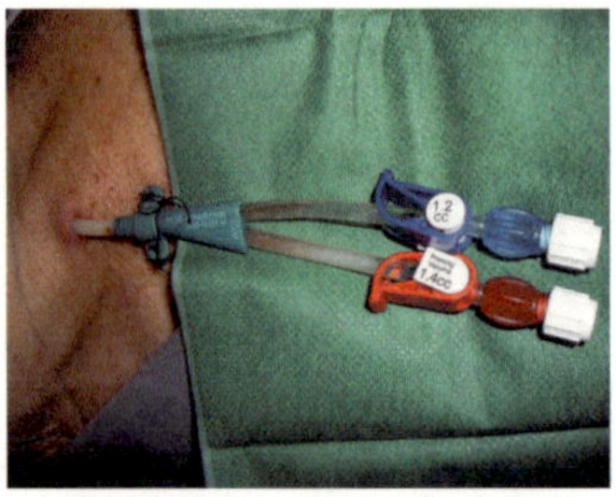

Fig. 1. Non cuffed internal jugular double lumen catheter

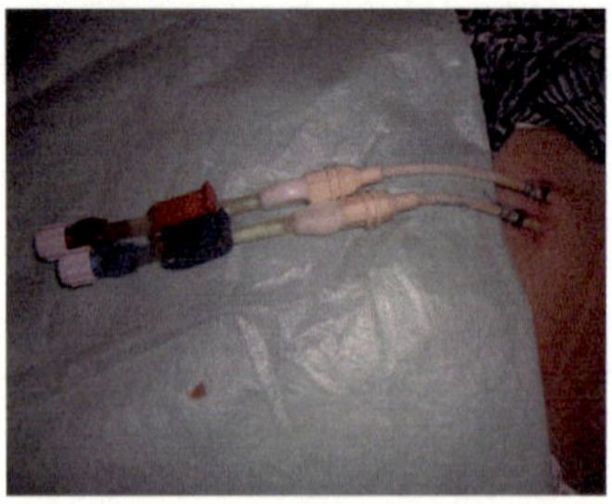

Fig. 2. Cuffed tunnelled internal jugular double lumen catheter

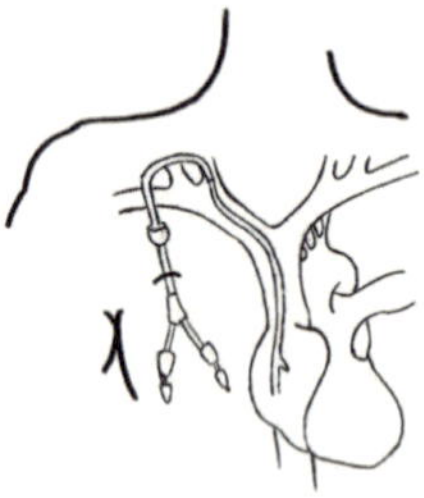

Fig. 3. Permanent cuffed jugular catheter

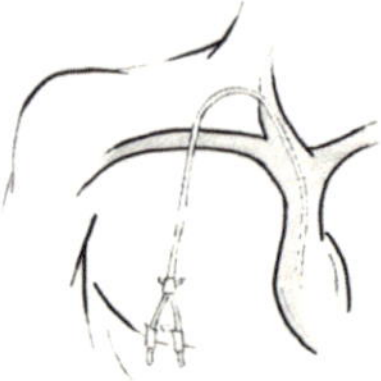

Fig. 4. Acute non-cuffed jugular catheter

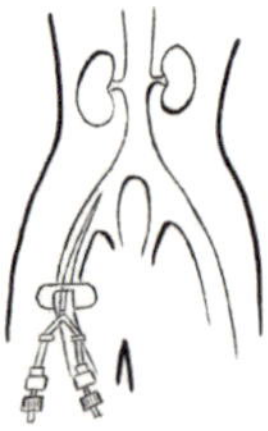

Fig. 5. Femoral non-cuffed catheter

Central veins such as jugular, subclavian or femoral, can be used as insertion routes of these catheters [42]. The femoral artery can be used as an access central vein when all other central veins have been excluded. For their insertion a modified Seldinger guide wire technique is used. In order to minimize immediate insertion complications, image guided assistance is recommended. Non-cuffed catheters are also suitable for use at the bedside of the patient [43, 44].

The 2006 National Kidney Foundation Dialysis Outcomes Quality Initiative (K/DOQI) guidelines recommend, after internal jugular or subclavian vein insertion, identifying radiographically any potential complications and confirming tip placement prior to either anticoagulation or catheter use [45]. Nowadays, the subclavian catheters should be generally avoided because of the high incidence of vein stenosis and thrombosis.

The maximum blood flow with this class of catheters is usually blood pump speeds of 300 mL/min, with an actual blood flow of 250 mL/min or less [46, 47]. Femoral catheters have to be at least 18 to 25 cm in length in order to have lower recirculation. The routine use-life of these catheters varies depending on the site of insertion. Generally speaking, internal jugular catheters are suitable for two to three weeks of use, while femoral catheters are usually used for a single treatment (ambulatory patients) or for three to seven days in bed bound patients [48]. However, the KDOQI guidelines suggest that non-cuffed, non tunnelled catheters should be used for less than one week. Tunnelled catheters should be placed for those who require dialysis for longer than one week [45]. More recently, a non-cuffed, non-tunnelled triple-lumen dialysis catheter has been developed. The purpose for third lumen is blood drawing and intravenous administration of drugs and fluid. In a multicenter, prospective study, blood flow rates and infectious complications were similar with double lumen catheter [49].

Infectious complications are the principal reason for catheter removal.

3.2 Permanent vascular access

Taking patient factors into consideration, such as life expectancy, comorbidities, the status of the venous and arterial vascular system, is very important in order to prescribe the appropriate access. Other factors are determined by the type of access itself, such as arteriovenous fistula (AVF), arteriovenous graft (AVG), or TC which have a different effect on circulatory system. Also, the duration of their functionality and the risk for infection and thrombosis are important factors to consider. Each type of surgical anastomosis has advantages and disadvantages [50]. In 2002 the American Association for Vascular Surgery and the Society for Vascular Surgery published reporting standards according to which three essential components of VA should be mentioned: conduit (autogenous, prosthetic), location and configuration (strait, looped, direct, etc.) [51].

3.2.1 Arteriovenous fistula

An AVF is the preferred type of vascular access; it has the lowest complication rates for thrombosis (one-sixth of AVGs) and infection (one-tenth of AVGs) [52, 53].

There are 3 types of AVFs:

- First type when artery and vein are connected in their natural position, either with a side-to-side or a side-artery-to-vein-end anastomosis.
- Second type, where a vein is moved to connect to an artery in end-to-side fashion to either bridge a larger anatomical distance, or to bring the vein to the surface where it is accessible for cannulation and requires a tunnel to position the vein in its new location.

- Third type where a vein is removed from its anatomical location and is connected to an artery and vein in end-to-end fashion.

Both second and third types require the formation of a tunnel [54] (Figure 6-9). End-to-end anastomoses are now rarely performed, since the complete disruption of the artery imposes a risk for peripheral ischemia and thrombosis. The most common surgical technique today is the side-to-end anastomosis. However, technical problems such as cutting the end of the vein in an oblique angle may create functional problems due to stenosis. An anastomosis more proximal in the arterial system should be smaller to prevent steal symptoms and limit maximal fistula flow, with the inherent complication of ischemic steal or heart failure [54]. Arteriovenous fistula creation is often performed under local anaesthesia, with low morbidity and requires time for maturation. Data from the Dialysis Outcomes and Practice Patterns Study (DOPPS) indicate that AVFs should mature at least 14 days before use [55]. Fistula size and flow increase over time of 8–12 weeks and the initial blood flow rates has a range of 200–300 mL/min.

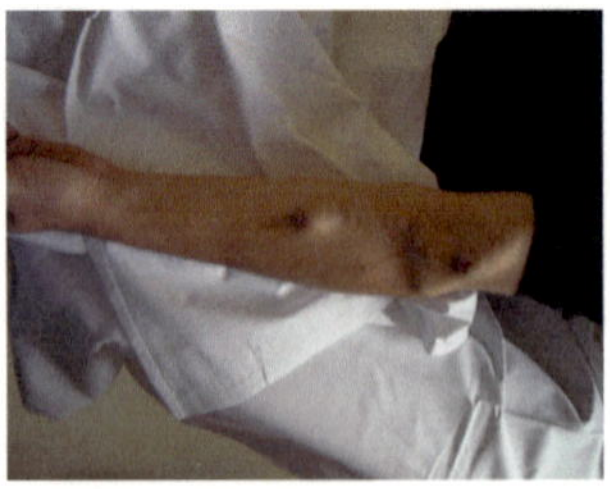

Fig. 6. Forearm AVF

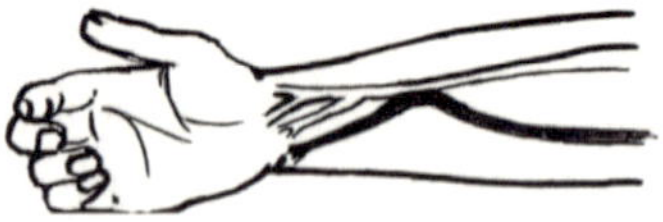

Fig. 7. Side to side forearm AVF

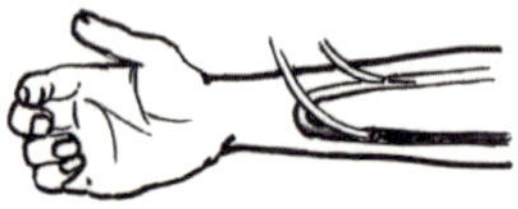

Fig. 8. End to end forearm AVF

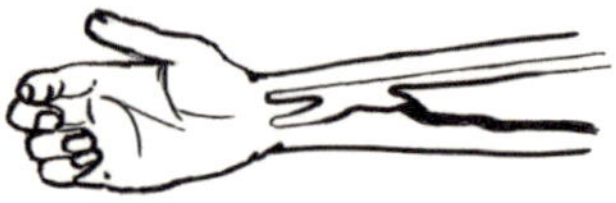

Fig. 9. Side to end forearm AVF

Placement of AVFs should be initiated when the patient reaches CKD stage 4, or within 1 year of the anticipated start of dialysis. A physical examination should document blood pressure differences between the upper extremities[56] and an Allen test should be performed as the lack of a well-developed palmar arch predispose for vascular steal symptoms in case the dominant artery is used for the VA creation [57].

Ultrasound must be done before surgical implantation because it can provide information for maximal surgical success by mapping arteries and veins; e.g. a preoperative arterial lumen diameter >2 mm is associated with successful fistula maturation [56], while a diameter of <1.6 mm predicts failure of the procedure [58]. Kidney Disease Outcomes Quality Initiative (KDOQI) Vascular Access guidelines, suggest that a working AVF should have a blood flow >600 mL/min, a diameter >0.6 cm, and be at a depth of 0.6 cm (between 0.5 and 1.0 cm) from the surface, 6 weeks after its creation. In fistulas that are successfully maturing, flow increases rapidly post-surgery, from baseline values of 30–50 mL/min to 200–800 mL/min within 1 week, generally reaching flows >480 mL/min at 8 weeks [59, 60]. The AVFs must be evaluated 4–6 weeks after placement, and experienced examiners (e.g., dialysis nurses) can identify non-maturing fistulas with 80% accuracy [61].

3.2.2 Arteriovenous graft

AVGs (Figure 10-12) were the most commonly used type of dialysis access in the U.S. [62]. However, they do not last as long as AVFs and they have higher rates of infection and thrombosis [52]. Grafts present a second choice of VA when AVF is not able to be performed because of vascular problems. They can be placed in the forearm, the upper arm, and the thigh, and can have a straight, curved or loop configuration. They may offer a large surface area for cannulation. AVGs can be cannulated about 2-3 weeks after placement, although there are studies suggesting that immediate assessment after placement for PTFE AVGs is possible [63, 64]. This interval is needed in order to allow the surrounding tissue to adhere to the PTFE conduit, to reduce the postsurgical oedema and the risk for local complications such as perigraft hematoma and seroma [65].

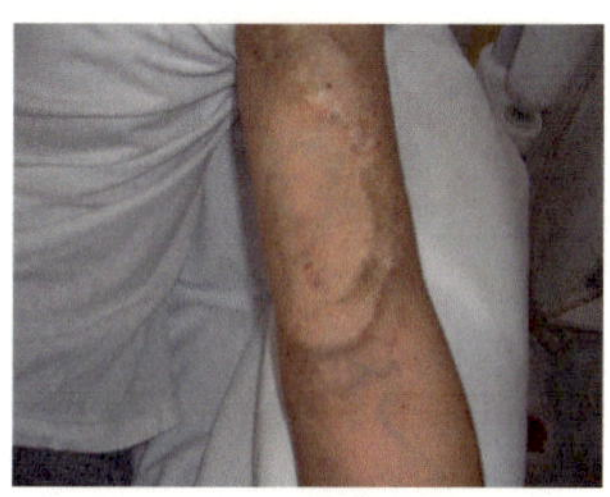

Fig. 10. Upper arm AVG

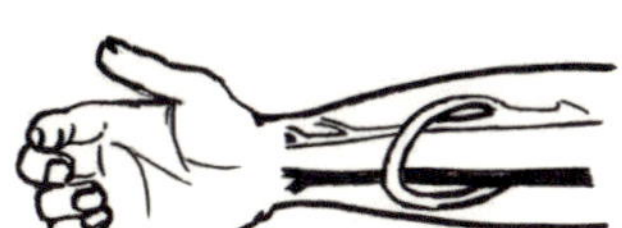

Fig. 11. Looped Forearm AVG

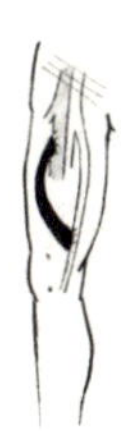

Fig. 12. Straight femoral AVG

3.2.3 Tunnelled hemodialysis catheter

TCs (Figure 2,3) are used when AVFs or AVGs are not possible to be created for several reasons such as multiple vascular surgeries, which lead to vascular thrombosis, or when patients have severe peripheral vascular disease or very low cardiac output. This is more frequently encountered in paediatric and very old patients.

Unfortunately, these are associated with the highest infection rate and they are not a very long-term access option. Studies have revealed that central venous catheters are colonized within 10 days of placement; however, colonization of the catheter biofilm does not correspond to positive blood cultures or clinical signs of bacteremia [66]. It seems that outcome of the infection treatment does not differ if, in addition to antibiotic therapy, the catheter will be guidewire changed or completely removed [67]. Recently Power A. et al published their experience with 759 TCs. The survival rate at 1, 2 and 5 years was 85%, 72% and 48% respectively. The infection rate was 0.34 per 1000 catheter days showing that with careful and appropriate use of TCs, they can provide effective and adequate long-term hemodialysis and rates of access related infection almost similar to AVGs' [68].

When conventional venous accesses have been exhausted and peritoneal dialysis is impossible, it is mandatory to use alternative procedures for VA in order to continue HD. Translumbar inferior vena caval CVCs belong to this category and it seems that they can offer relatively safe and effective long-term HD access [69]. Another alternative is the transhepatic hemodialysis catheters; they seem to be a potentially viable option with low rates of morbidity due to placement, high rates catheter-related maintenance and possibility of long-term functionality [70].

4. Hemodialysis vascular access in children

The choice of replacement therapy in children is variable. The registry of the North American Pediatric Renal Trials and Collaborative Studies (NAPRTCS) reports that of patients initiating renal replacement therapy in paediatric centres [71, 72]: one quarter of children underwent preemptive renal transplantation, one half were started on peritoneal dialysis and one quarter were started on hemodialysis. Kidney transplantation remains the preferred therapy for paediatric patients. Therefore, many of them receive maintenance HD through an indwelling catheter in perspective of short HD period [73]. In the United States, less than 800 paediatric patients receive maintenance HD therapy. The majority of smaller patients especially those less than 10kg or less than 2 years old, receive PD [74-76].

However, hemodialysis can be performed successfully in infants and very young children, as well [77]. Children who will undergo hemodialysis will need evaluation of their vasculature for placement of an arteriovenous (AV) fistula, arteriovenous graft, or cuffed double lumen catheter. The use of an AV fistula, which is the recommended type of vascular access in adults, is limited in children due to the size of their vessels. In the 2008 NAPRTCS annual report, vascular access for hemodialysis included external percutaneous catheter in 78% of patients, internal AV fistula in 12%, and internal and external AV shunt in 7.3 and 0.7 %, respectively [72]. K/DOQI has encouraged greater use of AV fistulas in larger children receiving hemodialysis who are not likely to receive a transplant within 12 months, with a goal of achieving more effective dialysis with fewer complications than the ones occuring with catheters. The choice of catheter size and configuration depends on the size of the patient. It is suggested that in children as small as 4 to 5 kg, a dual-lumen 8 Fr catheter can be well tolerated, and as the child becomes larger in size, a larger volume access can be placed [78]. Vascular access should be able to provide sufficient blood flow and adequate dialysis with a Kt/V greater than 1.2. A recommended flow rate of 3 to 5 mL/kg/min is acceptable in most patients due to the fact that flow rates in paediatrics vary by the size of catheter depending on the size of the patient, [79].

5. Vascular access complications and survival

Studies have shown a mortality risk dependent on access type, with the highest risk associated with central venous dialysis catheters, followed by AVGs and then AVFs [80, 81]. Additionally, patients who had a catheter as first VA, had more complications and higher mortality [82]. Same results have been presented by Ng LJ et al who examined hospitalization burden related to VA type among 2635 incident patients [83]. The CHOICE study examined mortality based on access type in 616 hemodialysis patients for up to 3 years of follow-up. Central venous catheters and AVGs were associated with approximately 50% and 26% increased mortality respectively, compared with AVFs with prevalence in men and elderly patients [84, 85]. Despite these findings and the KDOQI recommendations, dialysis access data from 2002–2003 showed that only 33% of prevalent hemodialysis patients in the US were being dialyzed via AVFs. On the contrary in Europe and Canada, the majority of the patients (74% and 53% respectively) were being dialyzed via AVFs [86].

Vascular access admissions continue to fall, with more procedures now performed in an outpatient setting, and are 45% below than in 1993. Among African American patients, the relative risk of an all-cause hospitalization or one related to infection is almost equal to that of Caucasians; the risk of a vascular access hospitalization, however, is 24 percent higher [87]. Thrombotic occlusion remains a major event, leading to permanent failure in 10% of AVFs and 20% of grafts each year. Interventional (percutaneous transluminal angioplasty and/or stent implantation) or surgical revision of thrombosed accesses has similar outcomes with a high rate of reinterventions. The elderly diabetic population with peripheral arteriosclerotic obstructive disease is in particularly prone to angio-access induced hand ischemia. [88]. It has been shown that patients with AVGs and TCs have higher levels of chronic inflammation than those with AVFs, and increased requirements in epoetin [89]. In our previous work with 149 hemodialysis patients who had undergone 202 vascular access procedures (177 Cimino-Brescia fistulae and 25 PTFE grafts) we found that the Cimino-Brescia fistula was used as the first choice of vascular access in all patients, except one in the elderly group. PTFE grafts were the second or third choice in 7 patients younger than 65 and 15 in the elderly group (p: NS). The only reason for technique failure was vascular thrombosis in both groups (p: NS). Other complications were: aneurysms (10/48 and 14/101, p: NS), infections (0/48 and 2/101 p: NS) and oedema (0/48 and 6/101, p: NS). (Table 1) Five-year technique survival of the first AV fistula in the two groups was 35% and 45% respectively (log-rank test, p: NS). (Figure 13) Our findings suggested that there was no difference in vascular access complications across age groups and the survival of the first AV fistula was independent of age [8]. Similar reports have been published by Swindlehurst N et all according to which the creation of permanent hemodialysis access in the elderly with AVF is not only possible but also proved to have a short hospital stay, high patency rates, and an acceptable rate of further intervention [90].

	Group A (age>60)	Group B(age<60)	P
Thrombosis	14/48	39/101	N.S.
Aneurysm	10/48	14/101	N.S.
Oedema	0/48	6/101	N.S.
Infection	0/48	2/101	N.S.

Table 1. Complications of vascular acces (Reference 8)

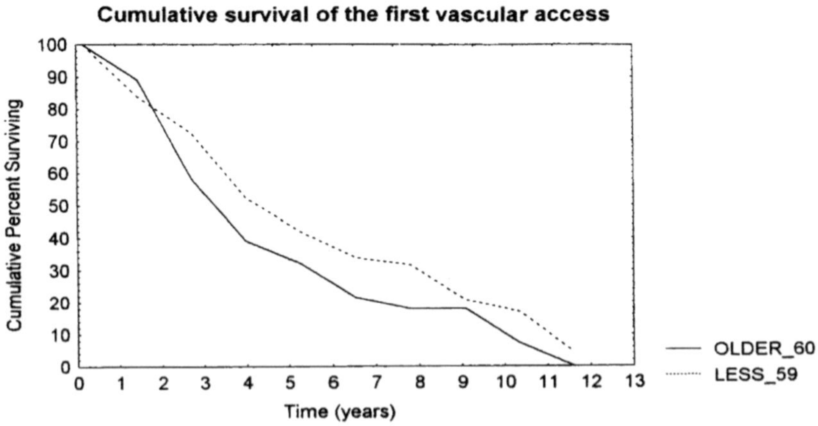

Fig. 13. Cumulative survival of first VA accord1ing to the patients' age(Reference 8)

In 2010 USRDS Annual Data Report, hospitalization in 2008 increased again, to a point 46% above their 1993 level. In 2007-2008, women treated with hemodialysis were 16 % more likely to be hospitalized, overall, than men. They also had a greater risk than men of cardiovascular, infectious and vascular access hospitalizations 11%, 14%, and 29% greater, respectively. Recently unpublished, our data are different than those we published in 1998. Our findings showed that among 189 patients, the female ones had had more possibility to start HD with double lumen catheter than the male ones, and also patients with heart failure independent of gender. Female patients had PTFE grafts as first vascular access (p=0,023) and the elderly patients had more complications and more vascular access procedures (p=0.026).

5.1 Non-tunnelled double lumen catheters complications

The non-tunnelled double lumen catheters' complications concern the early ones during the insertion and the late ones such as infection and thrombosis of the vessels.

The severity of acute complications varies with the site of insertion. The lowest rate is in the femoral position. A significant complication is perforation of the femoral artery. Bleeding usually resolves within minutes of direct compression and large femoral or retroperitoneal hematomas occur occasionally [91]. Subclavian insertion complications are more serious. Over-insertion of guide-wire can occasionally lead to atrial or ventricular arrhythmias but they are frequently transient [92]. Penetration or cannulation of the subclavian artery can lead to hemothorax, which may require a thoracotomy tube. The incidence of pneumothorax varies from less than 1 percent to more than 10 percent of insertions, depending on the skill and experience of the physician. Pericardial rupture and tamponade also have been described [93, 94]. There is less likelihood of arterial puncture or pneumothorax in ultrasound-guided catheter insertion [95]. Subclavian insertion from the left has an increased risk of pneumothorax and atrial perforation which can be presented with acute hemopericardium upon initiation of dialysis. Internal jugular vein is the preferred site of insertion because of subclavian stenosis and loss of the ipsilateral arm for future hemodialysis access. This complication appears to occur more often with subclavian (40 to 50 %) than with internal jugular insertions (up to 10 %) [96, 97]. At internal jugular insertions a carotid artery penetration may occur, but there is also a lower risk of pneumothorax (0.1 percent).

Prevention and treatment of catheter thrombosis are important clinical issues. To prevent formation of thrombus, both lumens of the double lumen catheter are instilled with heparin following hemodialysis [41]. Lytic agents such as urokinase and alteplase are effective in treatment of catheter thrombosis. Alteplase has effectiveness rates in thrombosis treatment comparable to the ones observed with urokinase [98]. Central vein catheters are associated with the development of central vein stenosis [99]. The K/DOQI guidelines therefore recommend avoiding placement in the subclavian vein, unless no other options are available. If central venous thrombosis is detected early, it responds well to directly applied thrombolytic therapy [99] or to percutaneous transluminal angioplasty when the fibrotic stenosis can be crossed with a guidewire [100]. The infection risks associated with temporary double lumen catheters include local exit site infection and systemic bacteremia, both of which require prompt removal of the catheter and appropriate intravenous antibiotic therapy [45, 101, 102]. Bacteremia generally results from either contamination of the catheter lumen or migration of bacteria from the skin through the entry site, down the hemodialysis catheter into the blood stream [103-105]. Skin flora, Staphylococcus and Streptococcus species, are responsible for the majority of infections.

There is conflicting evidence concerning the risk of infection based upon the site of insertion. In a large prospective randomized study (750 patients), the risk of infection was not reduced with jugular versus femoral venous catheterization [106]. But other prospective nonrandomized studies suggest, that the infection risk appears to sequentially increase for hemodialysis catheters inserted into the subclavian, internal jugular, and femoral veins, respectively [101, 107]. Coagulase-negative staphylococci, Staphylococcus aureus, aerobic gram-negative bacilli, and Candida albicans most commonly cause catheter-related bloodstream infection. In most cases of non-tunneled CVC-related bacteremia and fungemia, the CVC should be removed. The decision should be based on the severity of the patient's illness, documentation that the vascular-access device is infected, assessment of the specific pathogen involved, and presence of complications, such as endocarditis, septic thrombosis, tunnel infection, or metastatic seeding [108].

Overall, compared with the subclavian vein, the internal jugular vein remains the preferred access site in ambulatory patients. In the Intensive Care Unit, either femoral or internal jugular vein placement is satisfactory, with the use of ultrasound making internal jugular vein placement safer.

The best solution is to prevent the infection by proper placement technique, optimal exit site care and management of the catheter within the HD facility [41, 109].

5.2 Arteriovenous fistulas complications

Complications of AVFs can be divided into early and late causes.

Early causes include inflow problems due to small or atherosclerotic arteries, or juxta-anastomotic stenosis, so a pre-operative evaluation for suitable access sites has to been performed [110].

The aetiology of this acquired lesion is not entirely clear, but may be related to manipulating the free end of the vein, torsion, poor angulation, or loss of the vasa vasorum during anatomic dissection. More often than not, this lesion can be adequately treated with angioplasty [111, 112] or by surgical revision [113]. Outflow problems may include accessory veins that divert blood flow from the intended superficial vessel to deeper conduits, or central venous stenosis in patients with prior central venous catheters. Vessels, smaller than one-fourth of the fistula diameter, are usually not hemodynamically relevant. Juxta-anastomotic stenosis and accessory veins are the most common causes for early failure AVFs when pre-operative evaluations for suitable access sites have been performed [110].

Late causes for failure of AVFs include venous stenosis, thrombosis, and acquired arterial lesions such as aneurysms or stenoses. Venous stenosis may become apparent as flow decreases over time, worsening weekly Kt/V ([dialyzer clearance _ time]/body volume) or increasing recirculation. Native fistulas will not typically thrombose until flow is severely diminished. Thrombectomy of fistulas, although technically more challenging than in AVGs, is often successful and if flow is re-established, primary patency is longer than in grafts [114]. Aneurysms may form over the course of years as the fistula increases with increased flow and, unless associated with stenotic lesions, are more a cosmetic than functional concern. If the skin overlying the aneurysm is blanching or atrophic, or if there are signs of ulceration or bleeding, surgical evaluation should be obtained urgently [115]. Rupture of such aneurysms in high-flow fistulas can lead to exsanguination and death. (Figure 14)

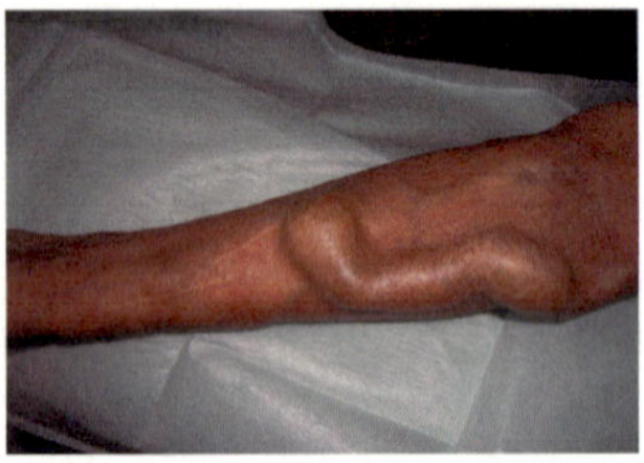

Fig. 14. Aneurysm in forearm AVF

5.3 Arteriovenous graft complications

Functional survival of AVGs is much sorter than AVFs. The natural course of AVGs is thrombosis due to venous stenosis caused by neointimal hyperplasia. The increased production of smooth muscle cells, myofibroblasts, and vascularisation within the neointima is the main cause of thrombosis. There is also angiogenesis and numerous macrophages in the tissue around the graft.[116, 117] Within the neointimal lesion, growth factors (GF) such as PDGF (platelet derived), VEGF (vascular endothelial), and basic FGF (fibroblast) are present.[117] Vascular endothelium is regulated by the presence of shear stress, [118, 119] and that flow within AVGs is likely to be different from native veins. Understanding the pathophysiology of neointimal hyperplasia would allow targeted therapy. Current studies are evaluating the role of radiation,[120] decoy peptides against transcription factors [121, 122] and local delivery of drugs with cell-cycle inhibitory effects (e.g., paclitaxel [123] and sirolimus). Cell-based strategies seek to take advantage of endothelial progenitor cells that release endogenous inhibitors of proliferation and thrombosis, such as nitric oxide (NO) and prostacyclin.[124] Venous stenosis in AVGs leads to decreased blood flow and thrombosis, at a rate of 1-1.5 times/patient/ year [52]. In most cases, thrombosis is associated with anatomical stenosis, which is mostly located in the venous anastomosis (60%), followed by the peripheral vein (37%), and within the graft (38%) [125]. Percutaneous angioplasty is safe and effective in treating venous stenosis [126] with a success rate from 80%-94%, and primary patency around 60% at 6 months and 40% at 1 year. Placement of self-expanding nitinol endovascular stents, appears to prolong patency in cases where focal lesions are resistant to repeated angioplasty [127]. Central stenosis is technically more difficult to treat, and stenotic lesions often recur within 6 months [54].

Thrombosis of an AVG is usually the result of multiple factors; such as the stenosis, hypotension, and the excessive compression for haemostasis. Haemodialysis' nurses have to be careful in order to avoid these factors. The risk for thrombosis increases with decreasing blood flow (BF). May RE et al found a 19% risk of thrombosis in 3-month period for an AVG with BF between 1010 and 1395 mL/min. This risk increased continuously with decreased BF; 1.67-fold at a BF of 650 mL/min, and 2.39-fold at a BF of 300 mL/min [128]. Graft thrombosis can be treated in outpatients by endovascular therapy. Angiographic search for a venous stenosis is always appropriate, and angioplasty is often indicated. Timely pharmacological thrombolysis or mechanical removal of the thrombus with a Fogarty catheter, and thrombo -aspiration or thrombectomy with a mechanical device [129] can prevent placement of a dialysis catheter.

AVG infections are serious complications and are the second leading cause of dialysis access loss. The incidence of hemodialysis-related bacteremia is more than 10-fold higher in AVGs than AVFs: 2.5 episodes per 1000 dialysis procedures versus 0.2 [130]. Patient have to be more careful for their hygiene because it seems to be the most important modifiable risk factor [131].

Pseudoaneurysms should be referred to a surgeon for resection when they are >2 times wider than the graft, rapidly increasing in size, or the overlying skin appears under duress (thin, bleeding, blanching) [132].

Ischemia, as a result of access placement is more common for AVGs than AVFs: vascular steal syndrome and ischemic monomelic neuropathy are two important clinical entities to distinguish.

Physiologic steal occurs in 73% of AVFs and 90% of AVGs, .Thus, in a radiocephalic fistula, arterial blood from the palmar arch may also deliver blood into the fistula. Unless there is the capacity for collateralization, this can lead to ischemia in the hand, ranging from complaints about cold hands to necrotic fingertips. Most of these complaints improve over time, but 1% of AVFs and up to 4% of AVGs require surgical revision [133]. Ischemic monomelic neuropathy is characterized by warm hands with a good pulse, but the hands are tender and swollen, usually immediately after surgery, and there is muscle weakness [134]. The cause is likely ischemia of the nerves and rapid surgical re-evaluation is needed. Nevertheless, there is evidence that the only differences between patients with PTFE older than 65 years old and younger ones are minor. Wound and skin complications and greater incidence of thromposis of VA associated with recombinant human erythropoietin have been reported (rHuEPO) [135].

5.4 Tunneled catheter complications

Early or late catheter dysfunctions are the functional complications of TCs. Kinking and unsuitable positioning of the catheter tip may be the cause of early dysfunction and can be addressed under fluoroscopic guidance. Among late causes of failure, are fibrin sheaths and thrombi around or at the catheter tip. Fibrinous sheaths can be disrupted by balloon angioplasty with improved flow through a new catheter in the same location. Symptomatic occlusions of the central veins usually require the removal of the catheter and system anticoagulation and must be weighed in the context of a continued need for dialysis and other available access options. Catheter use is linked to higher rates of infection and could compromise dialysis adequacy [136, 137]. Catheter related infections (CRI) are associated with increased all cause mortality and morbidity. 8-10% of MRSA bacteraemia in the UK occurs in patients receiving long term haemodialysis. It recently seems that the appropriately chosen antimicrobial lock solutions (ALS) reduce frequency of infections in HD patients [138]. Prophylaxis with gentamicin of the catheter lumens reduces bacterial infection morbidity and mortality related bacteremia of catheter without obvious bacterial resistance, making such use advisable [139]. Del Pozo et al in their prospective study showed that evaluation of tunnelled catheters with intra-catheter leukocyte culture helps in early HD catheters colonization, giving the possibility to eradicate biofilm without the removal of catheter [140].

6. Final remarks and conclusions

The radiocephalic and the humerobasilic AVF are the two types of VA with the longest duration of function, although a high rate of initial failure is seen with the radiocephalic AV fistula[141]. It is the preferred VA on account of the longest duration, its low complications rates and its ease of puncture [142-144].

Age, female gender, presence of diabetic nephropathy, start of dialysis with a catheter and failure to wait for initial maturation of the VA are risk factors and account for the majority of VA failures during RRT. Repeated VA failure has been identified as a risk factor for mortality [145].

The brachiocephalic AV fistula is the preferred type of VA, if the radiocephalic approach fails. In case of diabetic patients this seems to be the primary fistula if adequate vessels are not available, this is a frequent finding. Four year permeability rates of 80% have been reported [146]. In Rodriguez et al study, survival of brachiocephalic AV fistula was lower than radiocephalic; slightly more than one-half of patients have patent fistulae after 4 years and one -third after more than 8 years. It also shoed that more than two-thirds of patients in whom the first VA developed successfully did not have any subsequent VA failure, whereas initial failure increased the risk of subsequent failure. Female gender and presence of diabetes were risk factors related to VA failure [141].

The effort to create fistula first, has successfully increased the prevalence of AVFs [147]. However, the number of TCs has also increased, and those placed for bridging a patient to a functional AVF may stay in place longer [62]. Studies about fistula placement success from the US and European countries differ, significantly in the primary patency rate of AVFs at one year. US studies that include diabetic patients, report patency rates as low as 40%-43% [148, 149].

Konner et al reports a primary patency rate in diabetic patients of 69%-81%, depending on gender and age (results reported from 748 AVFs over 5 years) [150].

Chemla et al performed 552 AVFs in 4 years, achieving a primary patency rate at 22 months of 80% in 153 patients with radiocephalic fistulas [151].

Korsheed et al report that AVF formation resulted in a sustained reduction in arterial stiffness and BP as well as an increase in LVEF. These data state that the lower mortality of these patients with AVF, may be due to factors beyond VA associated infections and dysfunctions [152].
However, data from 1996 to 2006 collected from DOPPS indicate a growing use of catheters in many countries [153]. Also, our data in 2011 shows increased patency for TCs in female gender patients. Rayener et al report growing use of catheter according to DOPPS data. They also indicate that in facilities with the practice of early cannulation of AVF (within 4 weeks from their creation) and promptly performed VA surgeries with success in creating VA in older, diabetic women greatly enhance the odds of their patients for using a permanent access rather than TC [153]. In new dialysis patients, early referral to a nephrologist and early patient education strongly predict a successful functioning permanent VA at dialysis initiation and it also seems that the patients have better metabolic and clinical situation at the beginning of HD, lower long-term morbidity and higher survival for the first two years [154-158]. AV fistula is better when used for the first haemodialysis treatment compared to starting haemodialysis with a catheter [55, 159, 160]. Graft is, however, a better alternative than catheter for patients, where the creation of an attempted AVF failed or could not be created for different reasons [161].
In conclusion, as far as literature and our experience are concerned, arteriovenous fistula has to be the first choice in vascular access when suitable vessels are available. Arteriovenous grafts and Central Venous Catheters may be also a good alternative as fist choice when suitable vessels are not available or as a second choice when there is AVF failure. Female gender and old patients are more likely to start hemodialysis with a TC. Finally, a well matured vascular access is important for long access survival and early referral to nephrologists is mandatory.

7. Acknowledgements

Acknowledgements to Ioannis T. Papadakis Director of Nephrology Department Hippokration General Hospital and to the patients of Renal Unit who gave us the permission to add their pictures in our chapter. Also acknowledgements must be given to Mrs Sofia Andrikou for her designs of VA.

8. References

[1] Eggers, P.W., *Has the incidence of end-stage renal disease in the USA and other countries stabilized?* Curr Opin Nephrol Hypertens, 2011.

[2] Lee, H., et al., *Cost analysis of ongoing care of patients with end-stage renal disease: the impact of dialysis modality and dialysis access.* Am J Kidney Dis, 2002. 40(3): p. 611-22.

[3] Santoro, A., et al., *Vascular access for hemodialysis.* J Nephrol, 2006. 19(3): p. 259-64.

[4] Allon, M., *Implementing a vascular access programm: improved outcomes with multidisciplinary approaches, in Dialysis Access: A Multidisciplinary Approach,* S. Gray Richard J., Jeffrey J., Editor. 2002, Lippincott Williams & Wilkins: Philadelphia. p. 6-9.

[5] System, U.S.R.D., *2002 Annual Data Report.* Bethesda, National Institutes of Health, National Institute of Diabetes and Digestive Diseases, 2002.

[6] Feldman, H.I., S. Kobrin, and A. Wasserstein, *Hemodialysis vascular access morbidity.* J Am Soc Nephrol, 1996. 7(4): p. 523-35.

[7] Roy-Chaudhury, P., et al., *Vascular brachytherapy for hemodialysis vascular access dysfunction: exploring an unmet clinical need.* J Invasive Cardiol, 2003. 15 Suppl A: p. 25A-30A.

[8] Grapsa, E.J., et al., *Complications of vascular access in hemodialysis (HD)--aged vs adult patients.* Geriatr Nephrol Urol, 1998. 8(1): p. 21-4.

[9] *III. NKF-K/DOQI Clinical Practice Guidelines for Vascular Access: update 2000.* Am J Kidney Dis, 2001. 37(1 Suppl 1): p. S137-81.

[10] Schwab, S.J., et al., *Hemodialysis arteriovenous access: detection of stenosis and response to treatment by vascular access blood flow.* Kidney Int, 2001. 59(1): p. 358-62.

[11] Haas, G., *Versuche der Blutauswaschung am Lebenden mit Hilfe der Dialyse.* Klin Wochenschr, 1925. 4: p. 13-14.

[12] Kolff, W.J., *The artificial kidney.* J Mt Sinai Hosp N Y, 1947. 14(2): p. 71-9.

[13] Vienken, J., *'Bioengineering for life': a tribute to Willem Johan Kolff. Nephrol Dial Transplant,* 2009. 24(8): p. 2299-301.

[14] Kolff, W.J., *First Clinical Experience with the Artificial Kidney.* Ann Intern Med, 1965. 62: p. 608-19.

[15] Konner, K., B. Nonnast-Daniel, and E. Ritz, *The arteriovenous fistula.* J Am Soc Nephrol, 2003. 14(6): p. 1669-80.

[16] Aubaniac, R., *[A new route for venous injection or puncture: the subclavicular route, subclavian vein, brachiocephalic trunk].* Sem Hop, 1952. 28(85): p. 3445-7.

[17] Quinton, W., D. Dillard, and B.H. Scribner, *Cannulation of blood vessels for prolonged hemodialysis.* Trans Am Soc Artif Intern Organs, 1960. 6: p. 104-13.

[18] Seldinger, S.I., *Catheter replacement of the needle in percutaneous arteriography; a new technique.* Acta radiol, 1953. 39(5): p. 368-76.

[19] Shaldon Stanley M.A., M.D.C., M.R.C.P., Lecturer, Livio Chiandussi M.D. Padua, British Empire Cancer Campaign Research Fellow and Brenda Higgs M.B., B.SC. Lond., Senior House-Officer, *HAEMODIALYSIS BY PERCUTANEOUS CATHETERISATION OF THE FEMORAL ARTERY AND VEIN WITH REGIONAL HEPARINISATION.* The Lancet. 278(7207): p. 857-859.

[20] Cimino, J.E. and M.J. Brescia, *Simple venipuncture for hemodialysis.* N Engl J Med, 1962. 267: p. 608-9.

[21] Fogarty, T.J., et al., *A method for extraction of arterial emboli and thrombi.* Surg Gynecol Obstet, 1963. 116: p. 241-4.

[22] Brescia, M.J., et al., *Chronic hemodialysis using venipuncture and a surgically created arteriovenous fistula.* N Engl J Med, 1966. 275(20): p. 1089-92.

[23] Sperling, M., et al., *[Subcutaneous arteriovenous shunt for intermittent hemodialysis treatment].* Dtsch Med Wochenschr, 1967. 92(10): p. 425-6.

[24] Stolic, R.V., et al., *Correlation of mortality and location of arteriovenous fistula in hemodialysis patients.* Int J Artif Organs, 2011. 34(1): p. 26-33.

[25] Rohl, L., et al., *Direct arteriovenous fistula for hemodialysis.* Scand J Urol Nephrol, 1968. 2(3): p. 191-5.

[26] Girardet, R.E., et al., *Thirteen months experience with the saphenous vein graft arteriovenous fistula for maintenance hemodialysis.* Trans Am Soc Artif Intern Organs, 1970. 16: p. 285-91.

[27] Brittinger WD, S.M., Huber W et al. , *16 months experience with the subcutaneously fixed superficial femoral artery for chronic haemodialysis.* Proc EDTA 1970. 7: p. 408–412.
[28] Brittinger W-D, v.H.G., *Twittenhoff W-D et al., Implantation of a plastic valve into the superficialised femoral artery.* Proc EDTA 1971. 8: p. 521–525.
[29] Buselmeier, T.J., et al., *A totally new subcutaneous prosthetic arterio-venous shunt.* Trans Am Soc Artif Intern Organs, 1973. 19: p. 25-32.
[30] Baker, L.D., Jr., J.M. Johnson, and D. Goldfarb, *Expanded polytetrafluoroethylene (PTFE) subcutaneous arteriovenous conduit: an improved vascular access for chronic hemodialysis.* Trans Am Soc Artif Intern Organs, 1976. 22: p. 382-7.
[31] Mindich, B.P., et al., *Umbilical cord vein fistula for vascular access in hemodialysis.* Trans Am Soc Artif Intern Organs, 1975. 21: p. 273-80.
[32] Dardik, H., I.M. Ibrahim, and I. Dardik, *Arteriovenous fistulas constructed with modified human umbilical cord vein graft.* Arch Surg, 1976. 111(1): p. 60-2.
[33] Erben J, K.J., Bastecky J, Vortel V. , *Experience with routine use of sucblavian vein cannulation in haemodialysis.* Proc EDTA 1969. 6: p. 59–64.
[34] Schillinger, F., et al., *Post catheterisation vein stenosis in haemodialysis: comparative angiographic study of 50 subclavian and 50 internal jugular accesses.* Nephrol Dial Transplant, 1991. 6(10): p. 722-4.
[35] Dotter, C.T., M.P. Judkins, and J. Rosch, *Nonoperative treatment of arterial occlusive disease: a radiologically facilitated technique.* Radiol Clin North Am, 1967. 5(3): p. 531-42.
[36] Gracz, K.C., et al., *Proximal forearm fistula for maintenance hemodialysis.* Kidney Int, 1977. 11(1): p. 71-5.
[37] Konner, K., *Primary vascular access in diabetic patients: an audit.* Nephrol Dial Transplant, 2000. 15(9): p. 1317-25.
[38] Golding, A.L., A.R. Nissenson, and D. Raible, *Carbon transcutaneous access device (CTAD).* Proc Clin Dial Transplant Forum, 1979. 9: p. 242-7.
[39] Shapiro, F.L., et al., *Blood access without percutaneous punctures.* Proc Clin Dial Transplant Forum, 1980. 10: p. 130-7.
[40] Canaud B., D.S., *Vascular access for hemodialysis, in Reolacement of renal function by dialysis,* K.M.K. Horl H. W., Lindsay B.R., Ronco C., Winchester F.J., Editor. 2004, Kluwer academic publishers. p. 203-230.
[41] Schwab, S.J. and G. Beathard, *The hemodialysis catheter conundrum: hate living with them, but can't live without them.* Kidney Int, 1999. 56(1): p. 1-17.
[42] Fan, P.Y. and S.J. Schwab, *Vascular access: concepts for the 1990s.* J Am Soc Nephrol, 1992. 3(1): p. 1-11.
[43] Randolph, A.G., et al., *Ultrasound guidance for placement of central venous catheters: a meta-analysis of the literature.* Crit Care Med, 1996. 24(12): p. 2053-8.
[44] Work, J., *Vascular access for renal replacement therapy, in Intensive care in Nephrology,* H.R.B. P.T. Murray, J.B. Hall Editor. 2006, Taylor & Francis. p. 157-164.
[45] *Clinical practice guidelines for hemodialysis adequacy, update 2006.* Am J Kidney Dis, 2006. 48 Suppl 1: p. S2-90.
[46] Oliver, M.J., et al., *Randomized study of temporary hemodialysis catheters.* Int J Artif Organs, 2002. 25(1): p. 40-4.

[47] Little, M.A., P.J. Conlon, and J.J. Walshe, *Access recirculation in temporary hemodialysis catheters as measured by the saline dilution technique.* Am J Kidney Dis, 2000. 36(6): p. 1135-9.

[48] Cheesbrough, J.S., R.G. Finch, and R.P. Burden, *A prospective study of the mechanisms of infection associated with hemodialysis catheters.* J Infect Dis, 1986. 154(4): p. 579-89.

[49] Contreras, G., et al., *A multicenter, prospective, randomized, comparative evaluation of dual-versus triple-lumen catheters for hemodialysis and apheresis in 485 patients.* Am J Kidney Dis, 2003. 42(2): p. 315-24.

[50] Konner, K., *The initial creation of native arteriovenous fistulas: surgical aspects and their impact on the practice of nephrology.* Semin Dial, 2003. 16(4): p. 291-8.

[51] Sidawy, A.N., et al., *Recommended standards for reports dealing with arteriovenous hemodialysis accesses.* J Vasc Surg, 2002. 35(3): p. 603-10.

[52] Lameire, N. and R.L. Mehta, *Complications of dialysis.* 2000, New York: M. Dekker. xiv, 877 p.

[53] Sommer G. Bruce , H.M., *Vascular Access for Hemodialysis II.* 1991: p. 145-157.

[54] Hentschel, M.D., *Vascular Access for Hemodialysis.* Nephrology Rounds, 2008. 6(1).

[55] Rayner, H.C., et al., *Creation, cannulation and survival of arteriovenous fistulae: data from the Dialysis Outcomes and Practice Patterns Study.* Kidney Int, 2003. 63(1): p. 323-30.

[56] Silva, M.B., Jr., et al., *A strategy for increasing use of autogenous hemodialysis access procedures: impact of preoperative noninvasive evaluation.* J Vasc Surg, 1998. 27(2): p. 302-7; discussion 307-8.

[57] Beatherd, G.B., *A Practitioner's Resource Guide To Hemodialysis Arteriovenous Fistulas.* 2003: ESRD Network of Texas.

[58] Wong, V., et al., *Factors associated with early failure of arteriovenous fistulae for haemodialysis access.* Eur J Vasc Endovasc Surg, 1996. 12(2): p. 207-13.

[59] Yerdel, M.A., et al., *Effect of haemodynamic variables on surgically created arteriovenous fistula flow.* Nephrol Dial Transplant, 1997. 12(8): p. 1684-8.

[60] Malovrh, M., *Non-invasive evaluation of vessels by duplex sonography prior to construction of arteriovenous fistulas for haemodialysis.* Nephrol Dial Transplant, 1998. 13(1): p. 125-9.

[61] Robbin, M.L., et al., *Hemodialysis arteriovenous fistula maturity: US evaluation. Radiology,* 2002. 225(1): p. 59-64.

[62] USRDS, *2007 Annual Data Report.* 2007.

[63] Schild, A.F., et al., *Early cannulation prosthetic graft (FlixeneTM) for arteriovenous access.* J Vasc Access, 2011.

[64] Hakaim, A.G. and T.E. Scott, *Durability of early prosthetic dialysis graft cannulation: results of a prospective, nonrandomized clinical trial.* J Vasc Surg, 1997. 25(6): p. 1002-5; discussion 1005-6.

[65] Quinn B., D.C., C. G. Carstan, *Hemodialysis Access: Placement and Management of Complications, in Comprehensive Vascular and Endovascular Surgery,* J.L.M. J. W. Hallett, J. J. Earnshaw, J. A. Reekers, T. W. Rooke, Editor. 2009, Mosby ELSEVIER. p. 429-462.

[66] Raad, I., et al., *Ultrastructural analysis of indwelling vascular catheters: a quantitative relationship between luminal colonization and duration of placement.* J Infect Dis, 1993. 168(2): p. 400-7.
[67] Troidle, L. and F.O. Finkelstein, *Catheter-related bacteremia in hemodialysis patients: the role of the central venous catheter in prevention and therapy.* Int J Artif Organs, 2008. 31(9): p. 827-33.
[68] Power, A., et al., *Long-term Tesio Catheter Access for Hemodialysis Can Deliver High Dialysis Adequacy with Low Complication Rates.* J Vasc Interv Radiol, 2011.
[69] Power, A., et al., *Translumbar central venous catheters for long-term haemodialysis. Nephrol Dial Transplant,* 2010. 25(5): p. 1588-95.
[70] Younes, H.K., et al., *Transhepatic hemodialysis catheters: functional outcome and comparison between early and late failure.* J Vasc Interv Radiol, 2011. 22(2): p. 183-91.
[71] Seikaly, M., et al., *The 12th Annual Report of the North American Pediatric Renal Transplant Cooperative Study: renal transplantation from 1987 through 1998.* Pediatr Transplant, 2001. 5(3): p. 215-31.
[72] NAPRTCS. *NAPRTCS: 2008 Annual Report.* 2008; Available from: https://web.emmes.com/study/ped/announce.htm.
[73] *USRDS: the United States Renal Data System.* Am J Kidney Dis, 2003. 42(6 Suppl 5): p. 1-230.
[74] Verrina, E., V. Cappelli, and F. Perfumo, *Selection of modalities, prescription, and technical issues in children on peritoneal dialysis.* Pediatr Nephrol, 2009. 24(8): p. 1453-64.
[75] Fischbach, M., et al., *Hemodialysis in children: general practical guidelines.* Pediatr Nephrol, 2005. 20(8): p. 1054-66.
[76] Carey, W.A., et al., *Outcomes of dialysis initiated during the neonatal period for treatment of end-stage renal disease: a North American Pediatric Renal Trials and Collaborative Studies special analysis.* Pediatrics, 2007. 119(2): p. e468-73.
[77] Sadowski, R.H., W.E. Harmon, and K. Jabs, *Acute hemodialysis of infants weighing less than five kilograms.* Kidney Int, 1994. 45(3): p. 903-6.
[78] Goldstein SL, J.K., *Pediatric hemodialysis,* in *Pediatric Nephrology,* H.W. Avner ED, Niaudet P, Editor. 2003, Lippincott Williams & Wilkins. p. 1395-1410.
[79] Donckerwolcke, R.A. and T.E. Bunchman, *Hemodialysis in infants and small children.* Pediatr Nephrol, 1994. 8(1): p. 103-6.
[80] Pastan, S., J.M. Soucie, and W.M. McClellan, *Vascular access and increased risk of death among hemodialysis patients.* Kidney Int, 2002. 62(2): p. 620-6.
[81] Xue, J.L., et al., *The association of initial hemodialysis access type with mortality outcomes in elderly Medicare ESRD patients.* Am J Kidney Dis, 2003. 42(5): p. 1013-9.
[82] El Minshawy, O., T. Abd El Aziz, and H. Abd El Ghani, *Evaluation of vascular access complications in acute and chronic hemodialysis.* J Vasc Access, 2004. 5(2): p. 76-82.
[83] Ng, L.J., et al., *Hospitalization risks related to vascular access type among incident US hemodialysis patients.* Nephrol Dial Transplant, 2011.
[84] Astor, B.C., et al., *Type of vascular access and survival among incident hemodialysis patients: the Choices for Healthy Outcomes in Caring for ESRD (CHOICE) Study.* J Am Soc Nephrol, 2005. 16(5): p. 1449-55.

[85] Ocak, G., et al., *Haemodialysis catheters increase mortality as compared to arteriovenous accesses especially in elderly patients*. Nephrol Dial Transplant, 2011.

[86] Mendelssohn, D.C., et al., *Haemodialysis vascular access problems in Canada: results from the Dialysis Outcomes and Practice Patterns Study (DOPPS II)*. Nephrol Dial Transplant, 2006. 21(3): p. 721-8.

[87] System, U.S.R.D., *2010 Annual Data Report*. Bethesda, National Institutes of Health, National Institute of Diabetes and Digestive Diseases, 2010.

[88] Tordoir, J.H., F.M. Van Der Sande, and M.W. De Haan, *Current topics on vascular access for hemodialysis*. Minerva Urol Nefrol, 2004. 56(3): p. 223-35.

[89] Movilli, E., et al., *The kind of vascular access influences the baseline inflammatory status and epoetin response in chronic hemodialysis patients*. Blood Purif, 2006. 24(4): p. 387-93.

[90] Swindlehurst, N., et al., *Vascular access for hemodialysis in the elderly*. J Vasc Surg, 2011. 53(4): p. 1039-43.

[91] Raja, R.M., et al., *Comparison of subclavian vein with femoral vein catheterization for hemodialysis*. Am J Kidney Dis, 1983. 2(4): p. 474-6.

[92] Fan, P.Y., *Acute vascular access: new advances*. Adv Ren Replace Ther, 1994. 1(2): p. 90-8.

[93] Vanholder, R., et al., *Complications of subclavian catheter hemodialysis: a 5 year prospective study in 257 consecutive patients*. Int J Artif Organs, 1982. 5(5): p. 297-303.

[94] Edwards, H. and T.C. King, *Cardiac tamponade from central venous catheters*. Arch Surg, 1982. 117(7): p. 965-7.

[95] Geddes, C.C., et al., *Insertion of internal jugular temporary hemodialysis cannulae by direct ultrasound guidance--a prospective comparison of experienced and inexperienced operators*. Clin Nephrol, 1998. 50(5): p. 320-5.

[96] Hernandez, D., et al., *Subclavian vascular access stenosis in dialysis patients: natural history and risk factors*. J Am Soc Nephrol, 1998. 9(8): p. 1507-10.

[97] Cimochowski, G.E., et al., *Superiority of the internal jugular over the subclavian access for temporary dialysis*. Nephron, 1990. 54(2): p. 154-61.

[98] Daeihagh, P., et al., *Efficacy of tissue plasminogen activator administration on patency of hemodialysis access catheters*. Am J Kidney Dis, 2000. 36(1): p. 75-9.

[99] Schwab, S.J., et al., *Hemodialysis-associated subclavian vein stenosis*. Kidney Int, 1988. 33(6): p. 1156-9.

[100] Newman, G.E., et al., *Total central vein obstruction: resolution with angioplasty and fibrinolysis*. Kidney Int, 1991. 39(4): p. 761-4.

[101] Oliver, M.J., et al., *Risk of bacteremia from temporary hemodialysis catheters by site of insertion and duration of use: a prospective study*. Kidney Int, 2000. 58(6): p. 2543-5.

[102] Ishani, A., et al., *Septicemia, access and cardiovascular disease in dialysis patients: the USRDS Wave 2 study*. Kidney Int, 2005. 68(1): p. 311-8.

[103] Dahlberg, P.J., W.R. Yutuc, and K.L. Newcomer, *Subclavian hemodialysis catheter infections*. Am J Kidney Dis, 1986. 7(5): p. 421-7.

[104] Nielsen, J., H.J. Kolmos, and F. Espersen, *Staphylococcus aureus bacteraemia among patients undergoing dialysis--focus on dialysis catheter-related cases*. Nephrol Dial Transplant, 1998. 13(1): p. 139-45.

[105] Nielsen, J., S.D. Ladefoged, and H.J. Kolmos, *Dialysis catheter-related septicaemia--focus on Staphylococcus aureus septicaemia.* Nephrol Dial Transplant, 1998. 13(11): p. 2847-52.

[106] Parienti, J.J., et al., *Femoral vs jugular venous catheterization and risk of nosocomial events in adults requiring acute renal replacement therapy: a randomized controlled trial.* JAMA, 2008. 299(20): p. 2413-22.

[107] Kairaitis, L.K. and T. Gottlieb, *Outcome and complications of temporary haemodialysis catheters.* Nephrol Dial Transplant, 1999. 14(7): p. 1710-4.

[108] Mermel, L.A., et al., *Guidelines for the management of intravascular catheter-related infections.* J Intraven Nurs, 2001. 24(3): p. 180-205.

[109] George, A., et al., *Reducing dialysis associated bacteraemia, and recommendations for surveillance in the United Kingdom: prospective study.* BMJ, 2006. 332(7555): p. 1435.

[110] Beathard, G.A., *Strategy for maximizing the use of arteriovenous fistulae.* Semin Dial, 2000. 13(5): p. 291-6.

[111] Beathard, G.A., S.M. Settle, and M.W. Shields, *Salvage of the nonfunctioning arteriovenous fistula.* Am J Kidney Dis, 1999. 33(5): p. 910-6.

[112] Beathard, G.A., et al., *Aggressive treatment of early fistula failure.* Kidney Int, 2003. 64(4): p. 1487-94.

[113] Romero, A., et al., *Salvage of angioaccess after late thrombosis of radiocephalic fistulas for hemodialysis.* Int Surg, 1986. 71(2): p. 122-4.

[114] Turmel-Rodrigues, L., et al., *Treatment of stenosis and thrombosis in haemodialysis fistulas and grafts by interventional radiology.* Nephrol Dial Transplant, 2000. 15(12): p. 2029-36.

[115] Beathard, G.A., *Physical Examination: the forgotten tool, in Dialysis Access: A Multidisciplinary Approach,* S.J.J. Gray R. J., Editor. 2002, Lippincott Williams & Wilkins. p. 111-228.

[116] Swedberg, S.H., et al., *Intimal fibromuscular hyperplasia at the venous anastomosis of PTFE grafts in hemodialysis patients.* Clinical, immunocytochemical, light and electron microscopic assessment. Circulation, 1989. 80(6): p. 1726-36.

[117] Roy-Chaudhury, P., et al., *Venous neointimal hyperplasia in polytetrafluoroethylene dialysis grafts.* Kidney Int, 2001. 59(6): p. 2325-34.

[118] Paszkowiak, J.J. and A. Dardik, *Arterial wall shear stress: observations from the bench to the bedside.* Vasc Endovascular Surg, 2003. 37(1): p. 47-57.

[119] Corpataux, J.M., et al., *Low-pressure environment and remodelling of the forearm vein in Brescia-Cimino haemodialysis access.* Nephrol Dial Transplant, 2002. 17(6): p. 1057-62.

[120] Misra, S., et al., *BRAVO I: A pilot study of vascular brachytherapy in polytetrafluoroethylene dialysis access grafts.* Kidney Int, 2006. 70(11): p. 2006-13.

[121] Cai, X. and N.J. Freedman, *New therapeutic possibilities for vein graft disease in the post-edifoligide era.* Future Cardiol, 2006. 2(4): p. 493-501.

[122] Conte, M.S., et al., *Results of PREVENT III: a multicenter, randomized trial of edifoligide for the prevention of vein graft failure in lower extremity bypass surgery.* J Vasc Surg, 2006. 43(4): p. 742-751; discussion 751.

[123] Melhem, M., et al., *Development of a local perivascular paclitaxel delivery system for hemodialysis vascular access dysfunction: polymer preparation and in vitro activity.* Blood Purif, 2006. 24(3): p. 289-98.

[124] Rotmans, J.I., et al., *In vivo cell seeding with anti-CD34 antibodies successfully accelerates endothelialization but stimulates intimal hyperplasia in porcine arteriovenous expanded polytetrafluoroethylene grafts.* Circulation, 2005. 112(1): p. 12-8.

[125] Beathard, G.A., *Angioplasty for arteriovenous grafts and fistulae.* Semin Nephrol, 2002. 22(3): p. 202-10.

[126] Vesely, T.M., *Endovascular intervention for the failing vascular access.* Adv Ren Replace Ther, 2002. 9(2): p. 99-108.

[127] Sreenarasimhaiah, V.P., et al., *Salvage of thrombosed dialysis access grafts with venous anastomosis stents.* Kidney Int, 2005. 67(2): p. 678-84.

[128] May, R.E., et al., *Predictive measures of vascular access thrombosis: a prospective study.* Kidney Int, 1997. 52(6): p. 1656-62.

[129] Vesely, T.M., *Mechanical thrombectomy devices to treat thrombosed hemodialysis grafts.* Tech Vasc Interv Radiol, 2003. 6(1): p. 35-41.

[130] Taylor, G., et al., *Prospective surveillance for primary bloodstream infections occurring in Canadian hemodialysis units.* Infect Control Hosp Epidemiol, 2002. 23(12): p. 716-20.

[131] Kaplowitz, L.G., et al., *Prospective study of microbial colonization of the nose and skin and infection of the vascular access site in hemodialysis patients.* J Clin Microbiol, 1988. 26(7): p. 1257-62.

[132] KDOQI *Guideline 27:Treatment do pseuoaneurysm of dialysis AV grafts.*

[133] Schanzer, H., et al., *Treatment of ischemia due to "steal" by arteriovenous fistula with distal artery ligation and revascularization.* J Vasc Surg, 1988. 7(6): p. 770-3.

[134] Hye, R.J. and Y.G. Wolf, *Ischemic monomelic neuropathy: an under-recognized complication of hemodialysis access.* Ann Vasc Surg, 1994. 8(6): p. 578-82.

[135] Grapsa I., Oreopoulos D., *Dialysis in the elderly, in Replacement of renal function by dialysis,* K.M.K. Horl H. W., Lindsay B.R., Ronco C., Winchester F.J., Editor. 2004, kluwer academic publishers.

[136] Hoen, B., et al., *Risk factors for bacterial infections in chronic haemodialysis adult patients: a multicentre prospective survey.* Nephrol Dial Transplant, 1995. 10(3): p. 377-81.

[137] Combe, C., et al., *[Dialysis Outcomes and Practice Patterns Study: data on the use of central venous catheters in chronic hemodialysis].* Nephrologie, 2001. 22(8): p. 379-84.

[138] Jaffer, Y., et al., *A meta-analysis of hemodialysis catheter locking solutions in the prevention of catheter-related infection.* Am J Kidney Dis, 2008. 51(2): p. 233-41.

[139] Fdez-Gallego, J., et al., *Prophylaxis with gentamicin reduces bacterial infection morbidity and mortality related to permanent tunneled central venous catheter and does not cause bacterial resistance.* Nefrologia, 2011.

[140] Del Pozo, J.L., et al., *Intra-catheter leukocyte culture to monitor hemodialysis catheter colonization.* A prospective study to prevent catheter-related bloodstream infections. Int J Artif Organs, 2008. 31(9): p. 820-6.

[141] Rodriguez, J.A., et al., *The function of permanent vascular access.* Nephrol Dial Transplant, 2000. 15(3): p. 402-8.

[142] Kinnaert, P., et al., *Nine years' experience with internal arteriovenous fistulas for haemodialysis: a study of some factors influencing the results.* Br J Surg, 1977. 64(4): p. 242-6.

[143] Reilly, D.T., R.F. Wood, and P.R. Bell, *Prospective study of dialysis fistulas: problem patients and their treatment.* Br J Surg, 1982. 69(9): p. 549-53.

[144] Windus, D.W., *Permanent vascular access: a nephrologist's view.* Am J Kidney Dis, 1993. 21(5): p. 457-71.

[145] de Almeida, E., et al., *Survival in haemodialysis: is there a role for vascular access?* Nephrol Dial Transplant, 1997. 12(4): p. 852.

[146] Bender, M.H., C.M. Bruyninckx, and P.G. Gerlag, *The brachiocephalic elbow fistula: a useful alternative angioaccess for permanent hemodialysis.* J Vasc Surg, 1994. 20(5): p. 808-13.

[147] Beasley, C., J. Rowland, and L. Spergel, *Fistula first: an update for renal providers. Nephrol News Issues,* 2004. 18(11): p. 88, 90.

[148] Leapman, S.B., et al., *The arteriovenous fistula for hemodialysis access: gold standard or archaic relic?* Am Surg, 1996. 62(8): p. 652-6; discussion 656-7.

[149] Hodges, T.C., et al., *Longitudinal comparison of dialysis access methods: risk factors for failure.* J Vasc Surg, 1997. 26(6): p. 1009-19.

[150] Konner, K., et al., *Tailoring the initial vascular access for dialysis patients.* Kidney Int, 2002. 62(1): p. 329-38.

[151] Fassiadis, N., et al., *Does the surgeon's experience impact on radiocephalic fistula patency rates?* Semin Dial, 2007. 20(5): p. 455-7.

[152] Korsheed, S., et al., *Effects of arteriovenous fistula formation on arterial stiffness and cardiovascular performance and function.* Nephrol Dial Transplant, 2011.

[153] Rayner, H.C. and R.L. Pisoni, *The increasing use of hemodialysis catheters: evidence from the DOPPS on its significance and ways to reverse it.* Semin Dial, 2010. 23(1): p. 6-10.

[154] Stehman-Breen, C.O., et al., *Determinants of type and timing of initial permanent hemodialysis vascular access.* Kidney Int, 2000. 57(2): p. 639-45.

[155] Sesso, R. and M.M. Yoshihiro, *Time of diagnosis of chronic renal failure and assessment of quality of life in haemodialysis patients.* Nephrol Dial Transplant, 1997. 12(10): p. 2111-6.

[156] Arora, P., et al., *Prevalence, predictors, and consequences of late nephrology referral at a tertiary care center.* J Am Soc Nephrol, 1999. 10(6): p. 1281-6.

[157] Roubicek, C., et al., *Timing of nephrology referral: influence on mortality and morbidity.* Am J Kidney Dis, 2000. 36(1): p. 35-41.

[158] Pena, J.M., et al., *[Late nephrology referral influences on morbidity and mortality of hemodialysis patients. A provincial study].* Nefrologia, 2006. 26(1): p. 84-97.

[159] Pisoni, R.L., et al., *Vascular access use in Europe and the United States: results from the DOPPS.* Kidney Int, 2002. 61(1): p. 305-16.

[160] Ravani, P., et al., *Cardiovascular comorbidity and late referral impact arteriovenous fistula survival: a prospective multicenter study.* J Am Soc Nephrol, 2004. 15(1): p. 204-9.

[161] Ethier, J., et al., *Vascular access use and outcomes: an international perspective from the Dialysis Outcomes and Practice Patterns Study.* Nephrol Dial Transplant, 2008. 23(10): p. 3219-26.

5

Subjective Well-Being Measures of Hemodialysis Patients

Paulo Roberto Santos
Sobral School of Medicine, Federal University of Ceará
Brazil

1. Introduction

In recent years the frequency of intra-dialytic symptoms has been decreasing, improving the patient well-being during treatment sessions. This has mainly been due to technical advances, such as more reliable monitoring devices, better water quality, physiological bicarbonate-based dialysate and machines to control ultrafiltration. Nowadays during hemodialysis (HD), patients suffer less from hypotension, cramps, headache, dizziness, nausea and vomiting (Himmelfarb & Ikizler, 2010; Al-Hilali et al., 2004). However, instead of well-being during dialysis, this chapter examines the well-being of patients between sessions, in their daily lives, focusing on how they perceive their quality of life (QOL). Unfortunately, technical advances in HD have not brought changes in the characteristics of renal replacement therapy: severe dietary restrictions, lost time, dependence on a machine, common occurrence of clinical complications and high mortality. Treatment of end-stage renal disease (ESRD) with HD is thus inherently distressing, causing social and family changes, and interferes profoundly in patients' well-being (Cukor et al., 2007; Tsutsui et al., 2009; Low et al., 2008).

ESRD treated with HD should be highlighted among other chronic diseases concerning its treatment, evolution and life consequences. Treatment depends not only on polypharmacy, but also on artificial replacement of kidney function by a machine - still a deficient method that cannot prevent various complications: ostheodystrophy, atherosclerotic disease and risk for infections. This inefficacious replacement of kidney function causes these patients to have a twenty-fold higher chance of death than in the general population (Parmar, 2002). HD patients must adhere to a very restricted diet with controlled ingestion of water. In conventional HD, the patient is submitted to sessions of dialysis for approximately four hours three times a week in a renal unit (plus the time spent commuting to and from the renal unit), a time loss that influences employment, leisure and relationships. It is not surprising, then, that ESRD treated with HD affects QOL more intensely than heart failure, diabetes, chronic lung disease, arthritis and cancer (Mittal et al., 2001).

Therefore dialytic therapy is associated with powerful stressors. The literature shows that successful adaptation to dialysis depends more on personal stress modulators than on objective treatment variables (Tsay et al., 2005; Curtin & Mapes, 2001). Personal modulators are mainly subjective, due to psychology, personality and behaviour (Cukor et al., 2007). These subjective factors cannot be discovered by traditional medical measures like physical signs, laboratory and radiological data. The assessment of these subjective factors depends on patient reports. Health professionals have to know how patients are doing under dialysis if they want to offer better therapy. Growing awareness of this fact is reflected in the increasing number of randomized controlled trials and studies of new drugs and treatments that include patient-focused issues such as convenience, adherence difficulties, patients' feelings and preferences. How does my patient feel under dialysis? has become a central question.

It is a simple question. Indeed "how do you feel" is used in overall scores. But such a summary score does not comprise the complexity of well-being. Well-being comprises physical functioning, psychological aspects, social environment and spirituality. That is why validated instruments to measure QOL are so useful. They are multi-dimensional, comprising physical, psychological, emotional and social aspects affecting well-being. They are easy to administer and generate scores on a user-friendly numeric scale. This quantitative approach facilitates clinicians' interaction because they are accustomed to quantitative data. In summary, we need to be worried about well-being among HD patients, we already have reliable instruments to measure the main subjective variables involved in well-being, but health professionals trained in using subjective measures are lacking. The main objective of this chapter is to provide information about subjective measures in the area of dialysis.

This chapter first examines the subjective measures most used to assess the feelings of patients undergoing HD. The data are related to conventional HD (four-hour sessions three times a week). But the effects on patient well-being of other modalities (short daily or nightly dialysis) are also discussed. It also describes the main validated instruments to measure subjective aspects closely related to well-being, emphasizing QOL as a central measure. A complete list of instruments would be too exhausting, so it comments on those instruments which have provided relevant results in the field of ESRD and HD. It also presents data on recognized interactions of the type of variables associated with QOL, and whenever possible comments on my own results based on a characteristic sample from a renal unit located in a low-income area of Brazil. I think this sample is similar in many respects to all patients in the world, but with some particularities due to the area's prevailing socioeconomic status, which may be of interest to the reader. Finally, I express some personal views about how to improve QOL among HD patients. I believe opinions are still valuable in the present stage since there are no recommendations based on Level I or II evidence about interventions in order to improve QOL among dialysis patients.

2. What are subjective measures and their importance?

It is easiest to define subjective measures in contrast with objective measures. Traditionally in clinical practice, renal unit teams work with objective measures: physical signs, laboratory and radiological data. These measures are obviously independent of patients' feelings. In a group with high mortality like patients suffering from ESRD, physical signs, laboratory and radiological data serve to indicate poor control of the illness, need for treatment adjustments and risk of hospitalization and death. Meanwhile, subjective measures are generated from patients' reports. In this respect, administering questionnaires to patients elicits information that can be used to calculate subjective measures about patients' feelings, perceptions and judgements that cannot be discovered by objective measures or close observation of patients. It is well established that health professionals underestimate patients' feelings of well-being. Clinicians are often surprised to learn that patients with impairments and disabilities can perceive life as a good experience, in contrast to patients with more favourable clinical conditions, who can perceive poor QOL (Riis et al., 2005). Reports of family members, friends and caregivers usually do not match patients' real perceptions. Most instruments used for subjective measures show results on scales of how patients perceive their lives (as opposed to years of life remaining), how they feel (irrespective of clinical condition), and the ways they cope (independent of peers' opinions). There are several kinds of subjective measures concerning overall well-being: spirituality, depressive feelings, quality of life, sexual satisfaction and ways of coping. All these subjective measures should play a central role in medicine.

Subjective measures have become important, first, because they can predict clinically relevant outcomes. Spirituality, depressive feelings and QOL are now extensively validated indicators of withdrawal from therapy, hospitalization and death among HD patients (Koenig, 2001; Powell et al., 2003; Spinale et al., 2008; Lopes et al., 2002; Lowrie et al., 2003; Knight et al., 2003; Mapes et al., 2003; Revuelta et al., 2004). For example, withdrawal is the cause of 25% of deaths among HD patients in the United States (Cohen et al., 2003). Second, and most important, these measures have not only been validated as indicators, they have become a main outcome in dialysis treatment. Despite technical advances in dialysis therapy, mortality is still very high, at 15-25% a year (United States Renal Data System, 2003). With such high mortality rates, objective measures only reveal whether patients are in the expected mortality range, without shedding any light on how their life quality and how to improve it. In this scenario of high and stationary mortality, subjective measures have become a main outcome. The chance of improving the patient's remaining life, however short it may be, is the most important end-point of dialysis therapy. Therefore, QOL issues are increasingly being included in studies on HD, such as The Netherlands Cooperative Study on the Adequacy of Dialysis (NECOSAD) and the North Thames Dialysis Study (NTDS), and in the principal guides to clinical practice in dialysis: the Dialysis Outcomes and Practice Patterns Study (DOPPS) and Reduction of Morbidity and Mortality among Hemodialysis Patients (HEMO). The National Kidney Foundation (NKF), through its guidelines published as a series named K/DOQI, now recommends routine monitoring QOL level in clinical attendance of HD patients (Merkus et al., 2000; NKF, 2006). Moreover, besides the importance of subjective measures in the nephrology area, today randomized clinical trials and studies of new drugs and treatments place the survival variable alongside QOL and patients' convenience and well-being. In the final analysis, then, health professionals must increasingly pay attention to subjective measures.

In summary, subjective measures cannot be estimated by observation by either health professionals or families, nor can they be revealed by physical signs or laboratory/radiological data. They depend entirely on patient reports. But many questions arise in formulating subjective measurement techniques: What is important to ask? How can feelings and perceptions be put on a quantitative scale? What elements comprise well-being? All these questions have been addressed in recent studies. Knowledge has increased, to the point where doctors in clinical settings, without the help of specialists, can call on many validated instruments covering various dimensions of feelings. In short, the tools are available to measure patients' well-being to a reasonable degree of accuracy.

2.1 The central role of quality of life

Interest in QOL increased after the Second World War in the context of knowing how ownership of household appliances was influencing people's lives. However, in the medical field, this interest is more recent. A revision of medical papers detected an exponentially increasing number of articles on QOL during the 90s (Garrat et al., 2002).

The appearance of several validated questionnaires allowed quantitative measurement of QOL. The most popular instruments to measure QOL use numeric scales, making them attractive because clinicians are used to working with quantitative variables. These instruments solved the main problem of studying QOL. Measuring quality entails making subjective judgments about feelings, which can seem very complex to consider in daily medical practice. But when feelings, judgements and opinions are translated into scales, the resulting measurement can be associated with other traditional medical outcomes, like laboratory indicators and morbidity, mortality and adherence rates. This occurred in the 1990s, when QOL scores were validated as a powerful predictor of morbidity and death, not only in large trials, but also in small samples comprising patients from single renal units (Kalantar-Zadeh et al., 2001).

But multidimensionality is the main reason for the central role of QOL among other subjective measures. The World Health Organization's definitions of health and QOL as involving overall (physical, mental and social) well-being and not only the absence of disease were the basis for constructing all the instruments to measure QOL. Due to the broad scope of these definitions, QOL instruments try to capture a central value of life and to summarize perceptions of several life dimensions in a score. In practice, a QOL instrument must assess at least two levels: functioning (ability to perform daily living activities) and perceived well-being (emotional and mental well-being and satisfaction with social activities). These two levels combined in one instrument distinguish QOL measures from other subjective measures. Other measures focus on particular aspects of mental health (depression), personality (spirituality, coping style) and behaviour (sexuality). In contrast to the multidimensionality of QOL measures, the other subjective measures are one-dimensional and cannot capture the central value of life. In a simple view, other subjective measures are related to aspects of our lives and act as measures of well-being. These one-dimensional measures deserve being studied because they can serve as indicators for interventions to improve well-being. However, QOL is more than a measure, it covers the idea of a central life value, and as such QOL is an end-point, an aim of medical therapies.

3. Instruments for subjective measurement

In nephrology, most knowledge of QOL is based on results generated by the Medical Outcomes Study Questionnaire 36-Item Short Form Survey - SF-36 (Ware & Sherbourne, 1992). This is due to the fact the SF-36 has been chosen to measure QOL by important research groups, like the NECOSAD and NTDS, and by the main studies generating guidelines for clinical practice in dialysis, such as the DOPPS and HEMO. SF-36 is a generic instrument (it does not contain specific questions related to any kind of illness). It covers issues relating to eight dimensions of QOL: physical functioning, role-physical, bodily pain, general health, vitality, social functioning, role-emotional and mental health. It generates scores from 0 (worst) to 100 (best) for each dimension. There are population parameters of QOL assessed by the SF-36 for several countries, such as the United States, Canada, Australia, Spain, Sweden and England (Hopman et al., 2000; Mishra & Schofield, 1998; Jenkinson et al., 1999; Alonso et al., 1998; Sullivan & Karlsson, 1998). This enables making comparisons of QOL level between patients and healthy people. The SF-36 can be applied to people aged 14 years or older. It takes 20 to 30 minutes to administer, which is feasible in clinical daily practice. It can be administered by an interviewer, allowing inclusion of illiterate patients, an important portion of HD patients from underdeveloped areas. It can also be self-administered or given by telephone or computer. The major restriction is that the SF-36 does not cover two important dimensions of QOL: sleep and sexual activities. These two dimensions are well covered by the World Health Organization Quality of Life instrument (WHO-QOL), another generic instrument (WHOQOL Group, 1998). Use of the WHO-QOL is more limited in nephrology. It contains 100 items. The SF-36 and WHO-QOL also have brief versions with 12 items and 26 items, respectively.

Some researchers believe QOL among HD patients should be measured by a specific instrument (containing questions related to specific aspects of kidney disease). They argue that specific instruments can better expose difficulties direct related to ESRD and dialysis therapy, and may be more sensitive to detect changes over time. The KDQOL is a specific instrument to measure QOL. It was created in 1994 and has 134 items (Hays et al., 1994). However, the length of the questionnaire makes its clinical application difficult. The short version is used more (KDQOL-SF), containing 80 items divided into 19 dimensions: including the 36 items (eight dimensions) of the SF-36 and another 44 kidney-disease targeted items covering symptoms/problems, effects of kidney disease, burden of kidney disease, cognitive function, quality of social interaction, sexual function, sleep, social support, work status, patient satisfaction and dialysis staff encouragement. The scores on each dimension range from 0 (worst) to 100 (best). Its visibility in nephrology is due to its use in the United States Renal Data System.

The instrument called Evaluation of Individual Quality of Life (SEIQOL) is less used, but due to its particular method, I included it in this review (Moons et al., 2004). In the SEI-QOL, unlike the SF-36, WHO-QOL and KDQOL, patients choose and list the dimensions of QOL they judge relevant. This method facilitates identifying the dimensions of well-being the patient finds important. But it requires a complex process of abstract thinking, excluding a significant number of patients. Moreover, it is partly qualitative and partly quantitative and health professionals are not used to a qualitative approach. The SEIQOL covers three phases: first, patients are asked to name the five most important areas in their life; second, they are asked to score each area using a visual analog scale from 0 (could not be worse) to 100 (could not be better); and third, the named areas are ranked (weighted) and the total of the ranks cannot exceed 100%. The SEI-QOL results are obtained by multiplying the scores (0-100) and weights (0-100%). The method used by the SEI-QOL makes its administration in large samples difficult, but it can be useful in individual approaches.

As stated above, the main advantage of QOL measures is to cover several dimensions. But health professionals with less experience in evaluating QOL measures can be intimidated by the multiple scores from different domains. An overall well-being score would be easier. The QOL Scale (QOL SIS) is a single-item that I believe it can be used as a training score by inexperienced teams, and can serve to stimulate further consideration of using multidimensional instruments (Patel et al., 2002). The QOL SIS is an item contained in the McGill QOL questionnaire - MQOL (Cohen et al., 1995). The MQOL has several items, one of which directly asks patients about their overall assessment of their perceived QOL. This item can be used alone, in which case it produces the Feinstein Score (Lara-Munoz & Feinstein, 1999). The Feinstein Score ranges from 0 (very bad) to 10 (excellent). I strongly suggest that inexperienced renal unit teams test it as a preliminary approach to subjective measures.

Spirituality, defined as perception of meaning and purpose of life and not only as organized religion or a belief in a higher being, can be measured by validated instruments. The

Spiritual Well-Being Questionnaire (SWBQ) and Spiritual Belief Scale have only been used in a few studies with HD patients, but their results have clinical relevance. Spirituality was associated with QOL measures, satisfaction with life and perception of depression (Patel et al., 2002; Finkelstein et al., 2007). The SWBQ contains 20 items, five for each of four domains: personal, communal, environmental, and transcendental spiritual well-being (Gomez & Fisher, 2003). Respondents indicate how they feel in relation to 20 statements (items) over the past six months. All items are rated according to the 5-point Likert scale, ranging from "never" to "always do". The Spiritual Belief Scale was used in the study of Patel and associates (2002). The questionnaire has four items, each scored on a scale of 0 to 10. Two items measure the perceived importance of faith and its helpfulness in coping with ESRD and the other two items involve perception of the importance of attending religious services and its helpfulness in coping with ESRD.

The Beck Depression Inventory (BDI) is the standard instrument for screening clinical depression (Craven et al., 1988). The BDI covers 21 categories of symptoms. Each category has four levels of severity of that symptom, scored from 0 (little or no distress) to 3 (severe distress). The final score is the sum of the responses to the 21 symptom-items. The validated cut-off of score range of 14 to 16 corresponds to psychiatric diagnosis of major depressive disorder (Hedayati et al., 2006). As an alternative to the BDI, there is a short form (10 items) of the Epidemiological Studies Depression Screening Index (CES-D). The CES-D is not as widely validated as the Beck Depression Inventory, but has fewer questions, so it can be administered more quickly. It can be helpful as a screening tool of depression (Andresen et al., 1994). Each item of the CES-D is scored from 0 to 3 points and the total score ranges from 0 to 30. The CES-D was used in the DOPPS (score ≥ 10 as an indicator of probable depression) and was validated in comparison to the standard BDI (Lopes et al., 2004; Hedayati et al., 2006).

Erectile dysfunction among men is a well-established complication of dialysis. There are many studies in the literature on this theme. The International Index of Erectile Function (IIEF) is the standard instrument to assess male sexual functioning (Rosen et al., 1997). Most studies apply the six questions covering erectile function, but the instrument also covers orgasmic function (2 questions), sexual desire (2 questions), intercourse satisfaction (3 questions) and overall satisfaction (2 questions). The IIEF gives results according to four categories: no, minimum, moderate and advanced dysfunction. On the other hand, there is much less literature on the sexual aspects of women undergoing HD, although a validated instrument is available, the Female Sexual Function Index (FSFI). It is a 19-item questionnaire covering six domains of sexual function: desire, arousal, lubrification, orgasm, satisfaction and pain. The minimum score is 1.2 and the maximum is 36. A score < 26.55 indicates the presence of sexual dysfunction (Wiegel et al., 2005).

Coping is defined as the cognitive and behavioral efforts to manage, reduce or tolerate external and internal demands and conflicts among them (Lazarus & Folkman, 1984). In the context of ESRD, external demands are the various stressors associated with dialysis therapy. The coping method works as a modulator of stressors. The way patients cope with stress can determine how they will be affected by the problem. According to the theory of coping, patients' efforts may be to manage or alter the source of stress (problem-oriented coping) or to regulate stressful emotions (emotion-oriented coping) (Lazarus & Folkman, 1984). In other words, problem-oriented coping aims to make direct changes in a stressful situation whereas emotion-oriented coping seeks to ameliorate emotions associated with a problem. The Jalowiec Coping Scale (JCS) was the first version, with 40 items and results summarized in problem-oriented (15 items) and emotion-oriented (25 items) coping styles (Jalowiec & Powers, 1981). There is a second version of the JCS with 60 questions on coping strategies, classified into eight types: confrontative (10 items), evasive (13 items), supportive (5 items) and self-reliant (7 items) behaviors pertaining to problem-oriented coping; and emotive (5 items), palliative (7 items), optimistic (9 items) and fatalistic (9 items) behaviors pertaining to emotion-oriented coping (Jalowiec, 1991). The results are revealed by the frequency of each coping style or by scores (5-point Likert scale for each item). The JCS has been widely used among well and clinical populations, including studies of ESRD patients (Klang et al., 1996; Lindqvist et al., 1998; Yeh & Chou, 2007; Toimamueang et al., 2003; Lindqvist et al., 2000). In my group, we discern coping style as the principal measure of how intensely dialysis-associated stressors will affect HD patients. We are now working with the perspective that patient education in coping skills can be used to change the risk of poor QOL.

The instruments reported here have generated enough data in nephrology to have a panel of what and how subjective measures mediate patients' perceived QOL.

4. Variables associated with quality of life among hemodialysis patients

4.1 Objective measures

Objective measures are those associated with socio-demographic aspects and HD quality-of-care indicators. Most of socio-demographic variables are not modifiable, but quality of HD treatment can be modulated in practice by setting goals: hemoglobin of 11-12 g/dl, equilibrated $Kt/V \geq 1.2$, phosphorus of 3.5-5.5 g/L, and adequate nutrition. This section discusses the frequency and duration of dialysis sessions as objective variables in emerging modalities of short daily or nocturnal dialysis.

Age: Older age does not necessarily mean worse QOL among HD patients. Older patients compensate for physical deterioration by adjusting mental outlook aspects. This conclusion is supported by results showing that the main effects of age are on the physical domain of QOL rather than the mental domains (Deoreo, 1997; Singer et al., 1999; Lamping et al., 2000). Older people (> 65 years) perceive less decline of QOL and more satisfaction with life when compared to younger patients (Rebollo et al., 2001; Kimmel et al., 1995). In large samples from the HEMO Study as well as in small samples from single renal units, older patients on HD have better QOL than do younger patients (Unruh et al., 2008; Abdel-Kader et al., 2009). Maybe the larger gap between expected and actual QOL among younger patients makes the treatment restrictions more disturbing to them.

Gender: Among healthy people in countries like Canada, the United States and England, where the SF-36 has been used to estimate QOL in the general population, it has been found that men have better QOL than women (Ware, 1993; Jenkinson et al., 1999; Hopman et al., 2000). This gender difference is not found among HD patients (Kalantar-Zadeh et al., 2001). It seems that stressors associated with dialysis therapy, which are common to both genders, are powerful enough to overcome the gender aspects determining difference within the general population.

Race: African-American HD patients in the United States reported significantly better psychological well-being than non-African-Americans (Owen et al., 1998; Hicks et al., 2004; Unruh et al., 2004a). In countries like Brazil, with more miscegenation, it is difficult to classify patients according to race, so there are not extant studies of race-based differences.

Socioeconomic status: Brazil is a large country and has great regional socioeconomic disparities as well as local class differences. Most studies of HD samples are from the southeast region, which is the country's richest, where many universities are located. I work in northeast Brazil, which is a generally poor region. Last year in a chapter of a Brazilian book, I concluded that QOL level is lower among HD patients from low-income areas (Cruz & Cruz, 2010). A previous Brazilian study showed that QOL scores of high-socioeconomic HD patients tended to increase more over time than did the scores among low- and middle-class patients within a sample of eight dialysis units in the state of São Paulo (Sesso et al., 2003).

Travel time: Depending on the region, renal units can be very far from where patients live. In the north and northeast of Brazil, there are few renal units, and patients have to travel long distances to for dialysis (Ritt et al., 2007). In our renal unit, in the city of Sobral in northeastern Brazil, 80% of the patients undergoing regular HD live outside the city where the renal unit is located, in small towns within a radius of 144 miles. My research team has been unable to detect differences regarding laboratory values, adherence, QOL and depression according to the patient travel time. This may be because patients in our region who live in small rural communities are accustomed to traveling long distances to obtain government services of all types. However, in a large sample, longer travel time is associated to higher mortality and decreased QOL (Moist et al., 2008).

Anemia: With the spreading use of erythropoietin, several studies about the relationships between anemia control and QOL have been performed. The current recommendation is to achieve partial control of anemia (hemoglobin of 11-12 g/dl) due to potentially adverse cardiovascular events at higher hemoglobin levels (Besarab et al., 1998; Singh, 2008; Phrommintikul et al., 2007). Distinct approaches to patients with or without symptomatic cardiac disease concerning target hemoglobin are subject to debate, and the results are contradictory (Canadian Erythropoietin Study Group, 1990; Furuland et al., 2003). There are several studies showing better QOL with higher hemoglobin as well as showing no differences of QOL according to hemoglobin level. In a recent systematic review with meta-analysis, Clement et al. (2009) included only 11 studies from a total of 231 and concluded that hemoglobin levels in excess of 12 g/dl lead to small and not clinically meaningful improvements in QOL. The authors suggested, due to safety concerns, targeting treatment to hemoglobin levels in the range of 9-12 g/dl as opposed to hemoglobin > 12 g/dl.

Kt/V index: The dialysis dose, estimated by the Kt/V index, was a constant variable of interest in the early studies of QOL. The hypothesis was that higher dose would be associated with better QOL. With the exception of studies with small samples (Powers et al., 2000; Manns et al., 2002), no correlation between Kt/V and QOL was found (Kalantar Zadeh et al., 2001; Mittal et al., 2001). The advent of new membranes has rekindled interest in the relationships between high flux membranes and QOL. But once again, this time in a multi-center randomized trial, neither the dose (Kt/V 1.45 vs. 1.05) nor the dialysis membrane (high flux vs. low flux) demonstrated clinically meaningful benefits (Unruh et al., 2004b).

Malnutrition: There are several reports of associations between nutritional status and QOL through nutritional markers: creatinine, albumin, calf circumference and protein/energy intake (Ohri-Vachaspati & Seghal, 1999; Allen et al., 2002; Kalantar-Zadeh et al., 2001; Fujisawa et al., 2000; Raimundo et al., 2006). In our renal unit, we found different patterns of relationships between nutritional status and QOL according to gender: malnutrition and low protein intake correlated with low QOL among women but not among men.

Frequency and duration of dialysis sessions: An important current issue is the potential of more frequent and longer dialysis sessions to improve several clinical outcomes. As stated above, studies of dialysis dose and different membrane types in the context of conventional

HD have not shown an influence on QOL. In other studies, dialysis modalities with more frequent and longer dialysis sessions, like nocturnal (5 sessions weekly, 6 to 10 hours/session) or short daily dialysis (6 sessions weekly, 2 to 3.5 hours/session), in comparison with conventional HD, have been shown to have a positive influence on QOL (Lindsay, 2004; Culleton et al., 2007; Van Eps et al., 2010). However, everywhere in the world, but particularly in developing countries, the necessary economic and organizational changes will be the main obstacles to conducting more frequent dialysis on a large scale. This is certainly true in Brazil. First, current reimbursement by the National Health System is limited to thrice-weekly hemodialysis, so increased reimbursement to support more frequent and longer dialysis will be necessary. Second, daily HD will overtax the present capacity of renal units, so resources are needed to set up new and accessible satellite dialysis units.

4.2 Subjective measures

Objective measures are traditional and well-managed by clinicians. Nonetheless, QOL among HD patients remains poor. The increasing knowledge of subjective measures can be the key for more effective interventions to improve QOL.

Depression: The high prevalence - nearly 30% - and the role of depression in affecting well-being among HD patients are well established (Cukor et al., 2006). But there are limited studies focused on treatment of depression in HD patients. Serotonin reuptake inhibitors and psychotherapy can be indicated (Blumenfield et al., 1997; Kimmel & Peterson, 2006). But it is difficult to employ successful routines to treat depression in practice (Wuerth et al., 2003). Among HD patients, depressive feelings are associated with low QOL, and are predictors of both death due to any cause and withdrawal from dialysis (Lopes et al., 2004; Berlim et al., 2006; Drayer et al., 2006). Patients' social support interacts with depression, but once again subjective modulators have a central role. Better social support among individuals high in the personality trait of "agreeableness" was associated with a decrease in depressive symptoms, whereas social support had little effect on depression change for individuals ranked as low in "agreeableness" (Hoth et al., 2007).

Sexuality: Sexuality is a complex aspect of human lives because it comprises physiological needs and social demands. Dialysis therapy negatively affects sexual function both among men and women. Several well-known factors are associated with erectile dysfunction among men on HD: gonadal dysfunction; hyperprolactinemia; zinc, iodine and manganese deficiencies; hyperparathyroidism; uremic neuropathy; arteriosclerosis; anemia; and use of antihypertensives (Palmer, 1999). Some studies have found a prevalence of erectile dysfunction as high as 80% (Rosas et al., 2001). In the experience of my team, nearly half of young patients (20 to 50 years old) present erectile dysfunction and have significantly lower mental health assessed by the SF-36 when compared to patients with the same age range without erectile dysfunction. There are few studies on the sexuality of women undergoing HD. But similar to our experience among men, Seethala et al. (2010) found 46% sexual dysfunction among sexually active women on dialysis, assessed by the FSFI. But in contrast to men, sexual dysfunction among women has not been associated with low well-being, assessed by the Illness Effects Questionnaire (Seethala et al., 2010). No doubt, women must be studied more to confirm the differences between them and men concerning sexuality as a measure of well-being and QOL.

Spirituality: The relationship of spirituality, physical health and well-being is well documented in the literature (Levin & Vanderpool, 1991; Ellison, 1991; Powell et al., 2003).

In the nephrology area, there are reports of better QOL and less depression among dialysis patients with greater perception of spirituality and religiosity (Patel et al., 2002; Finkelstein et al., 2007). People identified as spiritual report better social support (Patel et al., 2002). Cumulative positive effects of social support and spirituality can explain lower mortality and better well-being (Spinale et al., 2008). Nevertheless, more studies on spirituality are necessary among HD patients. But it is promising that spirituality and social support could be targets of intervention. Strategies aiming at engaging patients in discussions about their spiritual concerns together with planning activities to involve patients' social support networks in treatment problems could improve subjective and objective outcomes.
Coping style: Common sense as well as scientific evidence shows that the way people face difficult situations is the main measure of the effects of stress in their lives. This explains why in clinical practice there are patients with many handicaps who still perceive their lives as pleasant, while others with fewer problems do not. This is also the basis of the importance of all subjective measures discussed here. Coping tests are simple and can be used by dialysis stuff without psychologists' help. Moreover, coping style is a modifiable variable, which can be changed by adaptation training programs. My study team found a correlation between emotion-oriented coping and poor QOL regarding the physical (physical functioning and role-physical) and mental (role-emotional and mental health) dimensions of the SF-36, in line with other studies of chronic disease patients, including the ESRD (Bombardier et al., 1990; Wahl et al., 1999; Dunn et al., 1994). In my view, coping is a potent measure and can be a suitable target for interventions to improve QOL. This personal view is addressed in more detail in the next section.

5. How to improve well-being among hemodialysis patients

When thinking about how to improve QOL among HD patients, two facts must be considered. First, despite a great number of studies, there are no recommendations possible based on Level I or II evidence (Madhan, 2010). The reason is that while there are many cross-sectional studies of QOL, there is a lack of interventional and randomized controlled trials. Second, there has been no improvement of QOL among dialysis patients in the past decade (Gabbay et al., 2010). Recent technical advances and treatment guidelines have not been associated with changes in QOL, although a study of a small sample showed it was possible to improve QOL associated with better quality-of-care indicators (Lacson et al., 2009). Thus, targeting the current quality-of-care indicators concerning anemia, nutrition, dialysis dose, phosphorus level and vascular access must be the first step. These indicators are well known by clinicians. But this first step is not enough. Dialysis associated stressors are powerful. So what else can be done? Faced with a lack of adequate evidence, opinion is what determines efforts to improve QOL. As an assistant nephrologist, medical professor and researcher on QOL and correlators, I suggest, based on my study results, that physiotherapeutic approaches along with psychological interventions can minimize the effects of dialysis on patients' well-being.
Dialysis patients have very low physical domains of QOL compared to healthy people. On the other hand, mental aspects are the same or even higher than in the general population (Perneger et al., 2003; Kusek et al., 2002). In my experience, the dimension role-physical (from the SF-36) consistently presents the lowest score among HD patients. Questions which generate role-physical score are related to difficulties in work and other daily activities

resulting from poor physical health. Thus, physical interventions, like physical conditioning programs, occupational activities and physiotherapeutic approaches must be tried on individuals and also as collective activities in renal units.

ESRD requires an individual to make a number of adjustments. To do so, patients need to understand their situation (cognitive effort) and modify their behavior (behavioral effort). The kinds of these efforts determine their coping style. I believe coping style is the principal measure between treatment-related stressors and outcomes. In my view, coping is the best variable for intervention and potentially the most correlated with QOL. I have detected emotion-oriented coping associated with poor QOL. Emotion-oriented coping is associated with passive personality traits, a sense of powerlessness and denial (Gilbar et al., 2005; Klang et al., 1996). Fortunately, coping is a modifiable variable. Patient education in coping skills can be used to change the risk of poor QOL (Tsay et al., 2005). I propose adaptation training programs aiming to improve patients' coping skills.

Finally, the emerging modalities with more frequent dialysis, like nocturnal or daily dialysis, are promising to enhance QOL. However, the implementation of sufficient renal units to offer this dialysis frequency demands time and resources. Moreover, these modalities may not be acceptable to some patients. It will be even more difficult to offer these modalities on a large scale in underdeveloped countries, where reimbursement of dialysis sessions is very low and there is lack of renal units that even offer conventional HD. Only time will tell whether more frequent dialysis will be standard treatment in the future.

6. Conclusion

Well-being is a main outcome in treatment of ESRD patients with dialysis. However, scientific evidence is lacking about interventions to improve well-being. The best way of assessing patients' well-being is to estimate the QOL level using validated instruments. Over the last decade neither technical advances nor quality-of-care guidelines have been enough to improve QOL among HD patients. Emerging knowledge about subjective measures associated with QOL can be the key for effective interventions. Clinicians must be familiar with subjective measures and use them in their daily practice to try to improve the well-being of patients undergoing HD. After 50 years of the widespread of dialysis treatment, the improvement of QOL among dialysis patients remains a formidable challenge.

7. References

Abdel-Kader K, Myaskovsky L, Karpov I, Shah J, Hess R, Dew MA & Unruh M. (2009). Individual quality of life in chronic kidney disease: influence of age and dialysis modality. *Clinical Journal of the American Society of Nephrology* 4(4): 711-718

Al-Hilali N, Al-Humoud HM, Ninan VT, Nampoory MRN, Ali JH & Johny KV. (2004). *Transplantation Proceedings* 36(6): 1827-1828

Allen KL, Miskulin D, Yan G, Dwyer JT, Frydrych A, Leung J, Poole D & the Hemodialysis (HEMO) Study Group. (2002). Association of nutritional markers with physical and mental health status in prevalent hemodialysis patients from HEMO study. *Journal of Renal Nutrition* 12(3): 160-169

Alonso J, Regidor E, Barrio G, Prieto L, Rodriguez C & Fuente L. (1998). Valores poblacionales de referencia de la versión española del cuestionario de salud SF-36. *Medicina Clínica* 111(11): 410-416

Andresen EM, Malmgren JA, Carter WB & Patrick DL. (1994). Screening for depression in well older adults: Evaluation of a short form of the CES-D (Center for Epidemiologic Studies Depression Scale) *American Journal of Preventive Medicine* 10(2): 77-84

Berlim MT, Mattevi BS, Duarte APG, Thomé FS, Barros EJG & Fleck MP. (2006). Quality of life and depressive symptoms in patients with major depression and end-stage renal disease: A matched-pair study. *Journal of Psychosomatic Research* 61(5): 731-734

Besarab A, Blton WK, Browne JK, Egrie JC, Nissenson AR, Okamoto DM, Schwab SJ & Goodkin DA. (1998). The effects of normal as compared with low hematocrit values in patients with cardiac disease who are receiving hemodialysis and epoetin. *The New England Journal of Medicine* 339(9): 584-590

Blumenfield M, Levy NB, Spinowitz B, Charytan C, Beasley CM Jr, Dubey AK, Solomon RJ, Todd R, Goodman A & Bergstrom RF. (1997). Fluoxetine in depressed patients on dialysis. *The International Journal of Psychiatry in Medicine* 27(1): 71-80

Bombardier CH, D'Amico C & Jordan JS. (1990). The relationship of appraisal and coping to chronic illness adjustment. *Behaviour Research and Therapy* 28(4): 297-304

Canadian Erythropoietin Study Group. (1990) Association between recombinant human erythropoietin and quality of life and exercise capacity of patients receiving haemodialysis. *British Medical Journal* 300(6724): 573-578

Clement FM, Klarenbach S, Tonelli M, Johnson JA & Manns BJ. (2009). The impact of selecting a high haemoglobin target level on health-related quality of life for patients with chronic kidney disease. *Archives of Internal Medicine* 169(12): 1104-1112

Cohen SR, Mount BM, Strobel MG & Bui F. (1995). The McGill Quality of Life Questionnaire: A quality of life measure appropriate for people with advanced disease. A preliminary study of validity and acceptability. *Palliative Medicine* 9(3): 207-219

Cohen LM, Germain MJ & Poppel D. (2003). Practical considerations in dialysis withdrawal. *The Journal of the American Medical Association* 289(16): 2113-2119

Craven JL, Rodin GM & Littlefield C. (1988). The Beck Depression Inventory as a screening device for major depression in renal dialysis patients. *International Journal of Psychiatry in Medicine* 18(4): 365-374

Cruz J & Cruz HMM (eds.). (2010). *Atualidades em nefrologia 11.* Sarvier: São Paulo

Cukor D, Peterson RA, Cohen SD, & Kimmel PL. (2006). Depression in end-satge renal disease hemodialysis patients. *Nature Clinical Practice Nephrology* 2(12): 678-687

Cukor D, Cohen SD, Peterson RA & Kimmel PL. (2007). Psychological aspects of chronic disease: end-stage renal disease as a paradigmatic illness. *Journal of the American Society of Nephrology* 18(12): 3042-3055

Culleton BF, Walsh M, Klarenbach SW, Mortis G, Scott-Douglas N, Quinn RR, Tonelli M, Donelly S, Friedrich MG, Kumar A, Mahallati H, Hemmelgam BR & Manns BJ. Effect of frequent nocturnal hemodialysis vs. conventional hemodialysis on left ventricular mass and quality of life. (2007). *The Journal of the American Medical Association* 298(11): 1291-1219

Curtin RB & Mapes DL. (2001). Health care management strategies of long-term dialysis survivors. *Nephrology Nursing Journal* 28(4): 385-394

DeOreo PB. (1997). Hemodialysis patient-assessed functional health status predicts continued survival, hospitalization and dialysis-attendance compliance. *American Journal of Kidney Diseases* 30(2): 204-212

Drayer RA, Piraino B, Reynolds III CF, Houck PR, Mazumdar S, Bernardini J, Shear MK & Rollman BL. (2006). Characteristics of depression in hemodialysis patients: symptoms, quality of life and mortality risk. *General Hospital Psychiatry* 28(4): 306-312

Dunn SA, Lewis SL, Bonner PN & Meize-Grochowski R. (1994). Quality of life for spouses of CAPD patients. *American Nephrology Nurses' Association Journal* 21(5): 237-247

Ellison CG. Religious involvement and subjective well-being. (1991). *Journal of Health and Social Behavior* 32(1): 80-99

Finkelstein FO, West W, Gobin J, Finkelstein SH & Wuerth D. (2007). Spirituality, quality of life and the dialysis patient. *Nephrology Dialysis Transplantation* 22(9): 2432-2434

Fujisawa M, Ichikawa Y, Yoshiya K, Higuchi A, Nagano S & Arakawa S. (2000). Assessment of health-related quality of life in transplant and hemodialysis patients using the SF-36 health survey. *Urology* 56(2): 201-205

Furuland H, Linde T, Ahlmen J Christensson A, Strombom U & Danielson BG. (2003). A randomized ontrolled trial of haemoglobin normalization with epoetin alfa in pre-dialysis and dialysis patients. *Nephrology Dialysis Transplantation* 18(2): 353-361.

Gabbay E, Meyer KB, Griffith JL, Richardson MM & Miskulin DC. (2010). Temporal trends in health-related quality of life among hemodialysis patients in the United States. *Clinical Journal of the American Society of Nephrology* 5(2): 261-267

Garrat A, Schmidt L, MacKintosh A & Fitzpatrick R. (2002). Quality of life measurement: bibliographic study of patient assessed health outcome measures. *British Medical Journal* 324(7351): 1417-1419

Gilbar O, Or-Han K & Plivazky N. (2005). Mental adjustment, coping strategies, and psychological distress among end-stage renal disease patients. *Journal of Psychosomatic Research*, 58(6): 471-476

Gomez R & Fisher JW. (2003). Domains of spiritual well-being and development and validation of the spiritual well-being questionnaire. *Personality and individual differences* 35(8): 1975-1991

Hays RD, Kallich JD, Mapes DL, Coons SJ & Carter WB. (1994). Development of Kidney Disease Quality of Life (KDQOL) instrument. *Quality of Life Research* 3(5): 329-338

Hedayati SS, Bosworth HB, Kuchibhatla M, Kimmel PL & Szczech LA. (2006). The predictive value of self-reported scales compared with physician diagnosis of depression in hemodialysis patients. *Kidney International* 69(9): 1662-1668

Hicks LS, Cleary PD, Epstein AM & Ayanian JZ. (2004). Differences in health-related quality of life and treatment preferences among black and white patients with end-stage renal disease. *Quality of Life Research* 13(6): 1129-1137

Himmelfarb J & Ikizler TA. Hemodialysis. (2010). *The New England Journal of Medicine* 363(19): 1833-1845

Hopman WM, Towheed T, Anastassiades T, Tenehouse A, Poliquin S, Berger C, Joseph L, Bronw JP, Murray TM, Adachi JD, Hanley DA & Papadimitropoulos E. (2000). Canadian normative data for the SF-36 health survey. *Canadian Medical Association Journal* 163(3): 265-271

Hoth KF, Christensen AJ, Ehlers SL, Raichle KA & Lawton WJ. (2007). A longitudinal examination of social support, agreeableness and depressive symptoms in chronic kidney disease. *Journal of Behavioral Medicine* 30(1): 69-76

Jalowiec A & Powers MJ. (1981). Stress and coping in hypertensive and emergency room patients. *Nursing Research* 30(1): 10-15

Jalowiec A. (1991). *Psychometric results on the 1987 Jalowiec coping scale.* Loyola University of Chicago: Chicago

Jenkinson C, Stewart-Brown S, Petersen S & Paice C. (1999) Assessment of the SF-36 version 2 in the United Kingdom. *Journal of Epidemiology and Community Health* 53(1): 46-50

Kalantar-Zadeh K, Kopple JD, Block G & Humphreys MH. (2001). Association among SF36 quality of life measures and nutrition, hospitalization, and mortality in hemodialysis. *Journal of the American Society of Nephrology* 12(12): 2797-2806

Kimmel PL, Peterson RA, Weihs KL, Simmens SJ, Boyle DH, Cruz I, Umana WO & Veis JH. (1995). Aspects of quality of life in hemodialysis patients *Journal of the American Society of Nephrology* 6(5): 1418-1426

Kimmel PL & Peterson RA. (2006). Depression in patients with end-stage renal disease treated with dialysis: Has the time to treat arrived? *Clinical Journal of the American Society of Nephrology* 1(3): 349-352

Klang B, Bjorvell H & Cronqvist A. (1996). Patients with chronic renal failure and their ability to cope. *Scandinavian Journal of Caring Sciences* 10(2): 89-95

Knight EL, Ofsthun N, Teng M, Lazarus JM & Curhan GC. (2003). The association between mental health, physical function, and hemodialysis mortality. *Kidney International* 63(5): 1843-1851

Koenig K. Religion and medicine IV. (2001). *International Journal of Psychiatry in Medicine* 31(3): 321-336

Kusek JW, Greene P, Wang S, Beck G, West D, Jamerson K, Agodoa LY, Faulkner M & Level B. (2002). Cross-sectional study health-related quality of life in African Americans with chronic renal insufficiency. *American Journal of Kidney Diseases* 39(3): 513-524

Lacson Jr E, Xu J, Lin S, Dean SG, Lazarus JM & Hakim R. (2009). Association between achievement of hemodialysis quality-of-care indicators and quality-of-life scores. *American Journal of Kidney Diseases* 54(6): 1098-1107

Lamping DL, Constantinovici N, Roderick P, Normand C, Henderson L, Harris S, Brown E, Gruen R & Victor C. (2000). Clinical outcomes, quality of life, and costs in the North Thames Study of elderly people on dialysis: a prospective cohort study. *Lancet* 356(9241): 1543-1550

Lara-Munoz C & Feinstein AR. (1999). How should quality of life be measured? *Journal of Investigative Medicine* 47(1): 17-24

Lazarus RS & Folkman S. (1984). *Stress, appraisal, and coping.* Springer Publishing: New York

Levin JS & Vanderpool HY. (1991). Religious factors in physical health and the prevention of illness. *Prevention in Human Services* 9(2): 41-64

Lindqvist R, Carlsson M & Sjoden P. (1998). Coping strategies and quality of life among patients on hemodialysis and continuous ambulatory peritoneal dialysis. *Scandinavian Journal of Caring Sciences* 12(4): 223-230

Lindqvist R, Carlsson M & Sjoden P. (2000). Coping strategies and health-related quality of life among spouses of continuous ambulatory peritoneal dialysis, hemodialysis, and transplant patients. *Journal of Advanced Nursing* 31(6): 1398-1408

Lindsay RM. (2004). The London, Ontario, Daily/Nocturnal Hemodialysis Study. *Seminars in Dialysis* 17(2): 85-91.

Lopes AA, Bragg J, Young E, Goodkin D & Mapes D. (2002). Depression as a predictor of mortality and hospitalization among hemodialysis patients in the United States and Europe. *Kidney International* 62(1): 199-207

Lopes AA, Albert JM, Young EW, Satayathum S, Pisoni RL, Andreucci VE, Mapes DL, Mason NA, Fukuhara S, Wikstrom B, Saito A & Port FK. (2004). Screening for depression in hemodialysis patients: Associations with diagnosis, treatment, and outcomes in the DOPPS. *Kidney International* 66(5): 2047-2053

Low J, Smith G, Burns A & Jones L. (2008). The impact of end-stage renal disease on close persons: a literature review. *Nephrology Dialysis Transplantation Plus* 1(2): 67-79

Lowrie EG, Curtin RB, Lepain N & Schatell D. (2003). Medical Outcomes Study Short Form-36: a consistent and powerful predictor of morbidity and mortality in dialysis patients. *American Journal of Kidney Diseases* 41(6): 1286-1292

Madham K. (2010). Quality of life. *Nephrology* 15 Suppl 1: S32-S34

Manns BJ, Johnson JA, Taub K, Mortis G, Ghali WA & Donaldson C. (2002) Dialysis adequacy and health related quality of life in hemodialysis patients. *American Society for Artificial Organs Journal* 48(5): 565-569

Mapes DL, Lopes AA, Stayathum S, McCullough KP, Goodkin DA, Locatelli F, Fukuhara S, Young EW, Kurokawa K, Saito A, Bommer J, Wolfe RA, Held PJ & Port FK. (2003). Health-related quality of life as a predictor of mortality and hospitlization: The Dialysis Outcomes and Practice Patterns Study (DOPPS). *Kidney International* 64(1): 339-349

Merkus MP, Jager KJ, Dekker FW, Haan RJ, Boeschoten EW & Krediet RT. (2000) Predictors of poor outcome in chronic dialysis patients: The Netherlands Cooperative Study on the Adequacy of Dialysis. *American Journal of Kidney Diseases* 35(1): 66-79

Mishra G & Schofield MJ. (1998). Norms for the physical and mental health component summary scores of the SF-36 for young, middle-aged and older Australian women. *Quality of Life Research* 7(3): 215-220

Mittal SK, Ahern L, MacKintosh A & Fitzpatrick R. (2001). Self-assessed physical and mental function of haemodialysis patients. *Nephrology Dialysis Transplantation* 16(7): 1387-1394

Moist LM, Bragg-Gresham JL, Pisoni RL, Saran R, Akiba T, Jacobson SH, Fukuhara S, Mapes DL, Rayner HC, Saito A & Port FK. (2008). Travel time to dialysis as a predictor of health-related quality of life, adherence, and mortality: The Dialysis Outcomes and Practice Patterns Study. *American Journal of Kidney Diseases* 51(4): 641-650

Moons P, Marquet K, Budts W & De Geest S. (2004). Validity, reliability and responsiveness of the Schedule for the Evaluation of Individual Quality of Life-Direct Weighting (SEIQoL-DW) in congenital heart disease. In: *Health and Quality of Life Outcomes*, march 11 2011, available from: www.hplo.com/content/2/1/27

NKF - National Kidney Foundation. (2006). Clinical Practice Guidelines and Clinical Practice Recommendations. 2006 updates: hemodialysis adequacy and peritoneal dialysis adequacy. *American Journal of Kidney Diseases* 44 Suppl 1: S1-S322

Ohri-Vachaspati P & Seghal AR. (1999). Quality of life implications of inadequate protein nutrition among hemodialysis patients. *Journal of Renal Nutrition* 9(1): 9-13

Owen WF, Chertow GM, Lazarus JM & Lowrie EG. (1998). Dose of hemodialysis and survival: differences by race and sex. *The Journal of the American Medical Association* 280(20): 1764-1768

Palmer BF. Sexual dysfunction in uremia. (1999). *Journal of the American Society of Nephrology* 10(6): 1381-1388

Parmar MS. (2002). Chronic renal disease. *British Medical Journal* 325: 85-90

Patel SS, Shah VS, Peterson RA & Kimmel PL. (2002). Psychosocial variables, quality of life, and religious beliefs in ESRD patients treated with hemodialysis. *American Journal of Kidney Diseases* 40(5): 1013-1022

Perneger TV, Leski M, Chopard-Stoermann C & Martin P. (2003). Assessment of heath status in chronic hemodialysis patients. *Journal of Nephrology*, 16(2): 252-259

Phrommintikul A, Hass SJ, Elsik M & Krum H. (2007). Mortality and target haemoglobin concentrations in anaemic patients with chronic kidney disease treated with erythropoietin: a meta-analysis. *The Lancet* 369(9559): 381-388

Powell LH, Shashabi L & Thoresen CE. (2003). Religious and spirituality: linkages to physical health. *American Psychologist* 58(1): 36-52

Powers KM, Wilkowski MJ, Helmandollar AW, Koenig KG & Bolton WK. (2000). Improved urea reduction ratio and KTV in large hemodialysis patients using two dialyzers in parallel. *American Journal of Kidney Diseases* 35(2): 266-274

Raimundo P, Ravasco P, Proença V & Camilo M. (2006). Does nutrition play a role in quality of life of patients under chronic haemodialysis? *Nutricion Hospitalaria* 21(2): 139-144

Rebollo P, Ortega F, Baltar JM, Álvarez-Ude F, Navascués RA & Alvarez-Grande J. (2001). Is the loss of health-related quality of life during renal replacement therapy lower in elderly patients than in younger patients? *Nephrology Dialysis Transplantation* 16(8): 1675-1680

Revuelta KL, López FJG, Moreno FA & Alonso J. (2004). Perceived mental health at the start of dialysis as a predictor of morbidity and mortality in patients with end-stage renal disease. *Nephrology Dialysis Transplantation* 19(9): 2347-2353

Riis J, Loewenstein G, Baron J & Jepson C. (2005). Ignorance of hedonic adaptation to hemodialysis: a study using ecological momentary assessment. *Journal of Experimental Psychology: General* 134(1): 3-9

Ritt GF, Braga PS, Guimarães EL, Bacelar T, Schiefer A, Kraychete AC, Gusmão ENA & Rocha PN. (2007). Renal replacement therapy in the State of Bahia: Evaluation of the distance between the patient's hometown and the nearest hemodialysis unit. *Jornal Brasileiro de Nefrologia* 29(2): 59-63

Rosas SE, Joffe M, Franklin E, Strom BL, Kotzker W, Brensinger C, Grossman E & Feldman HI. (2001). Prevalence and determinants of erectile dysfunction in hemodialysis patients. *Kidney International* 59(6): 2259-2266

Rosen RC, Riley A, Wagner G, Osterloh IH, Kirkpatrick J & Mishra A. (1997). The International Index of Erectile Function (IIEF): A multidimensional scale for assessment of erectile dysfunction. *Urology* 49(6): 822-830

Seethala S, Hess R, Bossola M, Unruh ML & Weisbord SD. (2010). Sexual function in women receiving maintenance dialysis. *Hemodialysis International* 14(1): 55-60

Sesso R, Rodrigues-Neto JF & Ferraz MB. (2003). Impact of socioeconomic status on the quality of life of ESRD patients. *American Journal of Kidney Diseases* 41(1): 186-195

Singer MA, Hopman WM & MacKenzie TA. (1999). Physical functioning and mental health in patients with chronic medical conditions. *Quality of Life Research* 8(8): 687-691

Singh AK. (2008). The controversy surrounding hemoglobin and erythropoiesis-stimulating agents: what should we do now? *American Journal of Kidney Diseases* 52 Suppl 6: S5-S13

Spinale J, Cohen SD, Khetpal P, Peterson RA, Clougherty B, Puchalski CM, Patel SS & Kimmel PL. (2008). Spirituality, social support, and survival in hemodialysis patients. *Journal of the American Society of Nephrology* 3(6): 1620-1627

Sullivan M & Karlsson J. (1998). The Swedish SF-36 health survey III. Evaluation of criterion-based validity: results from normative population. *Journal of Clinical Epidemiology* 51(11): 1105-1113

Toimamueang U, Sirivongs D, Limumnoilap S, Paholpak S, Phanphruk W & Chunlertrith D. (2003). Stress and coping strategies among renal transplant candidates in a Thai medical center. *Transplantation Proceedings* 35(5): 292-293

Tsay SL, Lee YC & Lee YC. (2005). Effects of an adaptation training programme for patients with end-stage renal disease. *Journal of Advanced Nursing* 50(1): 39-46

Tsutsui H, Koike T, Yamazaki C, Ito A, Kato F, Sato H, Tawada H & Oshida Y. (2009) Identification of hemodialysis patients' commom problems using the International Classification of Functioning, Disablity and Health. *Therapeutic Apheresis and Dialysis* 13(3): 186-192

United States Renal Data System - USRDS. (2003). Mortality and causes of death. Available from: www.usrds.org/2002/pdf/h.pdf

Unruh M, Miskulin D, Yan G, Hays RD, Benz R, Kusek JW, Meyer KB & the HEMO Study Group. (2004a). Racial differences in health-related quality of life among hemodialysis patients. *Kidney International* 65(4): 1482-1491

Unruh ML, Benz R, Greene T, Yan G, Beddhu S, DeVita M, Dwyer JT, Kimmel PL, Kusek JW, Martin A, Rehm-McGillicuddy J, Teehan B, Meyer KB & The Hemo Study Group. (2004b). Effects of hemodialysis dose and membrane flux on health-related quality of life in the HEMO Study. *Kidney International* 66(1): 355-366

Unruh ML, Newman AB, Larive B, Dew MA, Miskulin DC, Greene T, Beddhu S, Rocco MV, Kusek JW, Meyer KB & the Hemodialysis Study Group. (2008). The influence of age on changes in health-related quality of life over three years in a cohort undergoing hemodialysis. *Journal of the American Geriatrics Society* 56(9): 1608-1617

Van Eps C, Jeffries JK, Johnson DW, Campbell SB, Isbel NM, Mudge DW & Hawley CM. (2010). Quality of life and alternate nightly nocturnal home hemodialysis. *Hemodialysis International* 14(1): 29-38

Wahl A, Hanestad BR, Wiklund I & Moum T. (1999). Coping and quality of life in patients with psoriasis. *Quality of Life Research* 8(5): 427-433

Ware JE & Sherbourne CD. (1992). The MOS 36 Item Short Form Health Survey (SF-36) I. Conceptual framework and item selection. *Medical Care* 30(6): 473-83

WHOQOL Group. (1998). The World Health Organization quality of life assessment (WHOQOL): development and general psychometric properties. *Social Science and Medicine* 46(12): 1569-1585

Wiegel M, Meston C & Rosen R. (2005). The female sexual function index (FSFI): cross-validation and development of clinical cutoof scores. *Journal of Sex & Marital Therapy* 31(1): 1-20

Wuerth D, Finkelstein SH & Finkelstein FO. (2003). Chronic peritoneal dialysis patients diagnosed with clinical depression: results of pharmacological therapy. *Seminars in dialysis* 16(6): 424:427

Yeh SJ & Chou HC. (2007). Coping strategies and stressors in patients with hemodialysis. *Psychosomatic Medicine* 69(2): 182-190

6

Hemodialysis Access Infections, Epidemiology, Pathogenesis and Prevention

Nirosha D. Gunatillake, Elizabeth M. Jarvis and David W. Johnson
Department of Nephrology, Princess Alexandra Hospital, Brisbane Australia

1. Introduction

Renal replacement therapy (RRT), including various delivery types of haemodialysis, has revolutionised the care of patients with end stage renal disease (ESRD). The most common RRT modality is haemodialysis (ANZ Data 2010, Boddana et al., 2009). Access for dialysis is via arteriovenous fistulae (AVF), arteriovenous grafts (AVG) or via central venous dialysis catheters. The goal of access is to provide a means of accessing the vasculature to undertake RRT in order to deliver the optimal dialysis dose with the minimal associated morbidity and mortality. The National Kidney Foundation (NKF) Kidney Disease Outcome Quality Initiative (KDOQI, 2006) guidelines recommend an AVF prevalence rate of greater than 65%. Arteriovenous fistulae remain the preferred method of access due to improved survival rate and lower associated morbidity and associated medical costs (NKF-KDOQI, 2006). Despite all these measures, dialysis catheters remain commonly used for a variety of reasons. They are now well acknowledged as the harbinger of potential future significant morbidity and mortality.

As a result of the significant morbidity burden caused by dialysis catheters, there has been great interest in discovering new and inventive methods of reducing catheter-related infection. Out of this is borne the investigation of preventative measures outlined here. This is particularly important given the immunosuppressed nature of renal patients. The evidence for, and utility of measures, such as topical antimicrobial ointment application, antimicrobial catheter lock solutions, antibiotic impregnated catheters, differing AVF cannulation methods and catheter design, shall be explored below.

As we strive for improved outcomes in our patients many more patients are undertaking extended hours home haemodialysis. In those patients with the lowest risk accesses, questions have been raised as to the method of access cannulation and the spectre of increasing associated infectious events. The rope ladder technique involves regular rotation of cannulation sites whereas buttonhole technique uses the same cannulation sites and relies on formation of a track which is then repetitively accessed with blunt needles. This has been a very attractive method for home dialysis patients for a range of reasons. However, despite recent popularity with this technique, a number of studies including from our centre, have now shown that this technique is associated with increased septic events (Birchenough et al., 2008; Nesrallah et al., 2010; Van Eps et al., 2010; Van Loon et al., 2010).

2. Vascular access

Vascular access remains a predominant cause of morbidity in haemodialysis patients. There is significant global variation in the use of the different types of haemodialysis access. There have now been a number of studies examining trends of access use (Ethier et al., 2008; Pisoni et al., 2002) and further, epidemiological associations between access type and outcomes (Dhingra et al., 2001; Ishani et al., 2005; Moist et al., 2008; Pastan et al., 2002; Polkinghorne et al., 2004; Xue et al., 2003).

2.1 Geographical and temporal trends in access use

Pisoni et al., (2002) in the Dialysis Outcomes and Practice Patterns Study (DOPPS) confirmed significant variations in access practice between Europe and the United States. The practice comparison found that AVFs were much more common in prevalent patients in Europe, while AVGs and catheters were more commonly used in the US. Arteriovenous fistulae were used in 80% of the European prevalent population compared with only 24% of US prevalent populations and the use was associated with younger male patients with fewer co-morbidities. Use in incident patients varied from 66% in Europe to only 15% in the US. Conversely, AVGs and catheters were more common in incident patients in the US compared to Europe (2% versus 24% and 60% versus 31% respectively). Dialysis catheters were the first modality of access at commencement of dialysis in the US (Pisoni et al., 2002).

Trends in vascular access have changed over time but have shown a progression towards AVF use. Data from DOPPS I (1996-2001), DOPPS II (2002-2004) and DOPPS III (2005-2007) were compared and found that trends towards increasing AVF use were observed in Australia, New Zealand and the United Kingdom. Australia and New Zealand have traditionally had higher rates of AVF use. Arteriovenous fistulae in these countries, along with Japan and most European countries (excluding the United Kingdom, Belgium and Sweden), are used in over 70% of prevalent haemodialysis patients. The use of AVFs had increased significantly in the US in the same time from 24% in DOPPS I to 47% by DOPPS III (Ethier et al., 2008). Most recent data available shows that AVF use in the US is now greater than 57% (www.fistulafirst.org). In all the countries studied, AVG use remained stable or declined. The US showed the greatest decline in prevalent patient use, falling from 58% in DOPPS I to 29% in DOPPS III (Ethier et al., 2008).

Despite efforts to improve outcomes for ESRD patients, dialysis catheters remain a predominant form of vascular access well into the 21st century. Dialysis catheters were observed in greater than 20% of prevalent patients in the UK, Belgium, Sweden, Canada, and the US. A 2- to 3-fold increase in catheter use was observed in Italy, Germany, France and Spain by DOPPS III (Ethier et al., 2008). Catheter use will never be completely eliminated as they have a significant role in those patients who require urgent dialysis and for whom no other access exists. There is often regional variation in access practice patterns. The reasons for this appear to be multifactorial and include variables such as patient preference, surgical wait times, surgical expertise, as well as physician and nursing factors (Polkinghorne, et al., 2004).

2.2 Epidemiological aspects of access type

A number of studies have now shown an epidemiological association between access type and outcome. Use of venous catheters and AVGs over native AVFs has been shown to carry higher human costs. A number of studies have shown an association between catheter use and increased mortality from both infective and non-infective causes (Dhingra et al., 2001; Pastan et al., 2002; Polkinghorne et al., 2004). One study analysed a random sample of patients from the U.S. Renal Data System Dialysis Morbidity and Mortality Study (USRDS) Wave 1. Both diabetics and non-diabetics with catheters demonstrated similar trends in survival. The best overall survival was observed with AVF over AVG. The poorest survival was seen in patients with catheters (Dhingra et al., 2001). This increased mortality observed with AVGs and catheters has been replicated in a number of studies (Pastan et al., 2002; Polkinghorne et al., 2004; Xue et al., 2003). One of the largest investigations of access-related mortality included over 60,000 patients from the United States (Xue et al., 2003). The use of catheters at iniation of dialysis was associated with the greatest mortality risk (catheter hazard ratio [HR] 1.70, 95% CI 1.59-1.81; AVGs HR 1.16, 95% CI 1.08-1.24; AVF reference). . In this study, greater than 50% of patients commenced dialysis with a catheter.

A *prospective* study of almost 1000 patients in France looked at the risk factors for development of bacteraemia in chronic haemodialysis patients (Hoen et al., 1998). This again confirmed that the greatest risk factor for bacteraemia was use of a dialysis catheter, with an incidence of 0.93 episodes of bacteraemia per 100 patient months. Multivariate analysis confirmed vascular access as a major risk factor for bacteraemia. Catheter use for haemodialysis carried a relative risk of bacteraemia of greater than 7 times that of an AVF (relative risk [RR] 7.6, 95% CI 3.7-15.6). Arteriovenous grafts carried only a marginally higher relative risk compared to AVFs.

Access-related bacteraemia has also been shown to be an important factor in the subsequent development of cardiovascular-related morbidity and mortality. Where cause-specific mortality was assessed, increases in both infectious deaths (Dhingra et al., 2001; Ishani et al., 2005; Pastan et al., 2002; Polkinghorne et al., 2004) and cardiac deaths were also observed (Dhingra et al., 2001; Ishani et al., 2005). Interestingly, in one study, non-diabetics using catheters at the inception of dialysis had a worse survival rate than those patients using permanent vascular access, with the difference being detectable after only 2 months of observation. The overall relative risk of infection-related death was approximately 2-fold higher in patients with central venous catheters over those with AVFs and was more marked in diabetics than non-diabetics. The risk of death from cardiac causes was approximately 1.5-fold higher in those with dialysis catheters (Dhingra et al., 2001). A prospective cohort study of incident dialysis patients in the U.S scrutinised the association between access modality and bacteraemia, and also the association between bacteraemia and cardiovascular events (Ishani et al., 2005). Cox regression analysis (n=2358) demonstrated that initial dialysis access was the main antecedent of septicaemia or bacteraemia. Long term dialysis catheters, temporary dialysis catheters and AVGs displayed HRs of 1.95, 1.76 and 1.05, respectively. The presence of bacteraemia or septicaemia was associated with heightened risks of subsequent cardiovascular morbidity and mortality. In those without defined coronary artery disease, a bacteraemic episode conferred a greater risk of death or acute cardiovascular event than those with pre-existing cardiovascular disease.

A study undertaken in Australia examined incident haemodialysis patients between 1999 and 2002, and made further attempts to statistically adjust for the non-random nature of access selection. This study found that those patients starting dialysis with a dialysis catheter or AVG had a greater risk of dying in the first 6 months compared to those with AVF; catheters being the most life-limiting of all three. This trend continued with time. Dialysing via an AVF showed a mortality rate of 86 per 1000 person-years; AVGs had a

mortality rate of 146 per 1000 person-years and catheters had the highest mortality rate of 261 per 1000 person-years. Catheter use conferred 1.5- to 3-fold increased risks in both infectious and all-cause mortality. A similar trend in both increased infectious and all-cause mortality with AVGs was also observed but not significant on analysis (Polkinghorne et al., 2004).
Apart from catheter-related infectious mortality, proposed alternative mechanisms for the increased death rates in patients with catheters have included reduced dialysis doses delivered by central catheters and a higher prevalence of co-morbid conditions in patients who dialyse via catheters. However, the latter was not confirmed after controlling for vascular disease and congestive cardiac failure (Pastan et al., 2002). No patterns of catheter use associated with increasing age or existing co-morbidities were ascertained from the more recent DOPPS III analysis. The usage of dialysis catheters in younger (18-70 year old) non-diabetics increased 2-fold in the US and up to 3-fold in some European countries (France, Germany, Italy and Spain) (Ethier, et al., 2008).

3. Incidence, pathogenesis and bacteriology of access-related infections

Although the incidence of catheter-related bacteraemia is variable, the mean reported incidence is 3 episodes per 1000 catheter days (Dryden et al., 1991; Moss et al., 1990; Saad, 1999; Mokryzcki et al., 2000; Mokrzycki et al., 2001). Data from the HEMO study (Eknoyan et al., 2008) indicates that patients with central venous catheters have an increased relative mortality risk of 3.4 when compared with patients with AVFs (relative mortality risk of 1.4). The burden of catheter-related infection is high, with reported rates of metastatic infectious complications (e.g. osteomyelitis, endocarditis, septic arthritis or epidural abscess) of between 10% and 40% (Marr et al., 1997; Maya et al., 2007; Neilsen et al., 1998). *S. aureus* is responsible for the majority of vascular access infections, accounting for 70-90% of cases (Del Rio el at., 2009; Gould, 2007).

3.1 Catheter-related bacteraemia

Gram-positive species are the culprit organisms in 61-95% of cases of catheter-related bacteraemia. In the prospective study by Hoen et al (1998), the most common causative organism was *S. aureus*. Coagulase-negative staphylococcal bacteraemia was almost as common as that caused by *S. aureus*. *Escherichia coli* and other aerobic gram negative bacilli were the next most commonly isolated organisms. The presumed portal of entry for these organisms was via the vascular access. In this study, 6 deaths were directly attributable to bacteraemia. The most common causative organisms under these circumstances were *S. aureus* and *Pseudomonas* with equal occurrence, and other Enterobacteriaciae making up the remainder of isolated agents (Hoen et al., 1998).
Catheter-related bacteraemia may arise via two paths: (a) direct spread of microorganisms from the skin along the outside of the catheter leading to contamination of the bloodstream; or, (b) colonisation of the inner lumen of the catheter leading to the formation of biofilm and direct migration of organisms into the bloodstream. A biofilm is a multi-layered cell cluster with a strong propensity to adhere to polymer surfaces and provides a protected niche environment for microorganisms with physical barrier protection against antibiotics. Within the biofilm, bacteria exhibit increased growth rates, a higher cell density and more active gene transcription. This further contributes to the heightened resistance of bacteria to antibiosis (Fux et al., 2003). Even in the absence of

overt infection, microbial colonisation of catheters may engender a chronic inflammatory state, which in turn increases the risk of erythropoietin-resistant anaemia, malnutrition and cardiovascular disease (Barraclough et al., 2009).

3.2 Arterio-venous fistula bacteraemia

In those with AVF infection, *S. aureus* and *Staphylococcus epidermis* are most commonly responsible. Infection accounts for approximately one fifth of accesses being lost (Bhat et al., 1980). Microorganisms gain entry to the bloodstream during cannulation. In addition, the presence of pseudoaneuryms, peri-access haematomas, non-functioning clotted fistulae and manipulation of AVFs during non-dialysis interventions increase the risk of infection (Barraclough et al., 2009).

Recent evidence suggests that cannulation technique may have an important effect on the rates of bacteraemia related to AVFs. Over the last 30 years, the buttonhole cannulation technique has become increasingly popular. This technique involves repetitive cannulation of a small number of puncture sites, with the aim of creating a tunnel track into which the needles can be easily inserted. There are a number of benefits associated with using buttonhole cannulation for haemodialysis, particularly in the home environment. These benefits include easier and quicker needle insertion, less painful cannulation with the elimination of anaesthetic, reduction in "bad sticks", and reduction in hematoma formation (Doss et al., 2008; Hartig and Smyth, 2009). The alternative cannulation method, referred to as the rope ladder technique, involves needle puncture along the length of the fistula and is more inclined to give rise to small dilatations over the length of the fistula. However, several studies have suggested that the buttonhole technique is associated with an increased risk of access-related infection compared with the rope ladder method. Birchenough et al. (2008) established a positive correlation between use of the buttonhole cannulation technique and an increased risk for infection in adult patients on haemodialysis. Nesrallah et al. (2010) observed a significantly increased risk of *S. aureus* bacteremia infection with potentially fatal metastatic complications in patients receiving home nocturnal haemodialysis with buttonhole cannulation. They recommended advising prospective patients of the infection risks, and, in the absence of more rigorous studies, giving consideration to topical Mupirocin prophylaxis. Other studies have similarly reported increased access-related infection rates in association with buttonhole cannulation (Ludlow, 2010; Silva et al., 2010; Van Loon et al., 2010).

A subsequent retrospective observational cohort study in our unit involving 63 alternate nightly nocturnal haemodialysis and 172 conventional haemodialysis patients reported a statistically significant and clinically important increase in septic dialysis access events when nocturnal haemodialysis and buttonhole cannulation were used simultaneously (incidence rate ratio 3.0, 95% CI 1.04-8.66, $p=0.04$) (Van Eps et al., 2010). It is theorised that chronic bacterial colonisation of the buttonhole site may be the precursor to systemic infection, and that fibrosis surrounding the site may not provide as efficient a barrier as seen in those employing the rope ladder technique. This study highlights that increased infection control steps may be crucial in the setting of nocturnal haemodialysis and buttonhole technique.

4. Preventative measures against access-related infection

4.1 Aseptic technique

The method of handling the dialysis catheter is crucial. Stringent aseptic techniques must be employed, with KDOQI 2006 recommending washing the access site with antibacterial scrub and water followed by cleansing of the skin with 2% chlorhexidine/alcohol or 70% alcohol.

A multicentre prospective randomised trial (n=849) compared chlorhexidine-alcohol with povidone-iodine in the setting of post-operative surgical wounds and found that the chlorhexidine-alcohol preparation was associated with a significantly lower rate of surgical site infection (9.5% vs 16.1%, p=0.004, RR 0.59, 95% CI 0.41 - 0.85). However, in dialysis populations, there are only a few RCTs detailing the value of different antiseptic ointments. A small RCT studying povidone-iodine in subclavian catheters demonstrated a statistically significant improvement in exit site infections (5% vs 18%, p<0.02), tip colonisations and incidence of septicaemia compared with using sterile gauze dressings alone in the control group (Levin et al., 1991). The beneficial effect of povidone-iodine ointment was most marked in those with *S. aureus* nasal carriage (3-fold higher risk of subclavian catheter-related septicaemia, p<0.05). No significant increase in adverse effects was observed with povidone-iodine.

There is no particular dressing type that has shown benefit over another. A chlorhexidine-impregnated foam dressing has not been found to provide extra protection against infection in an open labelled study (Camins et al., 2010), despite previous evidence to the contrary in patients in an intensive care setting (Timsit et al., 2009).

Maximal sterile barrier precautions were further studied in a recent Korean study. Using multivariate analyses, they found that the use of maximally sterile barrier precautions (odds ratio 5.205 95% CI 0.015 - 1.130, p=0.23) and use of antimicrobial coated catheters (odds ratio 5.269 95% CI 0.073 - 0.814, p=0.022) were independent factors associated with a lower risk of acquiring a central venous catheter-related bacteraemic episode (Lee at al., 2008). In another single centre study, the institution of a catheter monitoring system and a formal maintenance program following catheter insertion was associated with a reduction in the occurrence of catheter-related bacteraemia by 33% (Yoo et al., 2001). A Cochrane systematic review of randomised controlled trials (McCann and Moore, 2010) reported that transparent polyurethane dressing did not reduce the risk of catheter-related exit site infection or bacteraemia compared to dry gauze.

4.2 Catheter care protocols

It is well accepted practice in the critical care sector to adopt a strictly protocolised approach to the care of central venous catheters (Beathard and Urbanes, 2008; Pronovost et al., 2010). Care bundles are commonly used in the intensive care unit. A "care bundle" is a set of evidence-based interventions that are administered to many intensive care patients, with the aim of risk reduction. There is no randomised trial evidence in the haemodialysis population, but prospective observational data has shown a marked reduction in bacteraemic episodes from 6.7 to 1.6 per 1000 catheter days over a twenty four month study period using an infection prophylaxis protocol based on NKF-K/DOQI guidelines (2001). The main focus of the protocol was strict cleansing of the catheter hub at the time of use in the dialysis facility to avoid any potential contamination. Other vital elements to catheter care include the technical placement of the catheter, exit site care and the handling of dialysis connections.

4.3 Topical antimicrobial agents

Use of topical antimicrobial agents has been associated with reduced rates of bacteraemic episodes and catheter loss of any cause (Rabindranath et al., 2009). Our group was one of the first to demonstrate that topical exit site application of mupirocin, an antibiotic active against Gram-positive organisms, resulted in significantly fewer catheter-related

bacteraemias (7 vs 35%, $p<0.01$) and a longer time to first bacteraemia (log rank score 8.68, $P<0.01$) (Johnson et al., 2002). The beneficial effect of mupirocin was entirely attributable to a reduction in staphylococcal infection (log rank 10.69, $P=0.001$) and was still observed when only patients without prior nasal *S. aureus* carriage were included in the analysis (log rank score 6.33, $P=0.01$). Median catheter survival was also significantly longer in the mupirocin group (108 vs 31 days, log rank score 5.9, $P<0.05$).
Recently, McCann & Moore (2010) published the results of their Cochrane systematic review in which they evaluated the benefits and harms of prophylactic topical antimicrobial agents on infectious complications among haemodialysis patients with central venous catheters. In a total of 10 randomised controlled trials involving 787 patients, the risk of catheter-related bacteraemia was reduced by topical exit site application of mupirocin (RR 0.17, 95%CI 0.07 - 0.43), polysporin triple ointment consisting of bacitracin, gramicidin and polymixin B (RR 0.40, 95% CI 0.19 - 0.86), and povidone-iodine ointment (RR 0.10, 95% CI 0.01 - 0.72). Mortalityrelated to infection was not reduced by any of these three agents.
In another meta-analysis topical antimicrobial agents reduced the rates of bacteraemia (risk rate ratio 0.22, 95% CI 0.12 - 0.40), exit site infection (RR 0.17, 95% CI 0.08 - 0.38), requirement for catheter removal and hospitalisation for infection compared with no antibiotics (James et al., 2008).
In spite of the demonstrated benefits of topical antimicrobial agents on catheter-associated infection rates, a real concern surrounding these agents is the potential risk of antibiotic resistance. Whilst these fears have not yet been realised, a number of groups have suggested that antimicrobial prophylactic therapy should be limited in duration and scope to minimise the possibility of promoting antimicrobial resistance. For example, a recent position statement issued by the European Renal Best Practice (ERBP) working group recommended the application of antimicrobial ointments (either mupirocin or polysporin ointment) after catheter placement only until the exit site has healed completely (Tordoir et al., 2007). They specifically advised against the use of these agents after the site has healed because of the fear of emerging resistance and *Candida* colonisation.

4.4 Antimicrobial locks

There is evidence that "locking" a catheter with a small amount of antimicrobial agent that remains within the catheter lumen can prevent bacteraemic episodes. These antimicrobial locks are thought to possess extra biofilm-removing properties. This is in contrast to heparin, which may serve to antagonise the antibacterial properties of certain antibiotics (Droste et al., 2003, Regamey et al., 1972) and may in fact promote biofilm formation (Shanks et al., 2006).
Nine randomised controlled trials looked at the potential role of antimicrobial locks versus the standard heparin lock. The mean baseline risk of catheter-related infection was 3.0 episodes per 1000 catheter days, with the catheter insertion duration ranging from 37-365 days (mean 146 days). Seven out of 9 trials used an antibiotic, 1 used taurolidine and 1 used 30% citrate. The different antimicrobial preparations included amikacin, cefazolin, cefotaxime, ciprofloxacin, EDTA, gentamicin, minocycline and vancomycin. Collectively, they showed a more than three-fold reduction in the occurrence of catheter-related bacteraemia, in addition to reductions in mortality and morbidity (Allon et al., 2008; Jaffer et al., 2008; Labriola et al., 2008;). Seven out of 9 of the studies reached statistical significance. The use of antimicrobial locks also significantly reduced the rate of catheter loss due to all complications (3 trials; n=399; RR 0.61, 95% CI 0.45-0.83) (Rabrinathan et al., 2009).

Unfortunately, most of these trials were of short duration, being limited to 12 months follow-up or less. Consequently, the long-term risk:benefit of antimicrobial locks is uncertain. Significant side effects of antimicrobial locks that have been documented in the above trials included hypocalcaemia (Power et al., 2009) digital parasthesiae (Power et al., 2009) and ototoxicity in 10% of those using gentamicin based catheter locks (Dogra et al., 2002). Moreover, there are significant concerns that long term use of antimicrobial locks may promote multiresistant organisms (MROs). An American unit using a gentamicin/heparin lock observed the appearance of gentamicin resistant bacteraemia after a period of 6 months (Landry et al., 2010). The most common complications following such bacteraemias were catheter removal and hospital admission. Thus, despite a 95% decrease in the rate of catheter-related bacteraemia, there was the emergence of gentamicin resistant gram negative infections with tunnelled catheters being the most common access in the group. After stopping the gentamicin antimicrobial lock, the resistance to gentamicin dropped after 18 months.

4.5 Non-antimicrobial locks

4.5.1 Citrate

The spectre of antibiotic resistance has led nephrologists to seek alternative catheter lock agents. Sodium citrate has been utilised as an alternative anticoagulant to intradialytic heparin. Anticoagulant activity is brought about by reducing the free plasma calcium concentration and thus retarding the coagulation cascade. A 30% citrate solution will have antimicrobial and antibacterial properties. Citrate does not promote bacterial resistance and therefore has been proposed as the ideal catheter lock solution (Bleyer, 2007).

Power et al. (2009) studied 232 haemodialysis patients randomised to either 46.7% sodium citrate or 5% heparin locks post-dialysis for a 6 month period. In both groups, the rate of catheter-related bacteraemia was 0.7 events per 1000 catheter days with no significant difference between groups. There was a statistically significant increase in catheter thrombosis in the citrate group ($p<0.001$). All patients had a tunnelled twin catheter single lumen Tesio catheter.

Weijiner et al. (2005) had previously shown an added benefit of Trisodium citrate 30% in a randomised controlled trial incorporating 291 randomised haemodialysis patients. In this group however, 98/291 (34%) and 193/291 (66%) possessed tunnelled cuffed catheters and non-tunnelled catheters respectively. Catheter-related infection rates were 1.1 per 1000 catheter days in the trisodium citrate 30% group versus 4.1 per 1000 in the heparin group ($p<0.001$). There was found to be no difference in the rate of thrombotic events. This study showed a risk reduction for catheter-related bacteraemia of 87% for tunnelled catheters ($p<0.001$) and 64% for non-tunnelled catheters ($p=0.05$). There were fewer deaths from bacteraemia in the trisodium citrate 30% group (0 vs 5, $p=0.028$). Exit site infections were also reduced.

A concern with use of citrate relates to its chelating properties that can lead to hypocalcaemia with subsequent risk of ventricular arrhythmias. The death of a patient in 2000 from cardiac arrest following installation of 46.7% sodium citrate into a haemodialysis catheter prompted a Food and Drug Association (FDA) warning about its use (Food and Drug Administration, 2009). Many haemodialysis centres therefore avoid high doses of citrate in catheter locks. There is ongoing interest in using lower concentrations of sodium citrate, either alone or in combination with taurolidine or ethanol.

4.5.2 Taurolidine

Taurolidine locks possess antimicrobial activity by producing methyl taurinamde products that bind to bacterial and fungal cell walls and cause damage. The antimicrobial effect is broad spectrum and has been shown to reduce the progression to biofilm production (Torres-Viena et al., 2000). There are no reports of antibiotic resistance.

A randomised controlled trial from the United Kingdom randomised subjects to receive either Taurolidine-Citrate lock (1.35% taurolidine & 4% citrate) or unfractionated heparin 5000units/mL. The primary outcome was time to first bacteraemic episode and secondary outcomes were total number of bacteraemic episodes and gram positive and gram negative infections. There was found to be no statistically significant difference in time to first bacteraemic episode (n=110). However, there was a significant reduction in gram negative infections (p=0.02). The main drawback to using Taurolidine-citrate locks is a greater need for thrombolytic therapy. Solomon et al. (2010) surmised that tauroldine-citrate usage impacted only infection of intraluminal origin and that better formulations with an improved anticoagulant profile should be sought. These findings echo those trends seen previously (Allon, 2003, Betjes and Van Agteren 2004; Taylor et al., 2008).

4.5.3 Ethanol

Ethanol is an effective disinfectant with a broad spectrum of activity against a host of micro-organisms. Its benefits include low toxicity, lack of antibiotic resistance, ready availability and low cost. Ethanol-containing catheter locks were initially used in oncology patients to maintain long term catheters and in those receiving total parenteral nutrition in order to manage catheter occlusion (Ball et al., 2003; Metcalf et al., 2004; Pennington and Pithie, 1987). As little as 60 minutes exposure to a 30% ethanol- 14% trisodium citrate locking solution has been show to effectively eradicate the common gram-positive and gram-negative bacteria colonising catheters (Takla et al., 2007). Maharaj et al. (2008) demonstrated an equally impressive effect on *Candida albicans* isolates within the same time frame. These antimicrobial benefits of ethanol appear to be associated with a neutral effect on the integrity of catheter material. A recent small study tested found no negative effect of a 30% ethanol-4% sodium citrate locking solution on catheters (Vercaigne et al., 2010). Guenu et al. (2007) similarly found no deterioration in silicone catheter viability following exposure to high concentrations of ethanol.

Our unit is currently conducting a randomised controlled trial of heparin versus ethanol lock for the prevention of catheter-associated infection (Broom et al., 2009). This is a single centre prospective open-label study comparing 3mL 70% ethanol catheter lock head to head with a standard heparin lock. Using time to first catheter-related bacteraemia as the primary outcome, the study will hopefully elucidate further the benefit of ethanol as a useful preventative measure against catheter-related infections.

4.5.4 Honey

The healing properties of honey have been recognised since antiquity. Ancient Greeks and Egyptians used honey to aid in the healing of burns and sores. During World Ward I German physicians used honey and cod liver oil together as a surgical dressing for battle wounds. The antimicrobial properties of honey are related to its very high sugar content, which kills bacteria through dessication, and enzymatic production of hydrogen peroxide (glucose + H_2O + $O_2 \rightarrow$ gluconic acids + H_2O_2). The enzyme glucose oxidase also confers acidity to the substance. The pH range of honey is 3.2-4.5, which is low enough to be inhibitory to many bacterial pathogens. Moreover, research has shown that peripheral B lymphocytes and T lymphocytes proliferate in the presence of honey concentrations as low as 0.1%, and that phagocytes are activated by honey at these same low concentrations (Abbas, 1997). Our unit has succeeded in showing the advantageous effects of Medihoney in a randomised controlled trial comparing thrice weekly exit site application of standardised antibacterial honey versus 2% mupirocin ointment on infection rates in patients with cuffed tunnelled central venous catheters (Johnson et al., 2005). Topical Medihoney led to comparable rates of catheter-related infection compared to those achieved with mupirocin, but conferred additional benefits including low cost, an excellent safety profile and lack of antibiotic resistance, especially mupirocin resistance.

4.6 Nasal eradication of *S. aureus*

Historically, nasal carriage of *S. aureus* has been associated with greater bacteraemic episodes with *S. aureus* in haemodialysis patients (Yu et al., 1986). Patients on chronic haemodialysis have been reported to have over twice the rate of *S. aureus* nasal colonisation as healthy controls. More recent data are in agreement with this, and it is widely believed that nasal colonisation provides a natural reservoir that facilitates ongoing habitation and propagation of *S. aureus* in human populations. (Elie-Turenne et al., 2010; Mermel et al., 2010). Nasal application of mupirocin has been proven to eradicate nasal carriage of *S.aureus* in up to 98.5% of cases (Taal et al., 2006). This strategy has been associated with a reduction in *S. aureus* bacteraemia compared to historical controls (Boelart et al., 1993), although again, use has been associated with the development of mupirocin resistance (Cavdar et al., 2004; Lobbedez et al., 2004). Currently however, there are no recommendations by the leading Nephrology bodies to perform routine eradication of nasal *S.aureus* in a bid to reduce catheter-related bacteraemia.

4.7 The role of catheter design, structure and placement

The first 30 days following catheter placement are vital to the prevention of bloodstream infection. During this period, technique should not be compromised as the main risk of entry is infection through medical staff interaction and the patient's normal skin microflora. After this time, the catheter is more vulnerable to internal sources of infection, possibly via the catheter hub, leading to subsequent haematogenous spread and bloodstream infection. Alternatively, infection at a distant internal site may lead to colonisation of the indwelling catheter (Knuttinen et al., 2009).

4.7.1 Tunnelled versus non-tunnelled catheters

The incidence of bacteraemia is greatly reduced in subjects using cuffed tunnelled catheters as opposed to non cuffed catheters. The majority of modern cuffed tunnelled catheters are made of either polyurethane or silicone. The cuffed portion, which lies in the subcutaneous tissue near the insertion site, creates a fibrous seal and provides an effective barrier against infection by preventing migration of bacteria down the outer surface of the catheter. Although there are no prospective randomised trials investigating infection-related morbidity between catheter types in the dialysis population, observed bacteraemia rates range from 0.16–0.86 per 100 days with non-tunnelled non-cuffed dialysis catheter to 0.016–0.27 per 100 days with tunnelled cuffed catheters. Evidence from the non-haemodialysis setting showed lower infection rates in tunnelled catheters (Andrivet et al., 1994; Timsit et al., 2007). Within a set of immunocompromised patients, the rates of bacteraemia were reduced by cuffed catheters (2% vs 5%), although this did not achieve statistical significance (Andrivet et al., 1994).

There is no clear evidence pointing to any differences in bacteraemia rates attained through usage of different catheter brands. Some groups have published data of long term tunnelled catheter usage (Tesio catheters, MedComp, Harleysville, Pennsylvania) highlighting bacteraemia rates similar to those achieved in arteriovenous fistulae. This particular group utilised strict protocols surrounding catheter care (Power et al., 2011). The four most commonly commercially available tunnelled catheters are the HemoSplit, Tesio twin catheter, Split-Catheter III and Permcath. A UK study examining catheter survival found that the Split Catheter III and Permcath fared worse than the HemoSplit and Tesio twin catheter. Infection rates were not specifically studied (Fry et al., 2008).

4.7.2 Catheter placement

There is no randomised trial evidence of any specific site of insertion conferring an increased risk of infection (Ruesch et al., 2002). In a large study of intensive care patients there was no statistically significant difference in the incidence of infection or duration of catheter amongst the insertion sites (Deshpande et al., 2005). Multivariate analyses from a number of studies have collectively suggested a higher rate of infection with the femoral vein location, with the infection risk with the jugular approach being greater than the subclavian approach (Breschan et al., 2007; Ishizuka et al., 2009, Ishizuka et al., 2008; Nagashima et al., 2006). These studies did not take into account baseline confounding variables.

4.7.3 Catheter devices

Trerotola et al.(2010) found no improvement in infection rates in tunnelled small bore central venous catheters with the insertion of a polyester cuff.

4.7.4 Antibiotic-impregnated catheters

Since the early 1990's, there have been different types of central venous catheter antibiotic coatings trialled primarily in the critical care setting. There are no RCTs of antibiotic impregnated catheters in the chronic haemodialysis population. Raad et al. (1997) compared minocycline and rifampicin coated catheters head to head with untreated uncoated catheters, and found a significantly reduced rate of catheter related bacteraemia (0% versus 5%, respectively). This was a double blinded study (n=281) where the antibiotic coated catheters had been pre-treated with tri-idodecyclmethylammoniumchloride surfactant. The minocycline and rifampicin components were both active against methicillin-sensitive and methicillin-resistant *S. aureus*, and also had reported activity against gram negative bacilli and *Candida* species. Within a multicentre study of intensive care units, Maki et al. (1997) found a higher degree of bacterial colonisation of the catheter material in the uncoated as compared to the antibiotic impregnated catheters.

Following these results, the United States CDC recommended the use of antibiotic coated catheters for those with a high rate of infection after full adherence to other infection control measures, such as maximal sterile barrier precautions. There was also a recommendation that in an adult with an expected need for a central venous catheter for more than five days an antibiotic impregnated catheter be used in preference.

More recently, a large retrospective study of central venous catheters in the critical care setting showed that there was a significant reduced incidence of catheter-related infection that was independent and complementary to the infection control precautions utilised. The incidence improved from 8.3 episodes of infection per 1000 patient days to 1.2 episodes per 100 patient days (Ramos et al., 2010). The body of evidence refers to only non-cuffed non-tunnelled catheters, and has not led to the wide availability of such devices in the chronic haemodialysis population.

4.8 Thrombolytic therapy

Catheter-related bacteraemia may arise via the formation of an intraluminal thrombosis, which may then act as a nidus for the development of bacterial biofilm (McGee et al., 2003; Jain et al., 2009). Recombinant tissue plasminogen activator has been shown to be useful in catheter thrombus (Clase et al., 2001; Macrae et al., 2005; Tumlin et al., 2010) and some paediatric studies have looked into its potential effect on bacteraemia rates in the haemodialysis population. It has been shown that the prophylactic use of a catheter lock containing tissue plasminogen activator plus antibiotic can reduce the incidence of catheter-related bacteraemia, and may improve the infection-free survival times of central catheters at high risk of infection (Onder et al., 2009).

4.9 Aspirin

In vitro and in vivo animal studies of infective endocarditis have demonstrated aspirin to have direct anti-staphylococcus effects. It is theorised that the salicylic component of aspirin, which is the major biometabolite, inhibits the expression of two key *S. aureus* virulence genes involved in endovascular pathogenesis. A retrospective observational study over 10 years in a single haemodialysis centre found a lower rate of catheter-associated *S. aureus* bacteraemia in patients using aspirin at a daily dose of 325mg (Sedlacek et al., 2007).

5. Conclusions

The goal of treatment of patients with end-stage kidney failure is to provide optimal dialysis while at the same time averting excess morbidity and mortality. It should always be borne in mind that this patient group is a vulnerable and relatively immunosuppressed cohort, often with appreciably significant co-morbidity. Evidence points towards the best outcome being achieved when dialysis is initiated using a native arteriovenous fistula, with the next best outcome with an arteriovenous graft. However, concomitant disease burden can make native access formation challenging.

The use of central venous catheters for dialysis purposes should be minimised and actively discouraged (ERBP Guidelines 2007, KDOQI 2006, CARI 2000) as they are associated with increased patient mortality, morbidity and cost of healthcare. The consequences of catheter-related bacteraemia may be life-threatening, and could reach a 10% mortality rate (Saxena et al., 2002) and also effect cardiovascular morbidity. For those individuals where haemodialysis catheters are hard to avoid, a proactive approach is appropriate, and various preventative measures should be considered. The use of a catheter care protocol may be beneficial. The concept of the "care bundle" may be an extremely useful tool in the haemodialysis environment. In many ways the dialysis patient often has multi-organ involvement and a stepwise, astringent, highly protocolised pathway is appropriate.

Institution of such protocols has resulted in a drastic reduction in catheter-related bacteraemia reported in some American intensive care units (Pronovost et al., 2006).

The use of antibiotic lock solutions and topical antimicrobial ointment (mupirocin, povidone-iodine and polysporin triple antibiotic) has been shown to be effective in reducing bacteraemia. The benefits of citrate locks have been demonstrated by two meta-analyses (Yahav et al., 2008; Labriola et al., 2008). However, there are tenable concerns regarding cardiac arrhythmias, which may be circumvented by using lower concentrations of citrate that may compromise their antimicrobial potency. Topical medical-grade honey has proved efficacious against exit site infection. Prophylactic antibiotic at the time of insertion is frequently administered, although this intervention has never been validated in randomised controlled trials (Ryan et al., 2004).

Antibiotic coatings are in wide usage in the critical care arena using non-cuffed non-tunnelled catheters, but their usage has not crossed over to the dialysis unit. Novel therapies, such as thrombolytic agents and aspirin, require larger randomised studies before their widespread use is advocated.

We now have an increasing number of possible interventions in our armentarium to help us offer the best care to our patients. However, much more evidence in the form of clinical trials is needed to further elucidate the efficacy of these preventative measures, and other potential treatments.

6. References

Abbas T. (1997) Royal treat. *Living in the Gulf*; 50-1.

Allon M. (2003). Prophylaxis against dialysis catheter related bacteraemia with a novel antimicrobial lock solution. *Clinical Infectious Disease*; 36: 1539-1544.

Allon M. (2008). Prophylaxis against dialysis catheter-related bacteraemia: a glimmer of hope. *American Journal of Kidney Disease*; 51: 165–168.

Andrivet P, Bacquer A, Ngoc CV & Ferme C. (1994). Lack of clinical benefit from subcutaneous tunnel insertion of central venous catheters in immunocompromised patients. *Clinical Infectious Diseases*; 18(2): 199-206.

ANZDATA Registry 2010 Report. (2010). The thirty third report. http://www.anzdata.org.au/anzdata/AnzdataReport/33rdReport/ANZDATA33rdReport.pdf

Ball PA, Brokenshire E, Parry B, Merrie A, Gillanders L, McIlroy K & Plank L. (2003). Ethanol locking as a possible treatment for microbial contamination of long-term central venous catheters. *Nutrition*; 19 (6): 570

Barraclough KA, Hawley CM, Playford EG & Johnson DW. (2009). Prevention of access-related infections. *Expert Reviews in Anti-Infective Therapy*; 7(10): 1185-200.

Beathard GA & Urbanes A. (2008). Infection associated with tunnelled haemodialysis catheters. *Seminars in Dialysis*; 21: 521-538.

Betjes MGH & Van Agteren M. (2004). Prevention of dialysis catheter-related sepsis with a citrate-taurolidine-containing lock solution. *Nephrology Dialysis Transplantation*; 19: 1546-1551.

Bhat DJ, Tellis VA, Kohlberg WI, Driscoll B & Veith FJ. (1980). Management of sepsis involving expanded polytetrafluoroethylene grafts for haemodialysis access. *Surgery*; 87(4): 445-50.

Birchenough E, Moore C, Stevens K, & Stewart S. (2010). Buttonhole cannulation in adult patients on haemodialysis: an increased risk of infection? *Nephrology Nursing Journal;* 37(5): 491-555.

Bleyer AJ. (2007). Use of antimicrobial catheter lock solutions to prevent catheter-related bacteraemia. *Clinical Journal of the American Society of Nephrology;* 2(5): 1073-1078.

Boddana P, Caskey F, Casula A & Ansell D. (2009). UK Renal Registry 11th Annual Report (December 2008): Chapter 14 UK Renal Registry and international comparisons. *Nephron Clinical Practice;,* 111 Suppl 1: c269-76.

Boelaert JR, Van Landuyt HW, Godard CA Daneels RF, Schurgers ML, Matthys EG, De Baere YA, Gheyle DW, Gordts BZ & Herwaldt LA. (1993). Nasal mupirocin ointment decreases the incidence of *Staphylococcus aureus* bacteraemias in haemodialysis patients. *Nephrology Dialysis Transplantation;* 8(3): 235-239.

Breschan C, Platzer M, Jost R, Schaumberger F, Stettner H & Likar R. (2007). Comparison of catheter-related infection and tip colonization between internal jugular and subclavian central venous catheters in surgical neonates. *Anesthesiology;* 107(6): 946–53.

Broom JK, O'Shea S, Govindarajulu S, Playford G, Hawley CM, Isbel NM, Campbell SB, Mudge DW, Carpenter S, Johnson BC, Underwood N & Johnson DW (2009). Rationale and design of the HEALTHY-CATH trial: A randomised controlled trial of Heparin versus EthAnol Lock THerapY for the prevention of Catheter Associated infecTion in Haemodialysis patients. *BMC Nephrology;* 10: 23

Camins BC, Richmond AM, Dyer KL & Zimmerman HN. (2010). A crossover intervention trial evaluating the efficacy of a chlorhexidine-impregnated sponge in reducing catheter-related bloodstream infections among patients undergoing haemodialysis. *Infection Control and Hospital Epidemio*logy; 31(11): 1118-23.

CARI *(Caring for Australasians with Renal Impairment) Guidelines. (2000). Dialysis Guidelines: Vascular Access.* Available at www.cari.org.au

Cavdar C, Atay T, Zeybel M, Celik A, Ozder A, Yildiz S, Gulay Z & Camsari T. (2004). Emergence of resistance in staphylococci after long-term mupirocin application in patients on continuous ambulatory peritoneal dialysis. *Advances in Peritoneal Dialysis;* 20: 67-70.

Clase CM, Crowther MA, Ingram AJ & Cina CS. (2001). Thrombolysis for restoration of patency to haemodialysis central venous catheters: a systemic review. *Journal of Thrombosis and Thrombolysis;* 11: 127-36.

Del Rio A, Cervera C, Moreno A, Moreillon P & Miro JM. (2009). Patients at risk of complications of *Staphylococcus aureus* bloodstream infection. *Clinical Infectious Disease;* 48(4): S246–S253.

Deshpande KS, Hatem C, Ulrich HL & Currie BP. (2005). The incidence of infectious complications of central venous catheters at the subclavian, internal jugular, and femoral sites in an intensive care unit population. *Critical Care Medicine;* 33: 13–20.

Dhingra RK, Young EW, Hulbert-Shearon TE, Leavey SF & Port FK. (2001). Type of vascular access and mortality in US haemodialysis patients. *Kidney International* 2001; 60(4): 1443–51.

Dogra GK, Herson H, Hutchison B, Irish AB, Heath CH, Golledge C, Luxton G & Moody H. (2002) . Prevention of tunnelled haemodialysis catheter-related infections using catheter-restricted filling with gentamicin and citrate: a randomized controlled study. *Journal of the American Society of Nephrology;* 13(8): 2133-9.

Doss S, Schiller B, Moran J. (2008). Buttonhole cannulation - an unexpected outcome. *Nephrology Nursing Journal;* 35(4): 417-419.

Droste JC, Jeraj HA, MacDonald A & Farrington K. (2003). Stability and in vitro efficacy of antibiotic-heparin lock solutions potentially useful for treatment of central venous catheter-related sepsis. *Journal of Antimicrobial Chemotherapy;* 51: 849–855.

Dryden MS, Samson A, Ludlam HA, Wing AJ & Phillips I. (1991). Infective complications associated with the use of Quinton Permcath for long-term central vascular access in haemodialysis. *Journal of Hospital Infection;* 19: 257–262.

Eknoyan G, Beck GH, Cheung AK, Daugirdas JT, Greene T, Kusek JW, Allon M, Bailey J, Delmez JA, Depner TA, Dwyer JT, Levey AS, Levin NW, Milford E, Ornt DB, Rocco MV, Schulman G, Schwab SJ, Teehan BP & Toto R; Hemodialysis (HEMO) Study Group. (2002). Effect of dialysis dose and membrane flux in maintenance haemodialysis. *New England Journal of Medicine;* 347: 2010–2019.

Elie-Turenne MC, Fernandes H, Mediavilla JR, Rosenthal M, Mathema B, Singh A, Cohen TR, Pawar KA, Shahidi H, Kreiswirth BN, & Deitch EA. (2010). Prevalence and characteristics of *Staphylococcus aureus* colonization among healthcare professionals in an urban teaching hospital. *Infection Control and Hospital Epidemiology;* 31: 574–580.

Ethier J, Mendelssohn DC, Elder SJ, Hasegawa T, Akizawa T, Akiba T, Canaud BJ & Pisoni RL. (2008). Vascular access use and outcomes: an international perspective from the dialysis outcomes and practice patterns study. *Nephrology Dialysis Transplantation;* 23: 3219–3226.

Fistula First Breakthrough Initiative (FFBI). (2007). Summary of the FFBI buttonhole technique environmental scan. http://www.fistulafirst.org.

Fry AC, Stratton J, Farrington K & Mahna K. (2008). Factors affecting long-term survival of tunnelled haemodialysis catheters—a prospective audit of 812 tunnelled catheters. *Nephrology Dialysis Transplantation;* 23(1): 275-281.

Fux CA, Stoodley P, Hall-Stoodley L & Costerton JW. (2003). Bacterial biofilms: a diagnostic and therapeutic challenge. *Expert Reviews in Anti-Infective Therapy;* 1: 667–683.

Gould IM. (2007). MRSA bacteraemia. *International Journal of Antimicrobial Agents;* 30(Suppl 1): S66–S70.

Guenu S, Heng AE, Charbonne F, Galmier MJ, Charles F, Deteix, Souweine B & Lartigue C. (2007). Mass spectrometry and scanning electron microscopy study of silicone tunnelled dialysis catheter integrity after an exposure of 15 days to 60% ethanol solution. *Rapid Commununications in Mass Spectrometry;* 21:229-236.

Hartig V & Smyth W. (2009). Everyone should buttonhole: a novel technique for a regional Australian renal service. *Journal of Renal Care;* 35(3): 114-9.

Hoen B, Paul-Dauphin A, Hestin D & Kessler M. (1998). *EPIBACDIAL: a multicenter prospective study of risk factors for bactaeremia in chronic haemodialysis patients.* Journal of the American Society of Nephrology; 9: 869-876.

Ishani R, Collins AJ, Herzog C & Foley R. (2005). Septicaemia, access and cardiovascular disease in dialysis patients: The USRDS Wave 2 Study. *Kidney International;* 68: 311-318.

Ishizuka M, Nagata H, Takagi K & Kubota K. (2009). Femoral venous catheterization is a major risk factor for central venous catheter-related bloodstream infection. *Journal of Investigative Surgery;* 22: 16–21.

Ishizuka M, Nagata H, Takagi K, Horie T, Furihata M, Nakagawa A & Kubota K. (2008). External jugular Groshong catheter is associated with fewer complications than a subclavian Argyle catheter. *European Surgical Research*; 40: 197–202.

Jaffer Y, Selby NM, Taal MW, Fluck RJ & McIntyre CW. (2008). A meta-analysis of haemodialysis catheter locking solutions in the prevention of catheter-related infection. *American Journal of Kidney Disease*; 51: 233–241.

Jain G, Allon M, Saddekni S, Barker JF & Maya ID. (2009). Does heparin coating improve patency or reduce infection of tunnelled dialysis catheters? *Clinical Journal of the American Society of Nephrology*; 4: 1787-90.

James MT, Conley J, Tonelli M, Manns BJ, MacRae J & Hemmelgarn BR. (2008). Meta-analysis: antibiotics for prophylaxis against haemodialysis catheter-related infections. Alberta Kidney Disease Network. *Annals of Internal Medicine*; 148(8): 596-605.

Johnson DW, MacGinley R, Kay TD, Hawley CM, Campbell SB, Isbel NM & Hollett P. (2002). A randomised controlled trial of topical exit-site mupirocin application in patients with tunnelled cuffed haemodialysis catheters. *Nephrology Dialysis Transplantation*; 17: 1802-1807.

Johnson DW, Van Eps C, Mudge DW, Wiggins KJ, Armstrong K & Hawley CM. (2005). Randomized, controlled trial of topical exit-site application of honey (Medihoney) versus mupirocin for the prevention of catheter-associated infections in haemodialysis patients. *Journal of the American Society of Nephrology*; 16: 1456–1462.

KDOQI 2006: National Kidney Foundation. (2006). Clinical practice guidelines and clinical practice for vascular access. http://www.kidney.org/professionals/kdoqi/guideline˙upHD˙PD˙VA/index.htm

Knuttinen M, Bobra S, Hardman J & Gaba R. (2009). A review of evolving dialysis catheter technologies. *Seminars in Interventional Radiology*; 26 (2): 106-114.

Labriola L, Crott R & Jadoul M. (2008). Preventing haemodialysis catheter-related bacteraemia with an antimicrobial lock solution: a meta-analysis of prospective randomized trials. *Nephrology Dialysis Transplantation*; 23: 1666–1672.

Landry DL, Braden GL, Gobeille SL & Haessler SD. (2010). Emergence of gentamicin-resistant bacteraemia in haemodialysis patients receiving gentamicin lock catheter prophylaxis. *Clinical Journal of the American Society of Nephrology*; 5 (10) : 1799-1804.

Lee D, Jung K & Choi Y. (2008). Use of maximal sterile barrier precautions and/or antimicrobial-coated catheters to reduce the risk of central venous catheter–related bloodstream infection. *Infection Control and Hospital Epidemiology*; 29(10): 947-950.

Levin A, Mason AJ, Jindal KK, Fong IW & Goldstein MB. (1991). Prevention of haemodialysis subclavian vein catheter infections by topical povidone-iodine. *Kidney International*; 40(5): 934–8.

Lobbedez T, Gardam M, Dedier H, Burdzy D, Chu M, Izatt S, Bargman JM, Jassal SV, Vas S, Brunton J & Oreopoulos DG. (2004). Routine use of mupirocin at the peritoneal catheter exit site and mupirocin resistance: still low after 7 years. *Nephrology Dialysis Transplantation*; 19(12): 3140-3143.

Ludlow V. (2010). Buttonhole cannulation in haemodialysis: improved outcomes and increased expense – is it worth it? *Canadian Association of Nephrology Nurses and Technologists Journal;* 20(1): 29-37.

Macrae JM, Loh G, Djurdjev, Shalansky S, Werb R, Levin A, Kiaii M. (2005). Short and long alteplase dwells in dysfunctional haemodialysis catheters. *Haemodialysis International*; 9: 189-95.

Maharaj AR, Zelenitsky SA & Vercaigne LM. (2008). Effect of an ethanol/trisodium citrate hemodialysis catheter locking solution on isolated of Candida albicans. *Haemodialysis International;* 12(3): 342-327.

Maki DG, Stolz SM, Wheeler S & Mermel LA. (1997). Prevention of central venous catheter-related bloodstream infection by use of an antiseptic impregnated catheter: a randomized, controlled trial. *Annals of Internal Medcine;* 127: 257-66.

Marr KA, Sexton D, Conlon PJ Corey GR, Schwab SJ & Kirkland K. (1997). Catheter-related bacteraemia and outcome of attempted catheter salvage in patients undergoing haemodialysis. *Annals of Internal Medicine;* 127: 275–280.

Maya ID, Carlton D, Estrada E & Allon M. (2007). Treatment of dialysis catheter-related Staphylococcus aureus bactaeremia with an antibiotic lock: a quality improvement report. *American Journal of Kidney Disease;* 50(2): 289-95.

McCann M & Moore ZE. (2010). Interventions for preventing infectious complications in haemodialysis patients with central venous catheters. *Cochrane Database Systematic Review;* 20(1): CD00689.

Mcgee DC & Gould MK. (2003). Preventing complications of central venous catheterisation. *New England Journal of Medicine;* 348: 1123-1133.

Mermel LA, Eells SJ, Acharya MK, Cartony JM, Dacus D, Fadem S, Gay EA, Gordon S, Lonks JR, Perl TM, McDougal LK, McGowan JE, Maxey G, Morse D & Tenover FC. (2010). Quantitative analysis and molecular fingerprinting of methicillin-resistant *Staphylococcus aureus* nasal colonization in different patient populations: a prospective, multicenter study. *Infection Control and Hospital Epidemiology;* 31: 592–597.

Metcalf SCL, Chambers ST & Pithie AD. (2004). Use of ethanol locks to prevent recurrent central line sepsis. *Journal of Infection;* 49: 20–22.

Moist LM, Trpeski L, Na Y & Lok CE. (2008). Increased haemodialysis catheter use in Canada and associated mortality risk: data from the Canadian Organ Replacement Registry 2001–2004. *Clinical Journal of the American Society of Nephrology;* 3: 1726–1732.

Mokrzycki MH, Jean-Jerome K, Rush H, Zdunek MP & Rosenberg SO. (2001). A randomized trial of minidose warfarin for the prevention of late malfunction in tunnelled, cuffed haemodialysis catheters. *Kidney International;* 59: 1935–1542.

Mokrzycki MH, Schroppel B, von Gersdorff G, Rush H, Zdunek M & Feingold R. (2000). Tunnelled cuffed catheter associated infections in haemodialysis patients seropositive for the human immunodeficiency virus. *Journal of the American Society of Nephrology;* 11: 2122–2127.

Moss AH, Vasilakis C, Holley JL, Foulks CJ, Pillai K & McDowell DE. (1990). Use of a silicone dual-lumen catheter with a Dacron cuff as a long-term vascular access for haemodialysis patients. *American Journal of Kidney Disease;* 16: 211-215.

Nagashima G, Kikuchi T, Tsuyuzaki H, Kawano R, Tanaka H, Nemoto H, Taguchi K & Ugajin K. (2006). To reduce catheter-related bloodstream infections: is the subclavian route better than the jugular route for central venous catheterization? *Journal of Infection and Chemotherapy;* 12: 363–5.

National Kidney Foundation KDOQI. (2001). Clinical practice guidelines and clinical practice for vascular access, update 2006. http://www.kidney.org/professionals/kdoqi/guideline˙upHD˙PD˙VA/index.htm

Nesrallah GE, Cureden M, Wong JHS & Pierratos A. (2010). Staphylococcus aureus bacteraemia and buttonhole cannulation: long-term safety and efficacy of mupirocin prophylaxis. *Clinical Journal of the American Society of Nephrology;* 5(6): 1047-53.

Nielsen J, Kolmos HJ & Espersen F. (1998). *Staphylococcus aureus* bacteraemia among patients undergoing dialysis—focus on dialysis catheter-related cases. *Nephrology Dialysis Transplantation;* 13: 139–145.

Onder AM, Chandar J, Billings A, Simon N, Gonzalez J, Francoeur D, Abitbol C & Zilleruelo G. (2009). Prophylaxis of catheter-related bacteremia using tissue plasminogen activator-tobramycin locks. *Pediatric Nephrology;* 24(11): 2233-43.

Pastan S, Soucie JM & McClellan WM. (2002). Vascular access and increased risk of death among haemodialysis patients. *Kidney International;* 62(2): 620–6.

Pennington CR & Pithie AD. (1987). Ethanol lock in the management of catheter occlusion. *Journal of Parenteral Nutrition;* 11: 507–5083.

Pisoni RL, Young EW, Dykstra DM, Greenwood RN, Hecking E, Gillespie B, Wolfe RA, Goodkin DA & Held PJ. (2002). Vascular access use in Europe and the United States: Results from the DOPPS. *Kidney International;* 61(1): 305–16.

Polkinghorne KR, McDonald SP, Atkins RC & Kerr PG. (2004). Vascular access and all cause mortality: a propensity score analysis. *Journal of the American Society of Nephrology;* 15(2): 477–86.

Power A, Duncan N, Singh SK, Brown W, Dalby E, Edwards C, Lynch K, Prout V, Cairns T, Griffith M, McLean A, Palmer A & Taube D. (2009). Sodium citrate versus heparin catheter locks for cuffed central venous catheters: a single center randomised control trial of sodium citrate versus heparin line locks for cuffed central venous catheters. *American Journal of Kidney Disease;* 53(6): 1034-1041.

Power A, Singh SK, Ashby D, Cairns T, Taube D & Duncan N. (2011). Long-term Tesio catheter access for haemodialysis can deliver high dialysis adequacy with low complication rates. *Journal of Vascular and Interventional Radiology;* 22(5): 631-637

Pronovost PJ, Holzmueller CG, Clattenburg L, Berenholtz S, Martinez EA, Paz JR& Needham DM. (2006). Team care: beyond open and closed intensive care units. *Current Opinion in Critical Care;* 12(6): 604-8.

Pronovost PJ, Goeschel CA, Colantuoni E, Watson S, Lubomski LH, Berenholtz SM, Thompson DA, Sinopoli DJ, Cosgrove S, Sexton JB, Marsteller JA, Hyzy RC, Welsh R, Posa P, Schumacher K & Needham D. (2010). Sustaining reductions in catheter related bloodstream infections in Michigan intensive care units: observational study. *British Medical Journal;* 4;340: 309-315

Raad I, Darouiche R, Dupuis J, Abi-Said D, Gabrielli A, Hachem R, Wall M, Harris R, Jones J, Buzaid A, Robertson C, Shenaq S, Curling P, Burke T & Ericsson C. (1997). Central venous catheters coated with minocycline and rifampin for the prevention of catheter-related colonization and bloodstream infections: a randomized, double-blind trial. *Annals of Internal Medicine;* 127: 267-74.

Rabindranath KS, Bansal T, Adams J, Das R, Shail R, MacLeod AM, Moore C & Besarab A. (2009). Systematic review of antimicrobials for the prevention of haemodialysis catheter-related infections. *Nephrology Dialysis Transplantation;* 24(12): 3763-74.

Ramos ER, Reitzel R, Jiang Y, Hachem RY, Chaftari AM, Chemaly RF, Hackett B, Pravinkumar SE, Nates J, Tarrand JJ & Raad II. (2010). Clinical effectiveness and risk of emerging resistance associated with prolonged use of antibiotic-impregnated catheters: More than 0.5 million catheter days and 7 years of clinical experience. *Critical Care Medicine;* 39 (2): 245 -251.

Regamey C, Schaberg D & Kirby WM. (1972). Inhibitory effect of heparin on gentamicin concentrations in blood. *Antimicrobial Agents and Chemotherapy*; 1: 329–332.

Ruesch S, Walder B & Tramer MR. (2002). Complications of central venous catheters: internal jugular versus subclavian access—a systematic review. *Critical Care Medicine*; 30: 454–60.

Ryan JM, Ryan BM & Smith TP. (2004). Antibiotic prophylaxis in interventional radiology. *Journal of Vascular and Interventional Radiology*; 15(6): 547-56.

Saad TF. (1999). Bacteraemia associated with tunnelled, cuffed haemodialysis catheters. *American Journal of Kidney Disease*; 34: 1114–1124.

Saxena AK, Panhotra BR, Uzzaman W, & Venkateshappa CK. (2002). The role of the *Staphylococcus aureus* nasal carriage and type of vascular access in the outcome of high-risk patients on haemodialysis. *Journal of Vascular Access*; 3(2): 74-9

Sedlacek M, Gemery JM, Cheung AL, Bayer AS & Remillard BD. (2007). Aspirin treatment is associated with a significantly decreased risk of *staphylococcus aureus* bactaeremia in haemodialysis patients with tunnelled catheters. *American Journal of Kidney Diseases;* 49: 401-408.

Shanks RM, Sargent L, Martinez RM, Graber M & O'Toole G. (2006). Catheter lock solutions influence staphylococcal biofilm formation on abiotic surfaces. *Nephrology Dialysis Transplantation*; 21: 2247–2255.

Silva GD, Silva RA, Niccolino AM, Pavanetti LC, Alasmar VL, Guzzardi R, Zanolli MB, Guilhen JC & Araujo ID. (2010). Initial experience with the buttonhole technique in a Brazilian haemodialysis center. *Journal of Brasilian Nefrology;* 32(3): 257-62.

Solomon LR, Cheesbrough JS, Ebah L & Al-Sayed T. (2010) . A randomized double-blind controlled trial of taurolidine-citrate catheter locks for the prevention of bacteraemia in patients treated with haemodialysis. *American Journal of Kidney Diseases;* 55 (6): 1060-1068.

Taal MW, Fluck RJ & McIntyre CW. (2006). Preventing catheter related infections in haemodialysis patients. *Current Opinion in Nephrology and Hypertension;* 15(6): 599-602.

Takla TA, Zelenitsky SA & Vercaigne LM. (2007). Effect of ethanol/trisodium lock on microorganisms causing haemodialysis related catheter infections. *Journal of Vascular Access;* 8(4): 262-7.

Taylor C, Cahill J, Gerrish M, & Little J. (2008). A new haemodialysis catheter-locking agent reduces infections in haemodialysis patients. *Journal of Renal Care;* 34(3): 116-120.

The European Renal Association - European Dialysis and Transplant Association. European best practice guidelines for haemodialysis (Part 1) ERA-EDTA. (2002). *Nephrology Dialysis Transplantation;* 17: (Suppl 7):1–111.

Timsit JF, Schwebel C, Bouadma L & Geffroy A. (2009). Chlorhexidine-impregnated sponges and less frequent dressing changes for prevention of catheter-related infections in critically ill adults: a randomized controlled trial. *Journal of the American Medical Association;* 25: 301(12): 1231-41.

Tordoir J, Canaud B, Haage P, Konner K, Basci A, Fouque D, Kooman J, Martin-Malo A, Pedrini L, Pizzarelli F, Tattersall J, Vennegoor M, Wanner C, ter Wee P & Vanholder R. (2007). EBPG on Vascular Access. *Nephrology Dialysis Transplantation;* 22 [Suppl 2]: ii88–ii117.

Torres-Viera C, Thauvin-Eliopoulos C, Souli M, DeGirolami P, Farris MG, Wennersten CB, Sofia RD & Eliopoulos GM. (2000). Activities of taurolidine in vitro and in experimental enterococcal endocarditis. *Antimicrobial Agents and Chemotherapy;* 44(6): 1720-1724.

Trerotola SO, Patel AA, Shlansky-Goldberg RD, Solomon JA, Mondschein JI, Stavropoulos SW, Soulen MC, Itkin M & Chittams J. (2010). Short-term infection in cuffed versus noncuffed small bore central catheters: a randomized trial. *Journal of Vascular and Interventional Radiology;* 21: 203–11.

Tumlin J, Goldman J, Spiegel DM, Roer D, Ntoso KA, Blaney M, Jacobs J, Gillespie BS & Begelman SM. (2010). A phase III, randomised, double-blind placebo-controlled study of tenecteplase for improvement of haemodialysis catheter function: TROPICS 3. *Clinical Journal of the American Society of Nephrology;* 5: 631-6.

United States CDC (Centers for Disease Control and Prevention). Guidelines for the prevention of intravascular catheter-related infections (2002). http://www.cdc.gov/mmwr/preview/mmwrhtml/rr5110a1.htm : 1–26.

Van Eps CL, Jones M, Ng T, Johnson DW, Campbell SB, Isbel NM, Mudge DW, Beller E & Hawley CM. (2010). The impact of extended-hours home haemodialysis and buttonhole cannulation technique on hospitalization rates for septic events related to dialysis access. *Haemodialysis International;* 14(4): 451-63.

Van Loon MM, Goovaerts T, Kessels AGH, van der Sande FM & Tordoir JHM. (2010). Buttonhole needling of haemodialysis arteriovenous fistulae results in less complications and interventions compared to the rope-ladder technique. *Nephrology Dialysis Transplantation;* 25: 225-30.

Vercaigne LM, Takla TA & Raghavan J. (2010). Long-term effect of an ethanol/sodium citrate solution on the mechanical properties of haemodialysis catheters. *Journal of Vascular Access;* 11(1): 12-6.

Weijmer MC, van den Dorpel MA, Van de Ven PJG, ter Wee P, van Geelen J, Groeneveld J, van Jaarsveld BC, Koopmans M, le Poole C, Schrander A, Sieger C & Stas KJ. (2005). Randomized, clinical trial comparison of trisodium citrate 30% and heparin as catheter-locking solution in haemodialysis patients. *Journal of the American Society of Nephrology;* 16: 2769-2777.

Xue J, Dahl D, Ebben J & Collins AJ. (2003). The association of initial haemodialysis access type with mortality outcomes in elderly Medicare ESRD patients. *American Journal of Kidney Diseases;* 42(5): 1013-1019.

Yahav D, Rozen-Zvi B, Gafter-Gvili A, Leibovici L, Gafter U & Paul M. (2008). Antimicrobial lock solutions for the prevention of infections associated with intravascular catheters in patients undergoing haemodialysis: systematic review and meta-analysis of randomized, controlled trials. *Clinical Infectious Diseases;* 47: 83–93.

Yoo S, Ha M, Chio D & Pai H. (2001). Effectiveness of surveillance of central catheter-related bloodstream infection in an ICU in Korea. *Infection Control and Hospital Epidemiology;* 22: 433–436.

Yu VL, Goetz A & Wagener M. (1986). *Staphylococcus aureus* carriage and infection in patients on haemodialysis. Efficacy of antibiotic prophylaxis. *New England Journal of Medicine;* 315: 91–96.

7

Acute and Chronic Catheter in Hemodialysis

Andrew S. H. Lai[1] and Kar Neng Lai[2]
[1]Department of Diagnostic Radiology
[2]Department of Medicine
Queen Mary Hospital, University of Hong Kong
Hong Kong

1. Introduction

Reliable and sustained access to the circulation is mandatory for the provision of long-term hemodialysis which is critical to the survival of patients with end-stage renal disease (ESRD). An ideal vascular access provides adequate blood flow to meet the hemodialysis prescription, with minimal complications due to infection or thrombosis. The natural arteriovenous fistula (AVFs) comes closest to meeting these criteria while arteriovenous grafts (AVGs) and central venous catheters (CVCs) present other vascular access options. In the United States, promoting a major shift in using fistula as first-choice vascular access has been strongly recommended by the 2001 Kidney Disease Outcome Quality Initiative (K/DOQI) vascular access guideline (NKF-DOQI 2001) and the "Fistula First" national initiative (Tonnessen et al 2005). Ideally, every patient would initiate dialysis with a mature fistula suitable for cannulation. In real clinical setting, this is not true due to combination of the following factors including (i) lacking nephrology follow-up at the time of ESRD, (ii) late nephrology referral, (iii) poor or no planning of fistula placement, (iv) inadequate fistula maturation and (v) poor vascular preparation due to prior venous cannulation.

In current practice, 20-50% of attempted AVFs fail to mature adequately. Despite a recent increase in the number of prevalent patients dialyzing with an AVF (47%) in the US following the fistula-first initiative, 28% of prevalent patients remain dependent on an AVG and 25% on a CVC. In Canada, recent data demonstrate that 50% of patients use an AVF, while 39% and 11% depends on a CVC or AVG, respectively (James et al 2009).

Sadly, hemodialysis CVCs are increasingly being introduced in patients requiring emergency or chronic renal replacement therapy. Table 1 outlines the advantages and disadvantages of CVCs. The percentages of patients undergoing dialysis with vascular catheters are increasing in Europe, ranging from 15% (Germany) to 50% (United Kingdom) of all hemodialysis patients. In the United States, up to 60% of patients start hemodialysis with CVCs (Pisoni et al 2002). Over the last decade, the number of patients using CVCs for hemodialysis doubled (Rayner et al 2004). According to the Dialysis Outcomes and Practice Patterns Study, 18% of patients with end-stage renal failure in the United States and 24% of those in Great Britain have been dialysed with such catheters (Quarello et al 2006). Table 2 summarizes the indication for using CVCs. Recent studies indicate that CVCs are used in 20-25% of incident (<6 months) chronic kidney disease (CKD) stage 5 patients and still used in 10-20% of prevalent hemodialysis patients (> 6 months) (Rayner et al 2004a, Moist et all 2007). The use of CVCs has been complicated by higher rates of thrombosis, dysfunction, and infection compared with AVFs. As a result of this, maintaining CVCs is associated with high costs (Lacson et al 2007). The increased use of CVCs requires a maximal precaution in its management and a stringent practice to reduce its risk and complications.

Advantages	Disadvantages
High success rate	High morbidity caused by thrombosis and infection
Insertion into multiple sites	Risks of permanent central venous stenosis or occlusion
Maturation time not required	Lower blood flow rates requiring a longer dialysis time
No venepuncture	
No hemodynamic consequences	
Easy replacement	
Functional for months (chronic tunneled CVC)	
Ease of correcting thrombotic complications	

Table 1. Advantages and disadvantages of central venous catheters for hemodialysis

- Pending maturation of arteriovenous fistula
- Providing temporary dialysis treatment for patients undergoing maintenance peritoneal dialysis but complicated by peritonitis such that the infection can be controlled and the peritoneum be rested
- Awaiting for living-related donor transplantation
- "Bridging dialysis" followed failed previous vascular or peritoneal access allowing planning of long-term access
- Permanent vascular access when other sites for arteriovenous fistula or grafts are exhausted

Table 2. Indications for central venous hemodialysis catheters

2. Types of central venous catheters

There are two main categories of hemodialysis catheters: (i) non-tunneled, uncuffed, designed for short-term venous access of up to three weeks and (ii) tunneled, cuffed catheters for longer use. An ideal CVC is biologically neutral and does not induce venous or catheter lumen thrombosis; its surface is coated with an agent, which prevents migration and multiplication of bacteria. It should enable continuous dialysis with the blood flow through the catheter > 350-400 ml/min. Moreover, it ought to be non-traumatic, soft, easy to insert, mechanically durable, bending-resistant, comfortable for the patient and inexpensive. A comparison of acute and chronic central venous catheters is shown in Table 3.

i. *Temporary acute catheters*

Acute untunneled CVCs are used in emergency situations (dialysis, plasma exchange, hemofiltration or hemoperfusion) or as a short-term bridging access (ideally < 7 days). The advantages of these catheters are their ease of insertion (even by the bedside), the ability to insert them in multiple sites in almost any patient and the lack of hemodynamic compromise associated with their use. Internal jugular vein is the preferred site as anatomically this provides the most direct route to the superior vena cava and right atrium. The vein should be localized by ultrasound (+/- Doppler). Insertion into the left internal jugular vein is associated with a higher incidence of central stenosis and poorer patency. For selected cases requiring short-term dialysis, the femoral vein can also be used. Subclavian vein should be discouraged as it may jeopardize the long-term arteriovenous access options with complication of subclavian stenosis. The catheters are usually inserted using the Seldinger technique. The catheter can be used immediately after confirming correct placement with fluoroscopy.

Acute	Chronic
For use of < 7 days	For use of > 3 weeks
Most are not tunneled and without a retention cuff - conical tip for easy insertion	Most are tunneled with a retention cuff - soft tip
Most are dual lumen with venous port 2-3 cm distal of arterial port	Thermoplastic polyurethane - larger internal diameter, biocompatible, nonthrombogenic
Polyurethane – stiff and withstanding high pressure	Carbothane - copolymer with strength for longevity and softness for flexibility
Silicone - larger lumen but needs a peel-away sheath	Silicone - larger lumen but needs a peel-away sheath, biocompatible, less thrombogenic

Table 3. Comparison between acute and chronic central venous catheters

To ensure continuous, independent blood flow, catheters are double-lumen. The distal part has two separate openings; one collecting the patient`s blood – "arterial", located 2-3 cm from the catheter end and the second one pumping the blood to the patient – "venous", placed at its end. Temporary catheters are usually made of stiff materials: polyurethane or polyvinyl, and thus are easier to introduce along the guidewire and a hemostasis valve is not needed. The sharp distal tip facilitates the insertion through the subcutaneous tissues. Compared to soft catheters, they are more resistant to bending in the vessel. At body temperature, after contact with the bloodstream, they become plastic, which reduces the risk of vessel damage. Temporary CVCs have no cuffsbut are quipped with dacron muffs. The insertion doe not require "tunnelization", thus fast access to the circulatory system can be provided. They vary in length, therefore the proper choice is easier depending the puncture site and availability of a central vessel. They may be used for several days or up to three weeks. Their main advantage is easy insertion into the vessel using the Seldinger technique with easy replacement not requiring expensive accessory devices, (which may not be always available) such as fluoroscopy or ultrasound. Generally, the blood flow through temporary CVCs is limited to 200-250 ml/min.

The newer catheters are made of silicone with bigger internal diameter which ensures the blood flow of 400 ml/min. Some of them are tunneled. Silicone is thermoset and thus the catheter is soft. Hence it has to be inserted using a dilator and peel-away sheath. Other materials include polyurethane which is thermoplastic and softens at body temperature. This reduces endothelial damage and thrombogenicity (Leblanc et al 1997). The tunneled catheters can be introduced either antegrade (skin to insertion site) or retrograde (insertion site to skin). The position of soft CVCs should be confirmed by fluoroscopy.

ii. Long-term tunneled catheters

Tunneled CVCs with cuffs are made of silicone, silastic or carbothane elastomer, polyurethane co-polymer and polycarbonate – these materials are softer and more plastic than those used in temporary catheters. Therefore, they are usually inserted using the Seldinger technique via peel-away sheath. Subcutaneous tunnelization and a cuff are to stabilize the catheter and prevent the spread of infections. The soft silastic elastomer enables the placement of the distal catheter tip in the right atrium, which should be confirmed by fluoroscopy. Bigger internal diameters (thicker catheters) provide better blood flows and a wider dilator or sequential dilator is frequently used.

The first model of a tunneled catheter was PermCath, an oval catheter with two circular canals. Subsequent models (e.g. Vas Cath) were designed with an internal septum dividing the internal lumen into two parts. The oval transverse section of the catheter facilitated its insertion through the peel-away sheath. The third popular option was the introduction of two catheters with a single lumen - Tesio or its modification. One collected the blood through the opening in the superior vena cava and the other one supplied blood through the opening in the right atrium. Other than the catheter body and lumen, the design of the shape of catheter tips is also emphasized for better blood flow, improved reliability and minimizing recirculation (Ash 2008).

The newest catheters implanted surgically are equipped with a subcutaneous port (Morgan 2001, Ross 2001), which reduces percutaneous device-related complications. In most cases, the port consists of a chamber made of a titanium, ceramics or other neutral plastic materials with silicone membrane and an attachable catheter. The silicone membrane enables repeated penetrations (about 1000-2000), depending on the product and size of the puncture needle. The entire system is placed under the skin, which prevents infections or accidental opening. There are different configurations of the catheter and port chamber from using two single catheters each attached to a single chamber port to a double-lumen catheter connected to a two-chamber port. The vascular port implantation is based on the same principles as those for central venous access except the ports are placed in a subcutaneous pocket. The port can be punctured with normal hemodialysis needles or needles with special make that does not cut an opening in the membrane. The main reason of low popularity of hemodialysis ports is their relatively high cost.

3. Percutaneous insertion of central venous catheter

As mentioned, the right internal jugular vein is the preferred site as the curve of the catheter is straight thus achieving the best result. If the left internal jugular vein is used, negotiation of the curve at the venous entry to the superior vena cava may require experience and care. Moreover, one must choose a longer catheter as compared with right jugular vein puncture. The length of catheter introduced from neck or thoracic access should enable its distal end to reach the right atrium when a soft catheter is used or be placed in the superior or inferior vena cava when the catheter is stiff. It is recommended to place hemodialysis CVCs under fluoroscopic screening to avoid trauma with the guidewire in the inferior vena cava during insertion and the distal part of catheter in the upper right atrium upon completion of placement (Lin et al 1998, Keenan 2002).

The first choice for catheterization is the right internal jugular vein, followed by the right external jugular vein, left internal jugular vein, left external jugular vein, and finally femoral veins or external iliac veins (Maya et al 2005). The vein should be localized by ultrasound and can be differentiated from the artery by Doppler. The probe should first be placed on the head of the sternomastoid muscle and then moves down towards the clavicle. The puncture site should be as low as possible but above the clavicle whereas the exit of the subcutaneous tunnel should preferably be below the clavicle.

Femoral and external iliac veins may be used for CVC insertion in bed-ridden patients or in the intensive care setting, particularly in patients requiring artificial lung ventilation, after head and neck trauma with numerous catheters and drains of the neck and thorax as well as those with tracheostomy (Zaleski et al 1999, Mathur et al 1993). Patients with kidney transplant potential should avoid femoral vein catheterization. With catheter insertion in the groin, meticulous hygiene of the puncture site is required. The patency period from the insertion to removal is markedly shorter in femoral vein access compared to catheters inserted through the internal jugular vein.

4. Catheterization-related complications

Irrespective of the type (non-tunneled or tunneled) or design (straight or with formed shape), their use is likely to be associated with complications (Table 4) (Morgan 2001, Ross 2001).

Early	Late
Inadvertent arterial puncture and central vessel perforation	Infection
Hemothorax	Central vein thrombosis
Pneumothorax	Catheter thrombosis formation
Pericardial tamponade	Central vein stenosis
Atrial perforation	Catheter dysfunction (can be early due to kinking)
Dissection/occlusion of carotid artery	Permanent vascular ingrowth
Arrthymias	
Air embolism	
Retroperitoneal hemorrhage (for femoral vein insertion)	
Primary failure - technical error	

Table 4. Complications of central venous catheters insertion

The incidence of complications reaches 5.9% with catheter insertion based only on topographic anatomy even with experienced clinicians (McDowell et al 1993). In contrast, the incidence of procedure-related complications in central venous catheterization under ultrasound guidance is only 0.8% (Trerotola et al 1997). Ultrasound-guided catheterization also limits the incidence of failures related to catheter insertion and reduces complications and necessity of multiple punctures of a vessel (Randolph et al 1996). Early complications which are mainly "surgical" include pneumothorax, pleural or mediastinal hemotoma, air embolism, thoracic tract injury, damage to nervous structures within the neck and thoracic region, puncture of the cardiac cavities, or cardiac arrest (Feldman et al 1996) (Figure 1). Non-surgical complications include cardiac arrhythmia and insertion site infection.

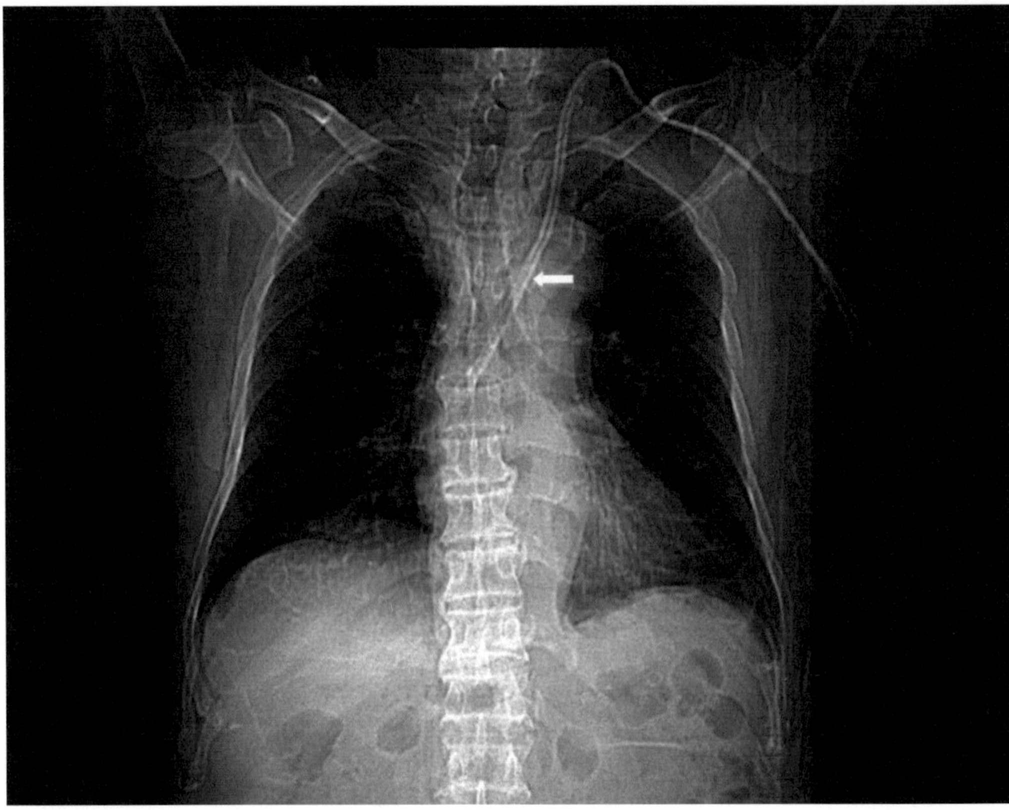

Fig. 1. Plain Chest Xray showing a CVC placed in the left internal jugular vein protruding out of the vessel wall (arrow)

Long-term complications are equally important. The common ones are thrombotic complications, vascular stenosis and catheter-related bacteremia (CRB). To reduce their complications, the internal surface of catheters is often coated with heparin. Coating or impregnation of catheters with silver salts and antibiotics reduces the colonization of bacteria.

4.1 Catheter dysfunction

The 2006 National Kidney Foundation K/DOQI guidelines defines access dysfunction as the inability to achieve blood flow (Qb) ≥ 300 ml/min during the first 60 minutes of hemodialysis despite at least one attempt to improve flow (National Kidney Foundation 2006). Since then, larger bore catheter design allows much higher Qb (> 400 ml/min) to be achieved at the same prepump pressure. Hence, waiting until Qb declines to 300 ml/min in these catheters may be inappropriate, missing the opportunity to detect catheter dysfunction earlier.

Early identification of catheter dysfunction enables prompt intervention and salvage. Catheter occlusion can be caused by kinking or malposition and these may be detected during the first hemodialysis session. Other causes of catheter dysfunction include leakage, drug precipitation, thrombus formation and growth of a fibrin sheath. Thrombus-related occlusion typically occurs late either with or without a fibrin sheath. The clinical features of different thrombotic occlusive complications are summarized in Table 5. Catheter dysfunction is frequently associated with recirculation that exerts a deleterious effect on dialysis efficiency and patient outcome (Leblanc et al 1997).

Complications	Features	Symptoms
Mural thrombus	Fibrin from vessel wall injury connected to fibrin-coated catheter leading to increased risk of venous thrombosis	Leakage of infusate from the insertion site, swelling, pain, tenderness, engorged vein
Intraluminal thrombus	Fibrin forms inside the catheter lumen causing partial or completion occlusion	Unable to infuse and/or withdraw blood
Fibrin sheath	Fibrin adheres to the external surface encasing the catheter and frequently extending the length of the catheter; thrombi trapped between sheath and catheter tip	Unable to infuse and/or withdraw blood
Fibrin tail or flap	Fibrin extends from the end of the catheter causing partial occlusion (fibrin tail acts as an one-way valve)	Able to infuse but not withdraw blood

Table 5. Different thrombotic occlusive complications related to central venous catheter for dialysis

Before the tunneled CVC thrombosis occurs, prophylactic inhibition of coagulation cascade should be considered. The earlier results of various antiplatelet agents and anticoagulation were not encouraging. Better patency has been maintained with catheter locking solutions between dialysis sessions. The standard protocol has been heparin instillation (1000 to 10000 units/ml) into the lumens in a volume sufficient to fill to the lumen tip (the lock). The heparin concentration is reduced because catheter lumens have increased in volume so as to reduce the possibility of unintentional systemic anticoagulation. Trisodium citrate with its antithrombotic and potentially antibacterial properties has also been tested as a locking solution. The American Society of Diagnostic and Interventional Nephrology Clinical Practice Committee recommends using a locking solution of 1000 units/ml heparin or 4% trisodium citrate to maintain CVC patency (Fuchs et al 1999).

Most recently, a Canadian multicenter study showed the once weekly use of recombinant plasminogen activator (1 mg in each lumen), as compared with heparin (5000 units/ml) thrice weekly, as a locking solution for CVC significantly reduced the incidence of catheter dysfunction and bacteremia (Hemmelgarn et al 2011).

4.2 Central thrombosis formation

Mural thrombosis in the superior vena cava and the right atrial wall associated with CVC placement is detected in one-third of patients but often remains asymptomatic [26]. Treatment by infusion of a fibrinolytic agent produces good results but angioplasty and stenting may be required for organized thrombosis.

4.3 Central vein stenosis

The incidence of central vein stenosis is considerable. As with fibrin sheath, central vein stenosis should be identified with a superior vena cavogram performed by removing the old catheter over the working guidewire followed by a pigtail catheter insertion (Figure 2). The management of central stenosis is evolving. Whenever found, endovascular balloon angioplasty should be attempted to a minimum of the contiguous uninvolved vein (Quinn et al 1995). Unfortunately, central vein stenosis tends to recur (Quinn et al 995, Kovalik et al 1994). The use of flexible stents has gained popularity recently despite the long term outcome is not well defined.

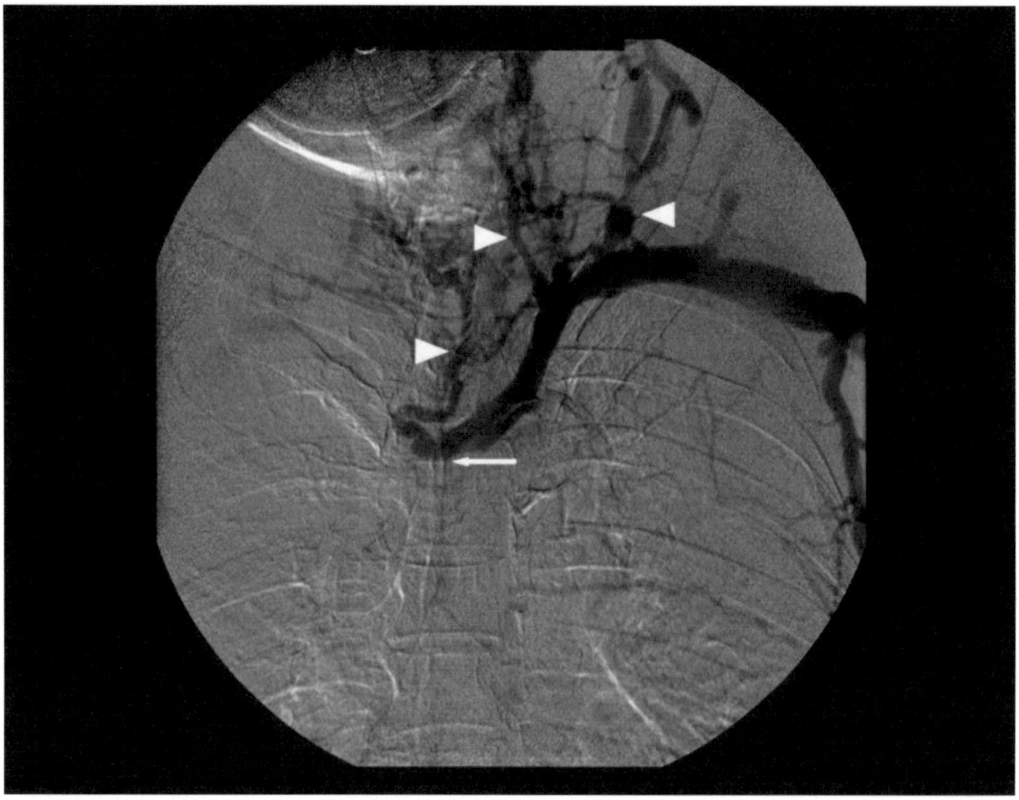

Fig. 2. Patient with a non-functioning left internal jugular vein hemodialysis catheter. Left subclavian venogram showed stenosis at proximal superior vena cava (arrow) with multiple collaterals in the neck (arrowheads).

4.4 Fibrin sheath

Fibrin sheaths account for 13-57% of catheter dysfunction (Suhocki et al 1996). The formation begins 24 hours after placement and it develops into a full-length sleeve after 5-7 days (Faintuch et al 2008). The sheath first occurs when fibrin adheres to the external surface before encasing the catheter and frequently extending the length of the catheter. The sheath seems to originate from the insertion site or the cuff and tends to migrate down the length of the catheter causing occlusion. Thrombi may also be trapped between sheath and catheter tip. A permcathogram done by injecting contrast through the catheter ports under fluoroscopic screening may show a persisting filling defect at the catheter tip or reflux of the contrast along the sheath in a retrograde direction (Figure 3). Fibrin sheaths may be treated by prolonged infusion of fibrinolytic agents (urokinase 30000 units/hour via each port x 4 hours or recombinant tissue plasminogen activator of 2.5 mg diluted in 50 ml normal saline at a rate of 17 ml/hour through each port x 3 hours), mechanical stripping using a snare inserted via the femoral vein by exchange of catheter over a guidewire (Suhocki et al 1996, Faintuch et al 2008, Goldberg et al 1985). Diverse degree of success in fibrin sheath stripping is reported from different centers.

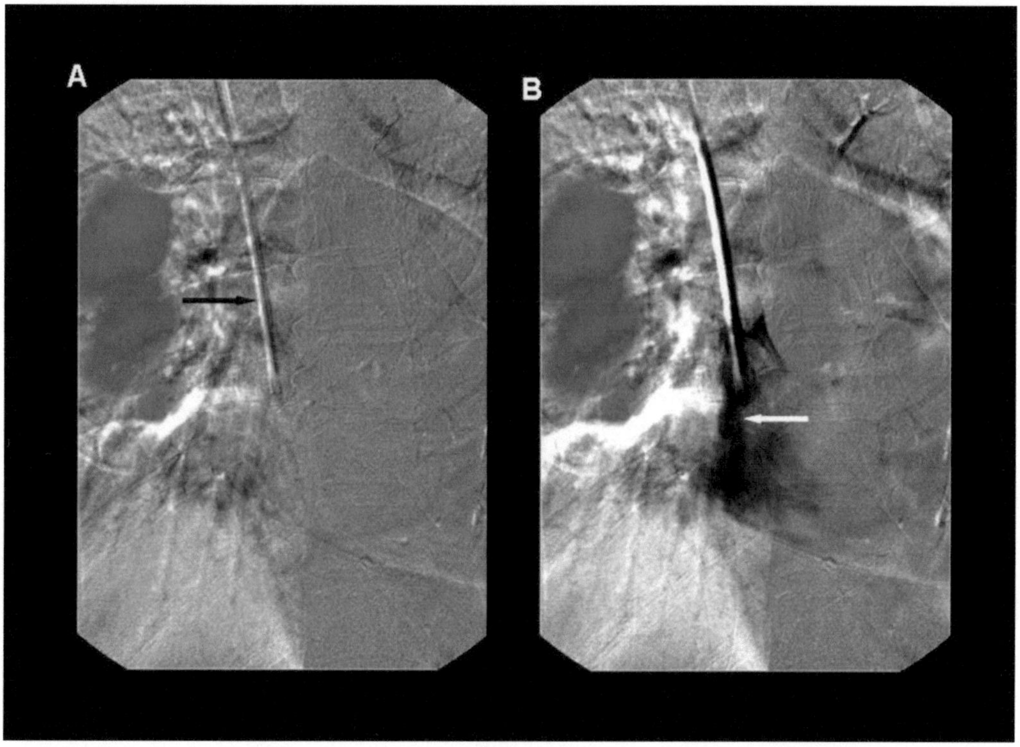

Fig. 3. (A) A fibrin sheath (arrow) formed inside the lumen of the CVC. (B) A permcathogram done showing a persisting filling defect (arrow) in the catheter lumen and reflux of the contrast at the catheter tip.

4.5 Catheter-related bacteremia

Catheter infection is a major cause of morbidity and mortality responsible for 6-28% of catheter failures (Bagui et al 2007). Diagnosis of catheter-related bacteremia (CRB) requires at least one of the following criteria: (a) clinical exit site infection with evidence of inflammation within 2 cm of sites; (b) definite organism grew from blood culture and catheter with no other apparent source of infection; (c) probable blood stream infection with defervescence after catheter removal when both blood and catheter tip infection is not confirmed in a symptomatic patients with no apparent source of infection; (d) possible blood stream infection in a symptomatic patients with defervescence after catheter removal, but remains culture negative.

The causative organisms are predominantly gram positive (~50%), gram negative bacilli (~25%) or polymicrobial (~20%). The most common occurrence is through the migration of skin organisms along the external surface of the catheter from the exit site wound or via the catheter lumen due to breakdown of aseptic technique. The organism can be embedded in a biofilm layer that confers protection from antibiotic therapy (Passerini et al 1992). Infection occurs when the organisms on the catheter exceed a certain quantitative threshold. Ninety percent of exit site infections respond to oral antibiotics without the necessity of catheter removal. Oral antibiotics can be used for minor infection but intravenous antibiotics should be administered if there is a discharge from the tunnel /exit site. If the infection fails to resolve with these measures, the catheter should be removed and replaced through a different track. Systemic sepsis or bacteremia carries a higher morbidity. K/DOQI guidelines recommend rapid removal of catheters in unstable patients with bacteremia or in stable patients if remain symptomatic 36 hours after achieving serum concentration of bactericidal antibiotics. In these cases, antibiotics should be administered for 14-21 days.

Reference	Type of locking solution	Intervention	Control
Dogra *et al.* 2002	Gentamicin	0.3	4.2
McIntyre *et al.* 2004	Gentamicin	0.3	4.0
Bleyer *et al.* 2005	Minocycline	0	0.472
Kim et al 2006	Gentamicin/Cefazolin	0.4	3.1
Saxena *et al.* 2006	Cefotaxime	1.7	3.6
Nori *et al.* 2006	Gentamicin	0	4.0
	Minocycline	0.4	4.0
Filiopoulos *et al.* 2011	Gentamycin	2.7	9.9
	Taurolidine/Citrate	3.7	9.9
Allon 2003	Taurolidine	0.6	5.6
Betjes and van Agteren 2004	Taurolidine	0	2.1
Weijmer *et al.* 2005	Citrate (30%)	1.1	4.1

Rate of CRB (per 1000 catheter-days)

Table 6. Catheter locking solutions for prophylaxis against catheter-related bacteremia (CRB)

Prophylaxis of catheter-related bacteremia has been studied with standard antibiotics or antimicrobial agents such as taurolidine and 30% citrate as catheter locking solution. Seven randomized clinical trials documented substantial efficacy of antibiotic locks (gentamicin, minocycline or cefotaxime) in prophylaxis against catheter-related bacteremia (Dogra et al 2002, McIntyre et al 2004, Bleyer et al 2005, Kim et al 2006, Saxena et al 2006, Nori et al 2006, Filiopoulos et al 2011). An additional four studies documented reduction in frequency of catheter-related bacteremia using taurolidine or citrate as locking solution (Filiopoulos et al 2011, Allon 2003, Betjes et al 2004, Weijmer et al 2005). These studies are summarized in Table 6.

4.6 Permanent vascular ingrowth

Tissue ingrowth into the catheter lumen occurs when the tissue entraps the catheter onto the endothelial surface of the vessel. There is no standard management for this problem. Surgical approach of a thoracotomy is required as cut down on to the internal jugular vein for catheter is not usually possible.

5. Other accesses for insertion of central venous catheter

If the jugular veins are not accessible for long-term placement, the subclavian vein opposite the dominating side can be used. The nephrologist must realize the risk of subclavian stenosis (Feldman et al 1996, Can 2008). The subclavian vein should never be catheterized on the side of the unhealed arteriovenous fistula.

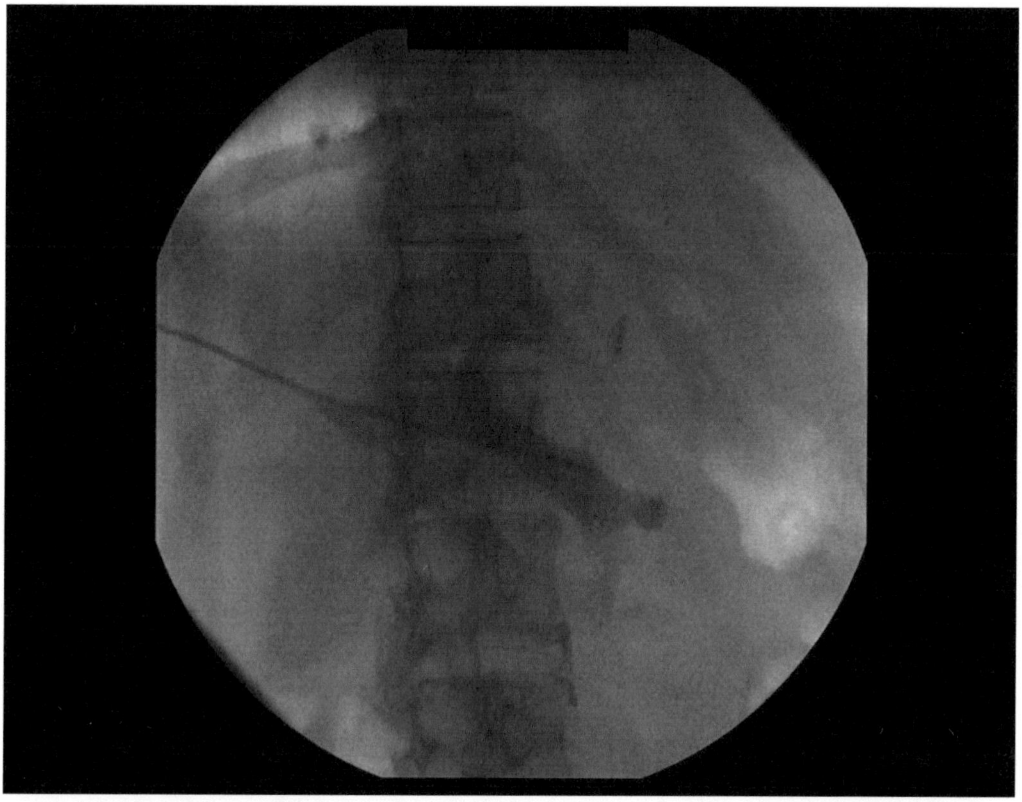

Fig. 4. Transhepatic placement of a Retrocath (45 cm long, 16Fr) into the portal vein. Contrast was injected to confirm the successful cannulation of the portal venous system.

Other alternative sites have been used for CVC placement when none of the typical central accesses is available. Such procedures must be conducted by an experienced interventional radiologist in a fully equipped facility. Alternative methods may be used: catheterization of the inferior vena cava, or hepatic, translumbar, renal, intercostal and mediastinal veins.

The translumbar approach to cannulation of the inferior vena cava, first described in 1971, has gained renewed attention as an alternative method for CVC access. High adequacy dialysis with low rates of catheter-related infection has recently reported from a single center study (Power et al 2009). The catheter care protocols, a policy of clinically appropriate catheter salvage with empirical broad-spectrum antibiotics and prior experience with translumbar catheter may also have the influenced outcome.

Transhepatic placement of hemodialysis catheter first described in 1994 can be associated with infrequent complications such as line sepsis, catheter migration, thrombosis and bleeding (Smith et al 204). These complications can be minimized when the procedure is performed by an interventional radiologist who is familiar with portal venogram (Figure 4)

(Yap et al 2010). In exceptional lack of options, transrenal access into the renal vein with consequent insertion of a tunneled catheter has been attempted (Murthy et al 2002).

6. Conclusion

Hemodialysis central venous catheters CVCs are commonly used in patients with renal failure requiring dialysis once other vascular options have been exhausted. Long-term catheters should be inserted using the Seldinger technique with a dilator and hemostasis valve under ultrasound guidance and fluoroscopic screening. Tunneled catheters with cuffs may be used both temporarily and permanently. The subcutaneous tunnel and cuff ensure stabilization of their position and limiting the migration of microorganisms on its external surface hence reducing the risk of infections. Finally, it must be emphasized that a well-functioning arteriovenous fistula is the best vascular access inducing the lowest number of complications.

7. Acknowledgement

Part of the work described in this paper was supported by the L & T Charitable Foundation & the House of INDOCAFE

8. References

Allon M: Prophylaxis against dialysis catheter-related bacteremia with a novel antimicrobial lock solution. *Clin Infect Dis* 2003; 36: 1539-1544.

Ash SR: Advances in tunneled central venous catheters for dialysis: design and performance. *Semin Dial* 2008; 21: 504-515.

Bagui A, Brook NR, Kaushik M, Nicholson ML. Tunnelled catheters for the hemodialysis patients. *Eur J Vasc Endovasc Surg* 2007; 33: 105-112.

Betjes M, Van Agteren M: Prevention of dialysis catheter-related sepsis with a citrate-taurolidine-containing lock solution. *Nephrol Dial Transplant* 2004;19:1546-1551.

Bleyer AJ, Mason L, Russell G, Raad II, Sherertz RJ: A randomized, controlled trial of a new vascular catheter flush solution (minocycline-EDTA) in temporary hemodialysis access. *Infect Control Hosp Epidemiol* 2005;26:520-524.

Can MR: Hemodialysis central venous catheter dysfunction. *Sem Dial* 2008; 21: 516-521.

Dogra GK, Herson H, Hutchison B, Irish AB, Heath CH, Golledge C, Luxton G, Moody H: Prevention of tunnelled hemodialysis catheter-related infections using catheter-restricted filling with gentamicin and citrate: a randomized controlled study. *J Am Soc Nephrol* 2002;13:2133-2139.

Faintuch S, Salazar GM: Malfunction of dialysis catheter: management of fibrin sheath and related problems. *Tech Vasc Interventional Rad* 2008; 11: 195-200.

Feldman HI, Kobrin S, Wasserstein A: Hemodialysis vascular access morbidity. *J Am Soc Nephrol* 1996; 7: 523-535.

Filiopoulos V, Hadjiyannakos D, Koutis I, Trompouki S, Micha T, Lazarou D, Vlassopoulos D: Approaches to prolong the use of uncuffed hemodialysis catheters: results of a randomized trial. *Am J Nephrol* 2011; 33: 260-268.

Fuchs S, Pollack A, Gilon D: Central venous catheter mechanical irritation of the right atrial free wall: a cause of thrombus formation. *Cardiology* 1999; 91: 169-172.

Goldberg JP, Contiguglia SR, Mishell JL, Klein MH: Intravenous streptokinase for thrombolysis of occluded arteriovenous access. *Arch Intern Med* 1985; 145: 1405-1408.

Hemmelgarn BR, Moist LM, Lock CE, Tonelli M, Manns BJ, Holden RM, LeBlanc M, Faris P, Barre P, Zhang J, Scott-Douglas N for the Prevention of Dialysis Catheter Lumen Occlusion with rt-PA versus Heparin (PreCLOT) Study Group: Prevention of dialysis catheter malfunction with recombinant tissue plasminogen activator. *New Engl J Med* 2011; 364: 303-312.

James MT, Manns BJ, Hemmelgarn BR, Ravani P: What's next after fistula first: Is an arteriovenous graft or central venous catheter preferable when an arteriovenous fistula is not possible? *Semin Dial* 2009; 22: 539-544.

Keenan SP: Use of ultrasound to place central lines. *J Crit Care* 2002; 17: 126-137.

Kim SH, Song KI, Chang JW, Kim SB, Sung SA, Jo SK, Cho WY, Kim HK: Prevention of uncuffed hemodialysis catheter-related bacteremia using an antibiotic lock technique: a prospective, randomized clinical trial. *Kidney Int* 2006;69:161-164.

Kovalik EC, Newman GE, Suhocki P, Knelson M, Schwab SJ: Correction of central venous stenosis: use of angioplasty and vascular wall stents. *Kidney Int* 1994; 45: 1177-1181.

Lacson E, Lazarus JM, Himmelgarb J, Ikizler TA, Hakim RM: Balancing fistula first with catheters last. *Am J Kidney Dis* 2007; 50: 379-395.

Leblanc M, Bosc JY, Paganini EP, Canaud B: Central venous dialysis catheter dysfunction. *Adv Ren Replace Ther* 1997; 4: 377-389.

Lin BS, Kong CW, Tarng DC, Huang TP, Tang GJ: Anatomical variation of the internal jugular vein and its impact on temporary haemodialysis vascular access: An ultrasonographic survey in uraemic patients. *Nephrol Dial Transplant* 1998; 13: 134-138.

Mathur MN, Storey DW, White GH, Ramsey-Stewart G: Percutaneous insertion of long-term venous access catheters via the external iliac vein. *Aust NZ J Surg* 1993; 63: 858-863.

Maya ID, Aldon M: Outcomes of tunnelled femoral hemodialysis catheter: Comparison with internal jugular vein catheters. *Kidney Int* 2005; 68: 2886-2889.

McDowell DE, Moss AH, Vasilakis C, Bell R, Pillai L: Percutaneously placed dual lumen silicone catheters for long-term hemodialysis. *Am Surg* 1993; 59: 569-573.

McIntyre CW, Hulme LJ, Taal M, Fluck RJ: Locking of tunnelled hemodialysis catheters with gentamicin and heparin. *Kidney Int* 2004;66:801-805.

Moist LM, Chang SH, Polkinghorne KR, McDonald SP, Australia and New Zealand Dialysis and Transplant Registry (ANZDATA): Trends in hemodialysis vascular access from the Australia and New Zealand Dialysis and Transplant Registry 2000-2005. *Am J Kidney Dis* 2007: 50: 612-621.

Moran JE, Ash SR for the ASDIN Clinical Practice Committee: Locking solutions for hemodialysis catheters: heparin and citrate: A position paper by ASDIN. *Semin Dial* 2008; 21: 490-492.

Morgan JE: Subcutaneous vascular access devices. *Semin Dial* 2001; 14: 452-457.

Murthy R, Arbabzadeh M, Lund G, Richard H, Levitin A, Stainken B: Percutaneous transrenal hemodialysis catheter insertion. *J Vasc Interv Radiol* 2002; 13: 1043-1046.

National Kidney Foundation: Clinical practice guidelines for vascular access: 2006 updated, *Am J Kidney Dis* 2006; 48 (suppl 1): S176-S285.

NKF-DOQI Clinical practice guidelines for vascular access: Updated 2000, *Am J Kidney Dis* 2001; 37 (suppl 1): S137-S181.

Nori US. Manoharan A, Yee J, Besarab A: Comparison of a low-dose gentamicin with minocycline as catheter lock solutions in the prevention of catheter-related bacteraemia. *Am J Kidney Dis* 2006;48:596-605.

Passerini L, Lam K, Costerton JW, King EG: Biofilms on indwelling vascular catheters. *Crit Care Med* 1992; 20: 665-673.

Pisoni RL, Young EW, Dykstra DM, Greenwold RN, Hecking E, Gillespie B, Wolfe RA, Goodkin DA, Held PJ: Vascular access use in Europe and the United States: results from the DOPPS. *Kidney Int* 2002; 61: 305-316

Power A, Singh S, Ashby D, Hamady M, Moser S, Gedroye W, Taube D, Duncan N, Carins T: Translumbar central venous catheters for long-term haemodialysis. *Nephrol Dial Transplant* 2009; 25: 1588-1595.

Quarello F, Forneris G, Borca M: Do central venous catheters have advantages over arteriovenous fistulas or grafts? *J Nephrol* 2006; 19: 265-279.

Quinn S, Schuman ES, Demlow TA, et al: Percutaneous transluminal angioplasty versus endovascular stent placement in the treatment of venous stenosis in patients undergoing haemodialysis: intermediate results. *J Vasc Interv Radiol* 1995; 6: 851-855.

Randolph AG, Cook DJ, Gonzales CA, Pribble CG: Ultrasound guidance for placement of central venous catheters: a meta-analysis of the literature. *Crit Care Med* 1996; 24: 2053-2058.

Rayner HC, Besarab A, Brown WW, Disney A, Saito A, Pisoni RL: Vascular access results from the "Dialysis Outcomes and Practice Patterns Study" (DOPPS): performance against "Kidney Disease Outcomes Quality Initiative (K/DOPQI) Clinical Practice Guidelines". *Am J Kidney Dis* 2004; 44: S 22-S26.

Rayner HC, Poisoni RL, Bommer J, et al: Mortality and hospitalization in haemodialysis patients in five European countries: results from the Dialysis Outcomes and Practice Pattern Study (DOPPS). *Nephrol Dial Transplant* 2004a; 19: 108-120.

Ross JR: Subcutaneous implantation of the LifeSite Hemodialysis Access System in the femoral vein. *J Vasc Access* 2001; 2: 91-96.

Saxena AK, Panhotra BR, Sundaram DS, Naguib M, Morsy F, Al-Ghamdi AM: Enhancing the survival of tunnelled hemodialysis catheters using an antibiotic lock in the elderly: a randomized, double-blind clinical trial. *Nephrology* 2006;11:299-305.

Smith TP, Ryan JM, Reddan DN: Transhepatic catheter access for hemodialysis. *Radiology* 2004; 232: 246-251.

Suhocki PV, Conion PJ, Knelson MH, Harland R, Schwab SJ; Silastic cuffed catheters for hemodialysis vascular access: thrombolytic and mechanical correction of malfunction. *Am J Kidney Dis* 1996; 28: 379-386.

Tonnessen BH, Money SR: Embracing the fistula first national vascular access improvement initiative. *J Vas Surg* 2005; 42: 585-586.

Trerotola SO, Johnson MS, Harris VJ, Shah H, Ambrosius WT, McKusky MA Kraus MA: Outcome of tunneled hemodialysis catheters placed via the right internal jugular vein by interventional radiologists. *Radiology* 1997; 203: 489-495.

Weijmer MC, Debets-Ossenkopp YJ, van der Vondervoort FJ, ter Wee PM: Randomized, clinical trial comparison of trisodium citrate 30% and heparin as catheter-locking solution in hemodialysis patients. *J Am Soc Nephrol* 2005;16:2769-2777.

Yap DH, Tso WK, Chu FS, Chan TM, Lai KN, Tang SC: Transhepatic placement of haemodialysis catheter: a solution for vascular access exhaustion. *Nephrology* 2010; 15: 661-662.

Zaleski GX, Funaki B, Lorenz JM, Garafalo RS, Moscatel MA, Rosenblum JD, Leef JA: Experience with tunneled femoral hemodialysis catheters. *Am J Roentgenol* 1999; 172: 493-496.

8

Complex Wounds in Patients Receiving Hemodialysis

Masaki Fujioka
Department of Plastic and Reconstructive Surgery, Clinical Research Center
National Hospital Organization Nagasaki Medical Center
Japan

1. Introduction

Patients receiving hemodialysis (HD) often have complex chronic wounds, which are hard to heal because of complications of other diseases, including DM, calciphylaxis, collagen disease, arteriosclerosis obliterans, chronic anemia, and weakness of the skin (Figures 1-3)[1-3]. Subsequent infection of necrotic skin tissue is associated with the risk of sepsis, which may be fatal if the blood access shunts become infected [4].

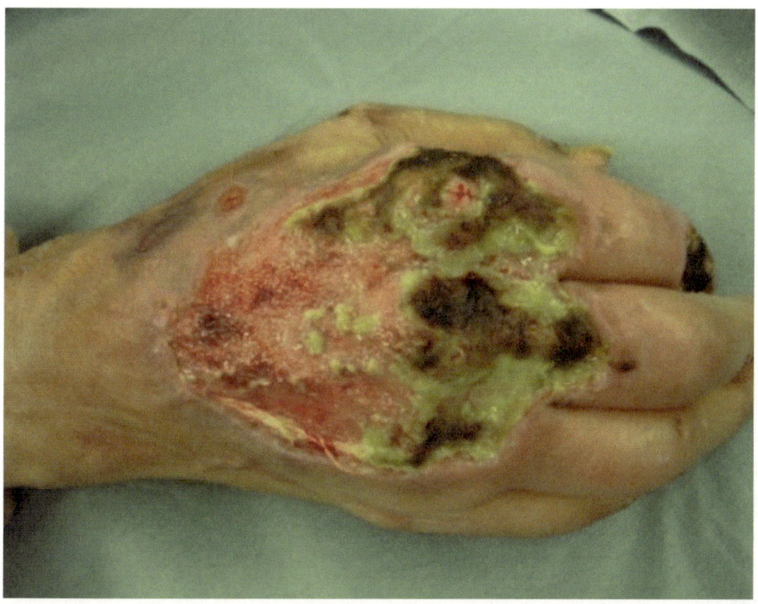

Fig. 1. (A) A 54-year-old woman was referred from an emergency unit for complex necrotic ulcer of the right hand with high fever. She had systemic lupus erythematosus and had been treated with 20 mg/ day of prednisolone for 40 years. She had received hemodialysis because of lupus nephritis for 34 years through a blood access shunt in the right elbow, which also showed inflammation. Debridement of the right hand was immediately performed.

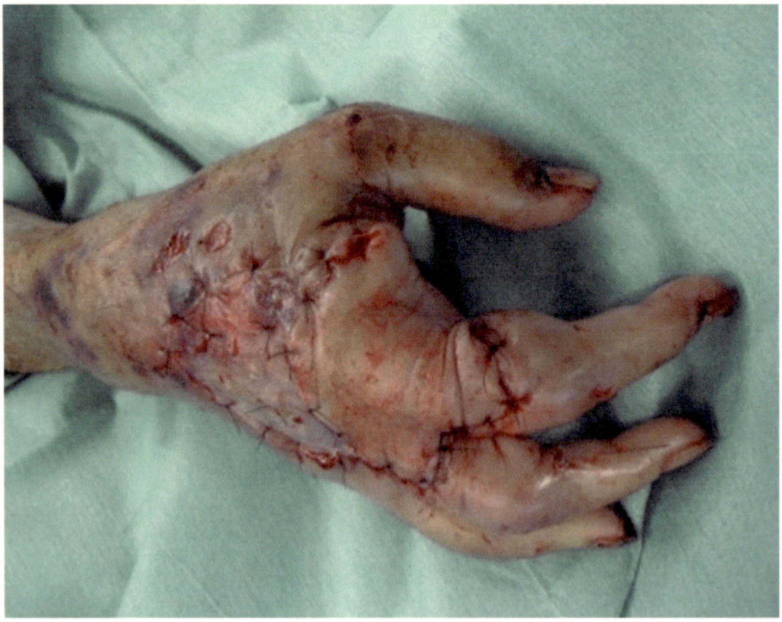

Fig. 1. (B) As the patient's wound improved over a period of 1 month, she underwent resurfacing surgery using local flap transfer and free skin grafting. The wound had completely resurfaced by 2 weeks after surgery.

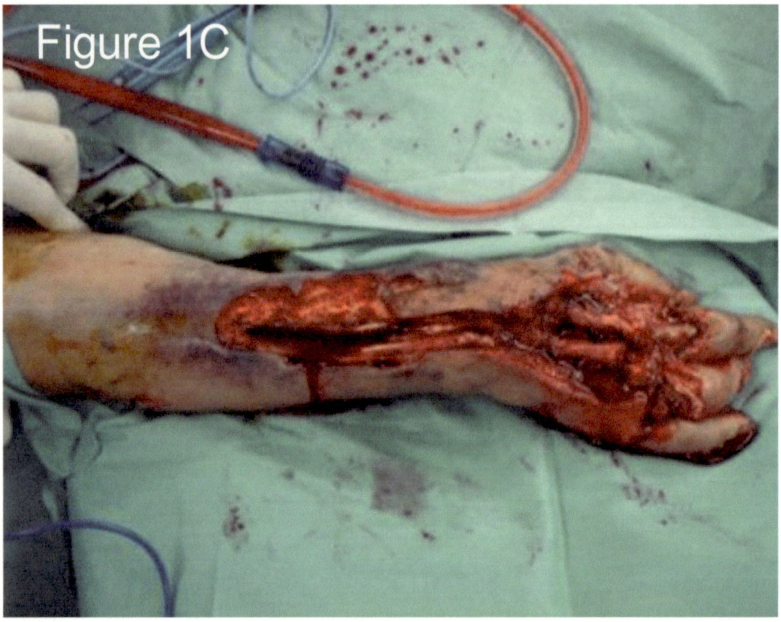

Fig. 1. (C) However, the wound aggravated and marked erythema expanded rapidly to the upper arm over the course of one day, which required immediate amputation of the infected hand at the forearm.

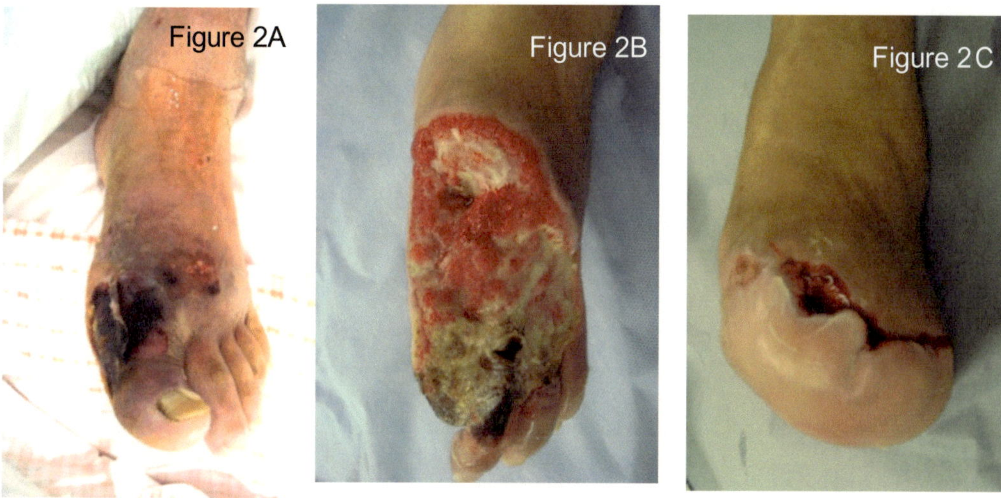

Fig. 2. (A) A 56-year-old man was referred from an emergency unit for a complex necrotic ulcer caused by a burn to the left foot with high fever. He had received hemodialysis because of diabetes mellitus for 4 years through a blood access shunt in the right elbow, which also showed inflammation. Amputation of the left big and 2nd toes was immediately performed. (B) As soft tissue necrosis progressed after debridement, and osteomyelitis occurred 1 month later, he underwent further amputation. (C) The wound improved over a period of 1 month with favorable granulation.

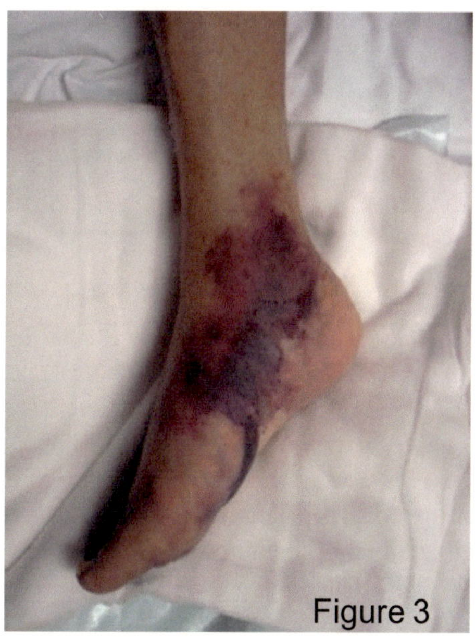

Fig. 3. A 65-year-old man was referred from an emergency unit for severe pain and a complex necrotic ulcer of the bilateral feet. He had arteriosclerosis obliterans, and had received hemodialysis because of chronic glomerulonephritis for 34 years. Right below-knee amputation was performed.

The number of patients requiring HD because of obesity-related renal diseases such as diabetes mellitus is increasing [5, 6]. This article focuses on the prevalence of complex wounds among patients with chronic renal failure (CRF) undergoing hemodialysis, and shows effective and successive treatments of these wounds.
We report our 6-year experience involving 30 patients receiving HD who had chronic skin ulcers. In addition, we investigated the differences in characteristics between patients receiving HD because of DM and those receiving HD due to other diseases.

2. How do complex wounds develop in patients receiving hemodialysis?

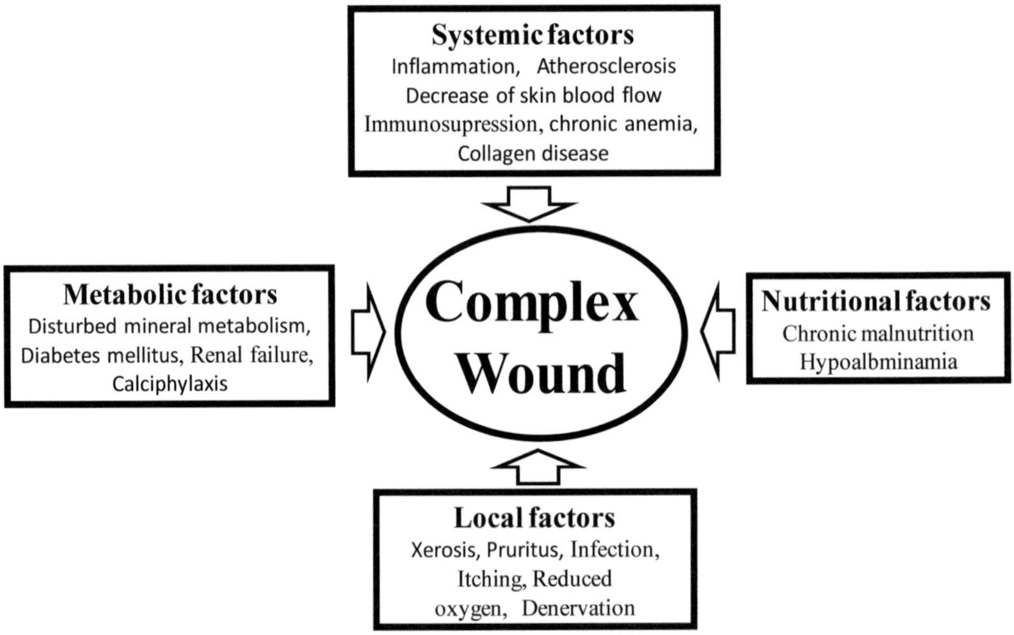

Fig. 4. Factors of complex wound development in patients receiving hemodialysis

Chronic renal failure affects practically all the systems of the body, causing neurological, gastrointestinal, cardiovascular, pulmonary, hematological, endocrine-metabolic, and dermatological disorders [7]. Among them, cutaneous disorders are one of the common problems in patients on long-term hemodialysis, which may not be only due to renal dysfunction, but may also be due to complications resulting from treatment. The commonest skin disorders are xerosis and pruritus [8, 9]. Recent epidemiological studies have demonstrated that the prevalence of pruritus among patients who are adequately dialyzed remains high, ranging between 42 and 75%[10-12]. Uremic pruritus is very frustrating for patients since no effective treatment for relief of the itching has been demonstrated. The pathophysiological mechanisms of pruritus are mainly unknown, despite several hypotheses being presented [13].
Furthermore, the skin of patients on hemodialysis is dry, and so the skin barrier structure and function are impaired [14]. The Observational Dialysis Outcomes and Practise Patterns

Study, collecting data from more than 29,000 HD patients, showed that 42% of HD patients experience moderate to extreme itching [15]. The impaired skin resistance and stimuli caused by scrunching because of itchy skin cause continuous inflammations, which contribute to local skin ulcers and the general development of malnutrition and cardiovascular disease [16]. In addition, disturbed mineral metabolism is associated with skin complaints in dialysis patients[17]. Other cutaneous manifestations include scaling (9.9%), pressure ulcer (2 .0%), and dermatitis (2%) [18, 19].

Regarding cutaneous infection, Bencini *et al.* reported that the incidence of fungal infection in patients undergoing hemodialysis was 67% [20]. CRF patients exhibit impaired cellular immunity due to a decreased T-lymphocyte cell count; this could explain the increased prevalence of fungal infections [21]. Other cutaneous infections include bacterial (13%) and viral (12%) infections, reportedly common in diabetics [9]. Difficulty healing wounds is a frequent problem in patients on HD because of their poor general conditions, including malnutrition, inflammation, and atherosclerosis syndrome [1]. Stein and Wiersum, in a retrospective analysis of 22,389 laparotomies, concluded that dysfunction played a significant role in the development and outcome of abdominal wound dehiscence [2]. Not only abdominal surgical wounds, but also all surgical sites sometimes develop poor wound adhesion causing a complex ulcer (Figure 5). Mistrík et al. reported at significant decrease in skin blood flow during the HD procedure and concluded that the skin blood flow may be impaired in HD patients, which leads to the development of difficulty in healing skin wounds [3]. Consequently, patients with end-stage renal disease were associated with higher resource use, complication rates, and mortality when they were injured [22].

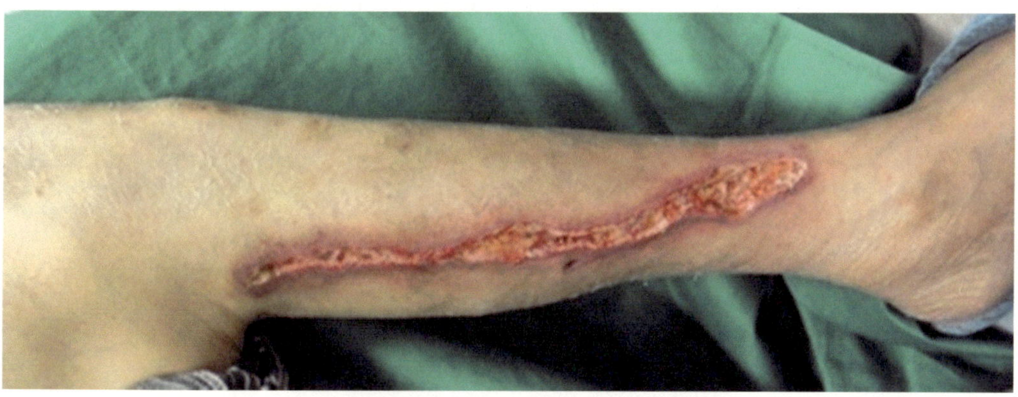

Fig. 5. Development of a complex leg ulcer because of wound dehiscence, following great saphenous vein harvest for vein grafting.

3. Profiles and clinical status of HD-receiving patients who develop extremity ulcers because of diabetes mellitus or other diseases

Thirty patients receiving HD who had chronic wounds of the limbs underwent surgical treatment in our unit from 2004 through 2010. The ages ranged from 52 to 89 years (mean, 66.5 years).

3.1 Causative disease in patients receiving HD

Patients receiving HD because of DM (57%) ranged in age from 53 to 74 years (mean, 62.4 ± 7.9 years), and patients receiving HD because of other diseases, including chronic glomerular nephritis (CGN), polycystic kidney, and systemic lupus erythematosus (43%), ranged in age from 52 to 69 years (mean, 61.3 ± 6.0 years) (no significant difference, Wilcoxon rank sum test). All diabetic patients were classified with type 2 diabetes mellitus. Serous calcium level of diabetic patients ranged from 7.1 to 9.3 mg/dl (mean, 8.5 ± 0.7 mg/dl), and that of non-diabetic patients ranged from 8.9 to 10.2 mg/dl (mean, 9.6 ± 0.5 mg/dl). There was no significant difference between the groups ($p=0.5$, Wilcoxon rank sum test). Inorganic phosphate levels of diabetic patients ranged from 2.4 to 4.2 mg/dl (mean, 3.7 ± 0.6 mg/dl), and that of non-diabetic patients ranged from 2.8 to 4.6 mg/dl (mean, 3.2 ± 0.8 mg/dl). There was no significant difference between the groups ($p=0.4$, Wilcoxon rank sum test).

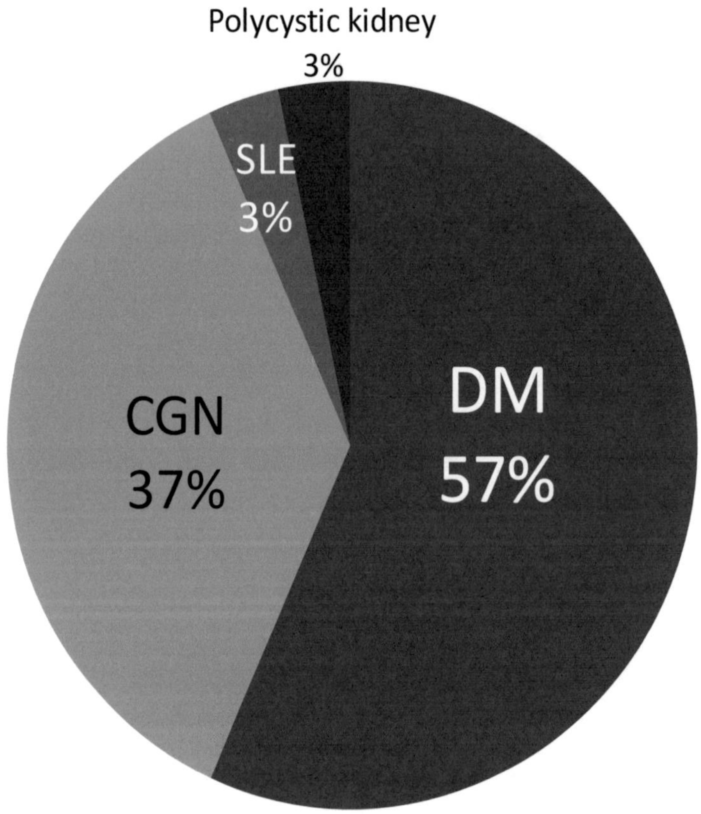

Fig. 6. Causative disease in patients receiving HD (N=30)

We investigated differences in the cause of wounds, size of wounds, need for immediate debridement, and interval between the start of HD and wound development, between patients with chronic renal failure due to DM and that due to other diseases (Tables 1, 2). All information was obtained from patients' medical records, examinations, and an interview at the first examination.

Patient number	Sex	Age	Causative disease	Wound diagnosis	Site of wound	Cause of wound	Wound size (cm)	Surgery	Infection and culture	Immediate debridement	HD duration (years)	Complication
1	M	53	DM	Ischemic skin necrosis	Rt. step	Ischemia	7×5	Amputation	MRSA	-	8	HT, ASO, Sepsis
2	F	68	DM	Ischemic skin necrosis	Rt. step	Ischemia	2×2	FSG	-	-	4	HT,ASO
3	M	56	DM	Burn	Lt. leg	Trauma	5×3	Amputation	MRSA	+	4	Angina, Sepsis
4	M	58	DM	Burn	Lt. shoulder	Trauma	28×25	FSG	MRSA	+	2	Mental disorder, Sepsis
5	F	70	DM	Necrotizing fasciitis	Lt. heel	Infection	11×5	FSG	MRSA	+	1	HT
6	F	55	DM	Osteomyelitis	Rt. finger	Infection	2×2	Amputation	MRSA	+	2	Sepsis
7	M	65	DM	Necrotizing fasciitis	Rt. leg	Infection	15×5	FSG	MRSA	+	1	HT
8	F	74	DM	Gangrene	Rt. thigh	Infection	5×3	FSG	MRSA	+	4	HT
9	F	75	DM	Ischemic skin necrosis	Rt. toe	Ischemia	2×2	Amputation	*Proteus mirabilis*	+	4	Cerebral infarction, HCV
10	F	68	DM	Chronic skin ulcer	Bil.toe	Trauma	2×2	FSG	-	+	4	
11	F	66	DM	Gangrene	Rt. leg	Infection	20×15	Amputation	*Streptococcus agalactiae*	+	1 month	Old MI, Heart failure, Sepsis
12	M	64	DM	Ischemic skin necrosis	Rt. finger	Ischemia	2×2	Amputation	-	-	4	
13	F	69	DM	Ischemic skin necrosis	Lt. toe	Ischemia	2×2	Amputation	-	-	6 months	ASO
14	M	68	DM	Chronic skin ulcer	Lt. toe	Trauma	2×2	Amputation	MRSA	-	5	Sepsis
15	F	52	DM	Chronic skin ulcer	Lt. toe	Trauma	30×15	FSG	MSSA	+	2	Mental disorder
16	M	75	DM	Pressure ulcer	Rt. leg	Trauma	10×7	Amputation	-	+	6	Sepsis
17	M	65	DM	Necrotizing fasciitis	scrotum	Infection	10×5	FSG	MRSA	+	4	

DM, diabetes mellitus. CGN, chronic glomerulonephritis. FSG, free skin grafting. SLE, systemic lupus erythematosus. MRSA, methicillin-resistant Staphylococcus aureus. HT, hypertension. ASO, arteriosclerosis obliterans

Table 1. Profiles and clinical status of patients undergoing HD with extremity ulcers due to diabetes mellitus.

Patient number	Sex	Age	Causative disease	Wound diagnosis	Site of wound	Cause of wound	Wound size (cm)	Surgery	Infection and culture	Immediate debridement	HD duration (years)	Complication
1	F	69	CGN	Skin necrosis	Rt. leg	Trauma	5 × 4	FSG	*Streptococcus constellatus*	-	4	Peritonitis
2	F	58	CGN	Postoperative skin necrosis	Rt. leg	Trauma	3 × 2	FSG	-	-	16	HT, Achilles' tendon rupture
3	F	62	CGN	Postoperative skin necrosis	Lt. thigh	Trauma	2 × 2	suturing	-	-	2	HT, hypothyroidism
4	M	65	CGN	Ischemic necrosis	Both legs	Ischemia	13 × 5	Amputation	MRSA	-	14	HT, ASO, Sepsis
5	M	65	Polycystic kidney	Ischemic skin necrosis	Rt. toe	Ischemia	3 × 2	Amputation	-	-	9	HT, ASO
6	F	52	SLE	Laceration	Lt. hand	Trauma	5 × 4	Amputation	MRSA	+	32	Chronic hepatitis, Sepsis, Steroid
7	M	67	CGN	Osteomyelitis	Lt. toe	Infection	2 × 2	Amputation	MRSA	-	9	Sepsis
8	M	89	CGN	Osteomyelitis	Lt. ankle	Infection	2 × 1.5	Debridement	MRSA	-	5	
9	F	70	CGN	Skin Ulcer	Lt. leg	Infection	8 × 5	Debridement	MRSA	-	4	Heart failure, HT
10	M	54	CGN	Skin necrosis	Rt. toe	Ischemia	2 × 1	Amputation	MRSA	-	26	Cerebral infarction
11	M	57	CGN	Pressure ulcer	Rt. hip	Ischemia	3 × 2	ischiectomy	MRSA	-	4	HT, Aortic dissection
12	F	86	CGN	Pressure ulcer	Lt .heel	Trauma	3 × 3	Flap	MRSA	-	2	Lip skin cancer, HT
13	F	70	CGN	Skin necrosis (hematoma)	Rt. step	Trauma	5 × 4	FSG	-	-	43	

DM, diabetes mellitus. CGN, chronic glomerulonephritis. FSG, free skin grafting. SLE, systemic lupus erythematosus.
MRSA, methicillin-resistant Staphylococcusa complex HT, hypertension. ASO, arteriosclerosis obliterans

Table 2. Profiles and clinical status of patients undergoing HD with extremity ulcers due to diseases other than diabetes mellitus.

3.2 Cause of wounds in patients with CRF due to DM or other diseases

Wounds in patients with CRF due to DM were caused by trauma (burns and pressure ulcers) in 6 cases (35.3%), infection in 6 cases (35.3%), and ischemia in 5 cases (29.4%). Wounds in patients with CRF due to other diseases were associated with trauma in 6 cases (46.5%), infection in 3 cases (23.2%), and ischemia in 4 cases (30.3%) (Figure 7).

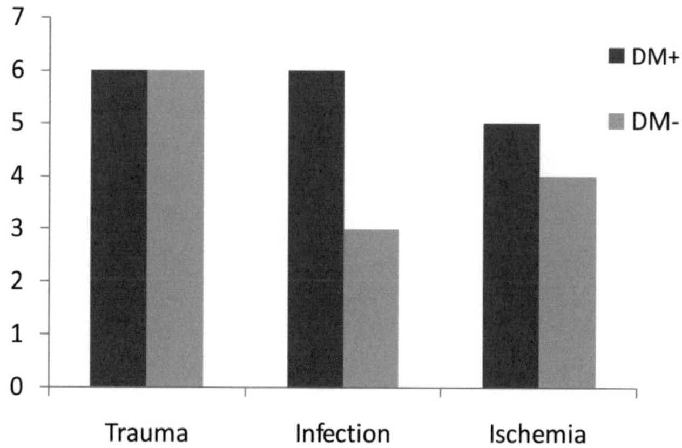

Fig. 7. Cause of wounds in patients with CRF due to DM or other diseases.

3.3 Differences in wound size in CRF caused by DM and other diseases

The size of wounds in patients with DM ranged in area from 4 to 450 cm^2 (mean, 69.5 ± 120.8 cm^2), and that in patients without DM ranged from 3 to 65 cm^2 (mean, 617.8 ± 18.9 cm^2) (no significant difference, Wilcoxon rank sum test) (Figure 8).

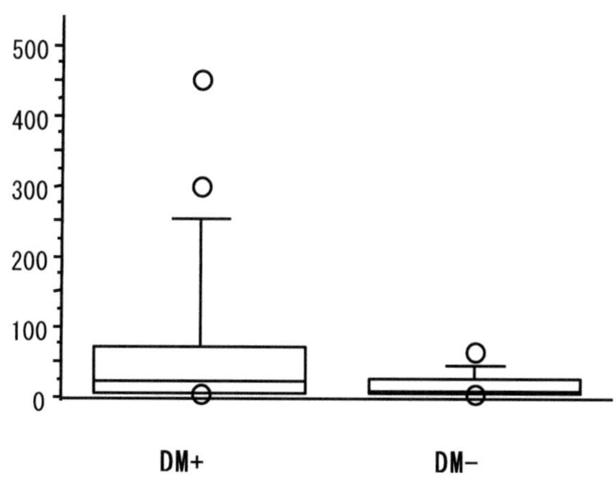

Fig. 8. Differences in size of wounds in CRF due to DM and other diseases.

3.4 Bacterial infection in patients receiving HD

Wound infection is common and difficult to control, because cutaneous surfaces are without protective barriers, through which patients receiving HD may easily acquire bacterial infection. Our study revealed that bacilli were cultured from 12 of 17 (70.6%) wounds in patients with DM. and 9 of 13 (69.2%) without DM. There was no significant difference in the frequency of bacterial isolation between the two groups (chi-square test). Concerning to the seriousness of infection, 13 of 17 wounds required immediate surgery including amputation and debridement in patients with DM, while, only 1 of 13 required immediate surgery in patients without DM. There was a significant difference between the groups ($p<0.05$, Chi-square test) (Figure 9). These results suggest that patients receiving HD because of diabetes are likely to develop more severe wound infections.

Methicillin-resistant *Staphylococcus aureus* (MRAS) was commonly isolated from these contaminated wounds, being isolated from 9 of 12 (75.0%) in the DM group, and 8 of 9 (88.9%) in the non-DM group.

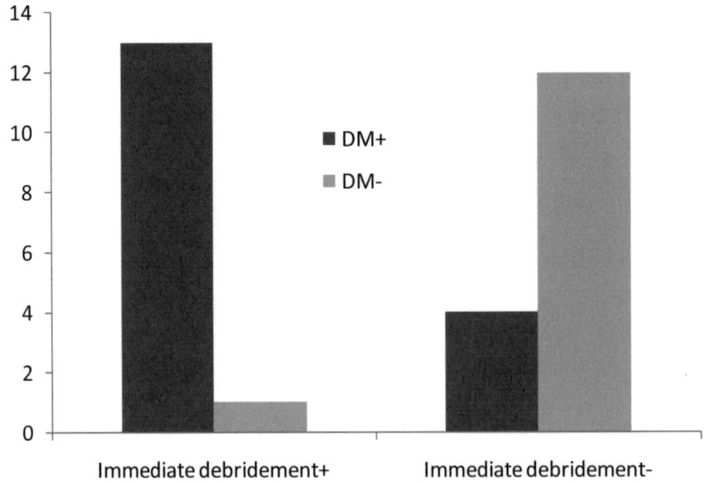

Fig. 9. Need of immediate debridement in patients with CRF due to DM or other diseases.

3.5 Interval between the start of HD and wound development

The interval between the start of HD and wound development in patients with DM ranged from 1 month to 8 years (mean, 3.2 ± 2.1 years), and that in patients without DM ranged from 2 to 43 years (mean, 12.4± 12.7 years). It was significantly shorter in patients with than in those without diabetes. ($p=0.017$, Wilcoxon rank sum test) (Figure 10).

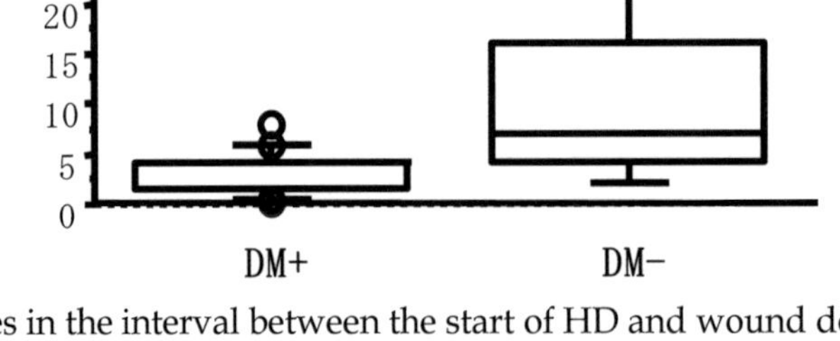

Fig. 10. Differences in the interval between the start of HD and wound development in CRF due to DM and other diseases.

4. Treatments of complex wounds in patients receiving HD

4.1 Immediate debridement and amputation aiming at infection control

Extremity ulcers in patients receiving HD are often difficult to heal. Nonetheless, patients with severely ischemic limbs due to maintenance HD are markedly increasing in number [1,2]. They often require multiple surgeries because arteriosclerosis obliterans usually progresses, which causes other ischemic ulcers (Figures 2, 11, 12).

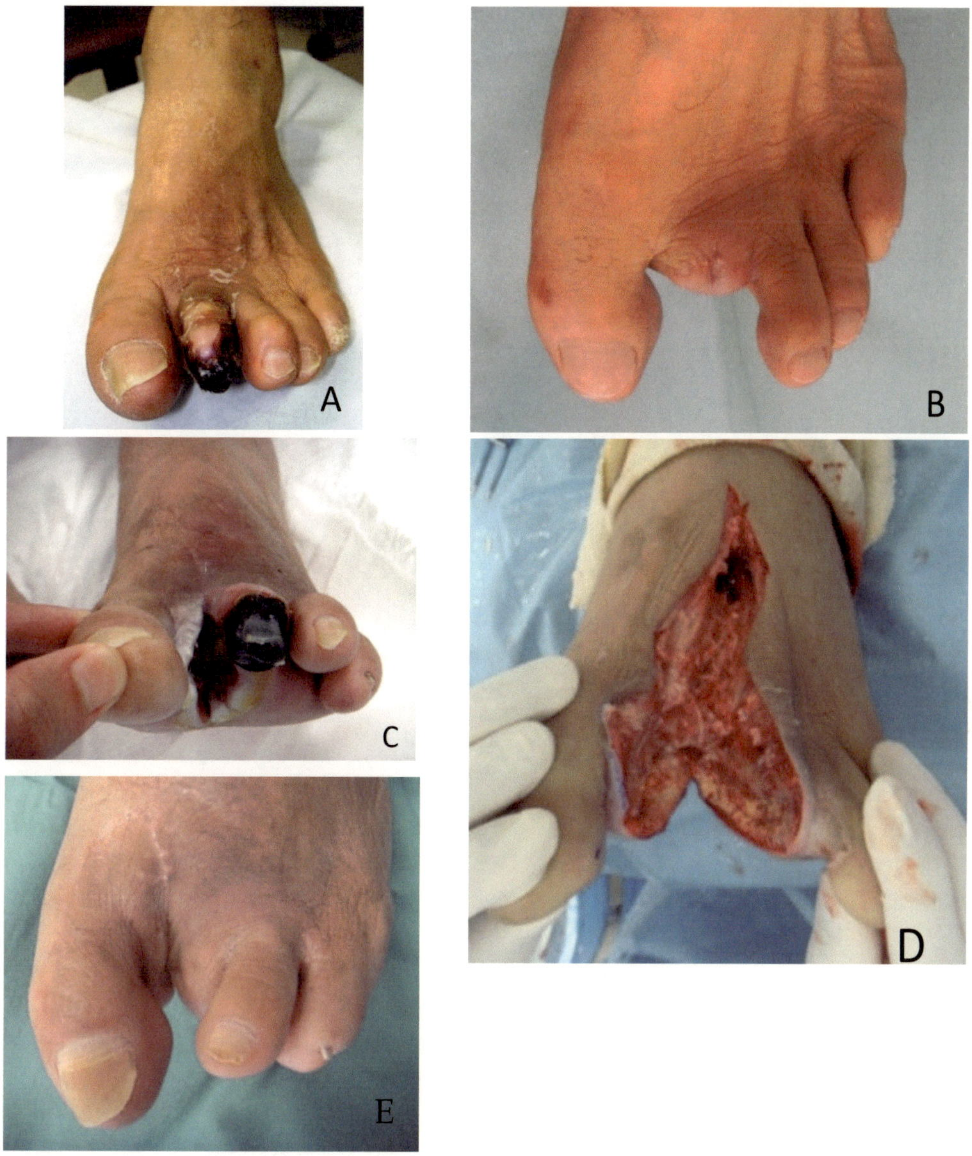

Fig. 11. (A) A patient with an ischemic foot due to maintenance HD developed necrosis of the left 2nd toe. (B) The ulcer was resolved by amputation. (C) However, he developed another site of necrosis with infection (arrow) on the third toe. (D) The patient underwent immediate debridement and osteotomy. (E)The wounds healed satisfactorily.

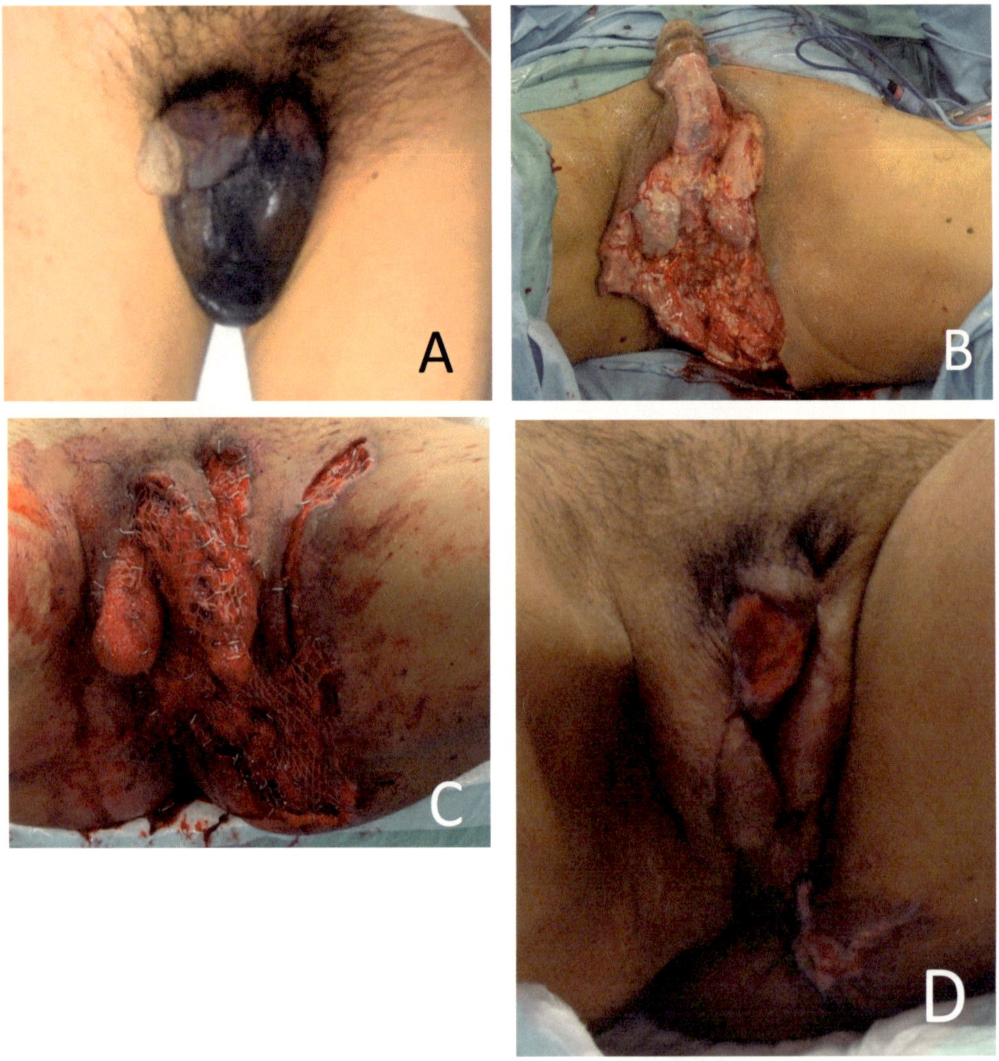

Fig. 12. (A) A case of Fournier's gangrene. A patient receiving HD due to DM developed progressive infection and necrosis of the scrotum and penis. (B) He underwent immediate debridement. (C)The wound was resurfaced with a mesh graft 2 weeks later. (D) However, necrosis of the penis progressed, and so the patient underwent amputation of the penis

Amputations of limbs or fingers are sometimes performed for these complex ulcers, because patients receiving HD are thought to present with immunocompromised conditions, and aggressive life-threatening infections such as sepsis require immediate surgical debridement in order to salvage the blood access line and their life (Figure 13). Only administrating antibiotics for the contaminated wound containing necrotic tissue is of no use and worsens the condition of patients, because antibiotic agents cannot reach the non-vascularized and infected necrotic mass. Immediate surgical debridement is the only recommended way to resolve these soft tissue infections (Figure 14) [23, 24]. Surgical amputation is sometimes the only way to resurface these wounds, especially for some ischemic necrotic wounds including total finger or foot dry necrosis. In our study, 14 patients underwent finger or limb amputation, with 9 due to complicated sepsis and 5 due to dry necrosis associated with arteriosclerosis obliterans.

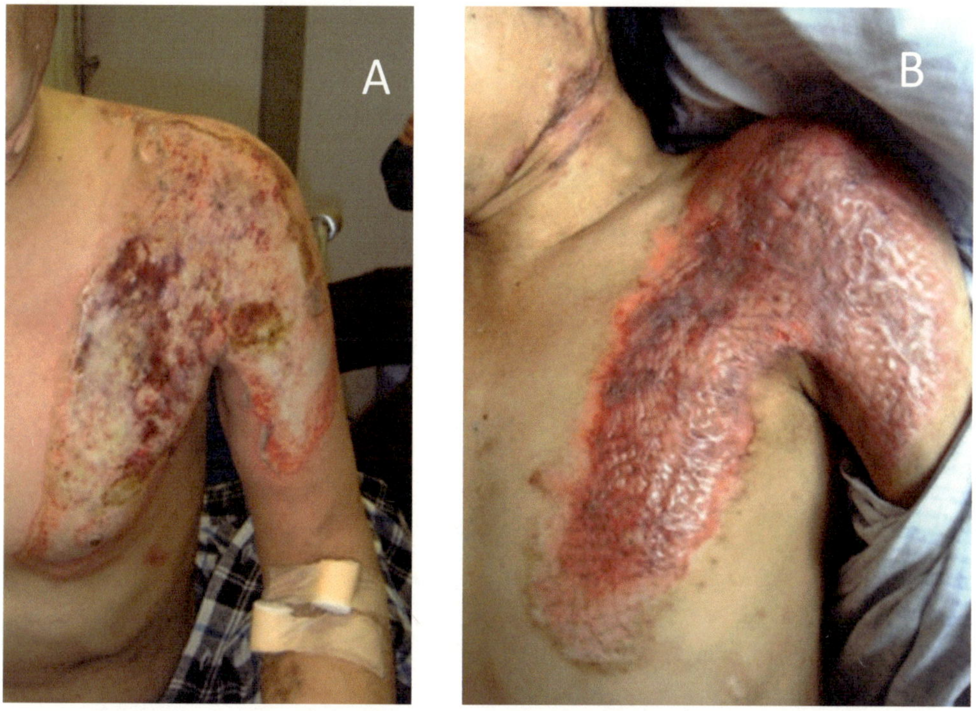

Fig. 13. (A) A 63-year-old man who suffered a burn visited our medical center 4 days after injury. He had received hemodialysis because of diabetes mellitus for 2 years. The blood access shunt in the left elbow, shown in the picture. On the first examination, the burn wound was covered with necrotic eschar with infection, and the patient showed burn wound sepsis with high fever. Debridement and free skin grafting were immediately performed. (B) The burn wound had resurfaced 3 weeks after surgery.

It is commonly believed that the development of ischemic limb ulcers in patients with CRF is influenced by underlying advanced diabetic microangiopathy [25]. Although we have investigated severe extremity ulcers requiring surgical treatment, the present study indicates that the development of ulcers in patients with DM is not only associated with ischemia but is also strongly influenced by infection, because 11 of 13 patients with DM had infectious conditions such as gangrene, osteomyelitis, necrotizing fasciitis, and/ or sepsis. On the other hand, the development of ulcers in patients without DM was mainly due to ischemia and trauma. Only 2 patients developed MRSA sepsis originating from secondary wound infection, and they underwent amputation.

The interval from the start of HD to wound development in patients with was significantly shorter than that in those without DM. Generally, ulcers in patients with CRF and DM are thought to develop because of peripheral neuropathy, which reduces protective sensations [26]. In addition, several investigators have reported incidences of peripheral arterial occlusive disease in patients receiving HD ranging from 2.5 to 19.0% [27, 28]. Because of these neurovascular disorders, extremity ulcers develop more easily in patients with DM than in those with other diseases.

These infectious wounds often result in higher mortality rates because blood access shunts, especially when an artificial vessel is grafted, are easily infected. Bacteria from the wounds usually diffuse proximally along the subcutaneous flow of lymph or blood and can cause shunt infections, which lead to the loss of blood access channels and life-threatening sepsis. All our patients with infectious wounds (14 cases) required immediate debridement, including amputation to prevent such unfavorable general infections, because aggressive local inflammatory reactions had already developed (Figure 14). Thirteen of these patients had DM.

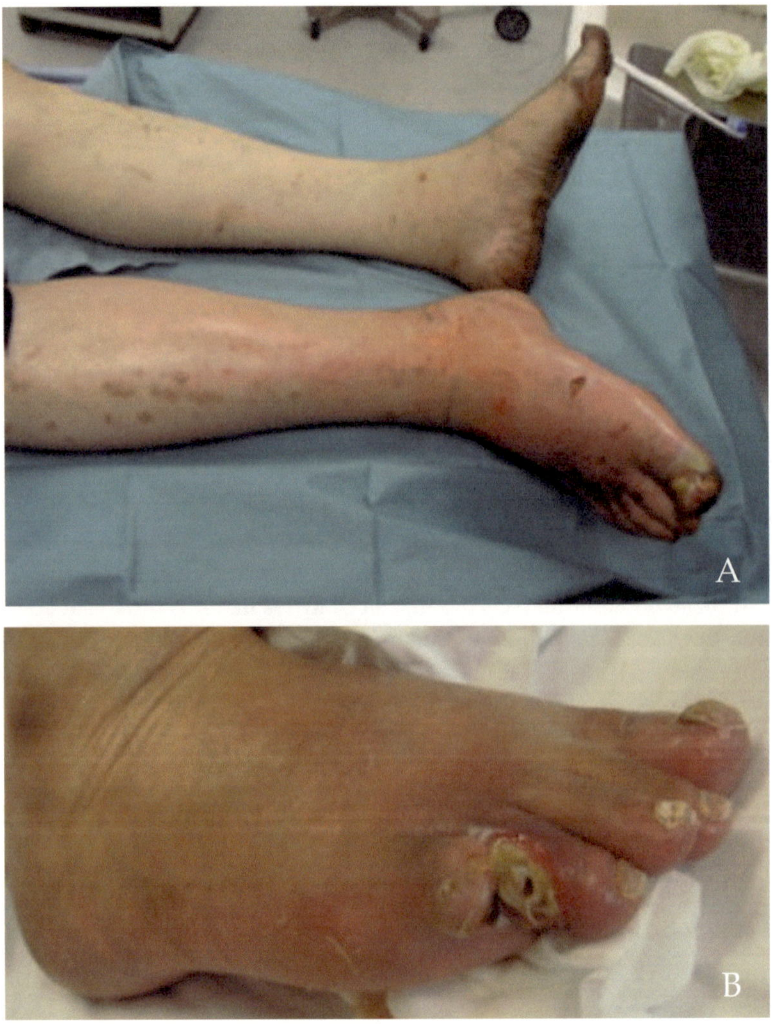

Fig. 14. (A) A 65-year-old man developed necrotizing fasciitis of the right leg, with pain and high fever. He had received hemodialysis because of diabetes mellitus for 1 year. The blood access shunt in the right elbow showed inflammation. Below-knee amputation was immediately performed. (B) A 52-year-old man developed a complex necrotic ulcer on the right foot with a high fever. He had received hemodialysis because of diabetes mellitus for 2 years. His blood access shunt in the left elbow also showed inflammation. Amputation of the fifth toe was immediately performed.

MRSA was isolated from almost all chronic wounds in patients with DM, which also suggested that HD-receiving patients with DM tend to bear multi-drug-resistant organisms, and, thus, strict infection control is required to prevent outbreaks.

The control of infection after aggressive debridement is the most important point to heal the wound and prevent the recurrence of infection. When initial debridement is insufficient and local infection recurs, further debridement is required. Wound infection cannot be controlled in the presence of necrotic tissue. If a patient shows relapsed wound infection without necrosis and foreign bodies remaining in the wound, cleansing the wound using continuous irrigation employing suction and irrigation system is recommended. This was also adapted for the treatment of osteomyelitis (Figure 15) [29]. It is concluded that when a risk of recurring an infection remains after primary debridement, two-stage management, involving late second stage surgery included secondary debridement and stable reconstruction, should be considered.[30]

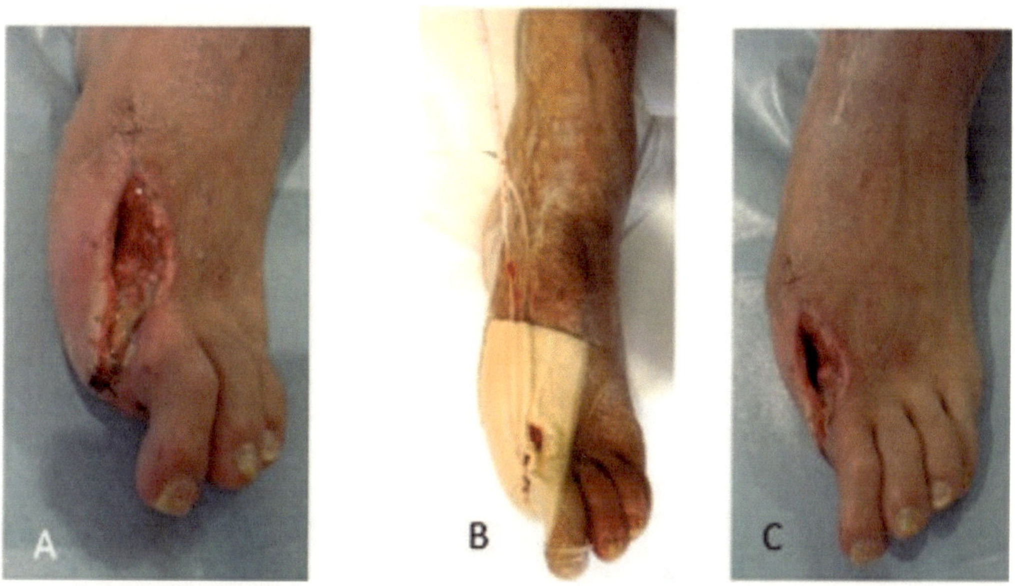

Fig. 15. (A) A patient receiving HD because of DM for 3 years developed osteomyelitis of the left big toe, and underwent debridement and wound closure. However, the soft tissue infection relapsed 5 days later. (B) He underwent secondary debridement and continuous irrigation, using a suction and irrigation system. (C) Three weeks later, the wound was covered with abundant granulation tissue with no infection. The wound closed spontaneously.

5. Wound bed preparation for patients receiving HD

After the debridement of necrotic tissue, the wound bed needs to be prepared to receive either a graft or flap. [31] The resurfacing of wounds is one of the most important procedures, because such wounds will cause further infection, exudates, odors, and bleeding, which decrease the patient's quality of life. Chronic ulcers may sometimes prevent the patient from living at home. [32] Wound bed preparation has allowed uncomplicated wounds to heal quickly. [23, 33-37] The management of chronic wounds has progressed from assessing the status of a wound to understanding the underlying molecular and cellular abnormalities that prevent the wound from healing. The concept of wound bed preparation offers a systematic approach to remove barriers to healing such as tissue (non-viable), infection/inflammation, moisture (imbalance), and edge (non-advancing or undermining) and enhancing the effects of advanced therapies. [35, 36] Wound bed preparation is an essential element of wound management that advances endogenous healing as well as the efficacy of topical and other wound therapy.[38] Wound bed preparation techniques will allow complex wounds to grow abundant granulation tissue. When a wound is covered with suitable granulation and no contamination is observed, free skin grafting should be performed as soon as possible (Figure 16). In cases of bone- or tendon-exposed wounds, some flaps are required to resurface the wounds, because grafted skin will not take directly on tendon or bone (Figure 17).

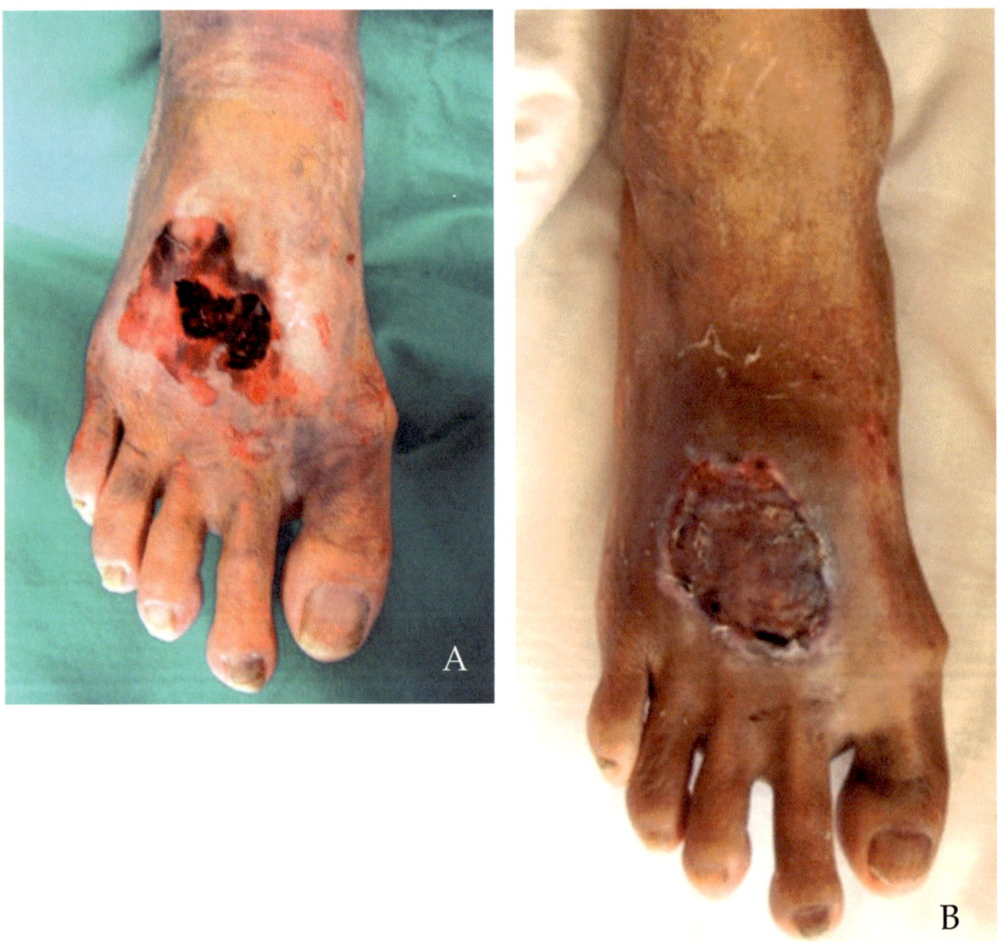

Fig. 16. (A) A 86-year-old female suffered a hematoma due to falling on a step. She had received hemodialysis because of chronic glomerulonephritis for 43 years. (B) Three weeks after the treatment of the wound bed, abundant granulation tissue was observed. She underwent a free skin graft, and the wound resurfaced favorably.

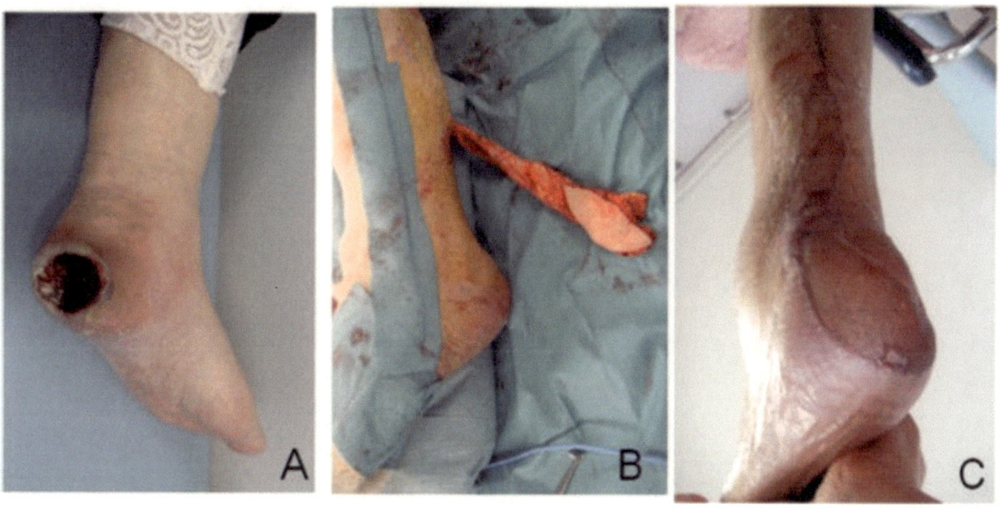

Fig. 17. (A) An 86-year-old female suffered from a bone-exposed wound due to a pressure ulcer on the heel. She had received hemodialysis because of chronic glomerulonephritis for 2 years. (B) She underwent reversed sural flap surgery. (C) The wound was completely resurfaced. She regained the ability to walk.

6. Several adjuvant and devices in the management of hard-to-heal wounds

In this section, several adjuvant and devices are presented, including growth factor, bioengineered tissues, and a negative pressure system, which are combined for the improved clinical treatment of complex wounds. [24]

Firstly, several growth factors have been used clinically to prepare favorable wound beds. Of these growth factors, basic fibroblast growth factor (bFGF) is the only angiogenic cytokine currently available in Japan.[39] Treatment with bFGF allows chronic ulcers to heal more quickly (Figure 18). [40] Secondly, artificial dermis, which is composed of atelocollagen sponge and a silicone membrane, is beneficial for these wounds because of its unique characteristics (Figure 19). Atelocollagen sponge allows the early infiltration of mononuclear cells and fibroblasts, leading to the rapid resolution of inflammatory reactions and more favorable growth of granulation tissue. On the other hand, the silicone membrane protects against a loss of fluid, protein, and electrolytes, which helps maintain a suitable environment for wound healing. [41, 42] Formerly, resurfacing tendon- or bone-exposed wounds required vascularized flaps, showing high morbidity at the donor site, skilful micro- or plastic surgeons, microsurgical instruments, and much time, because a free skin graft would not take on unfavorable wound beds, such as in the presence of infected granulation and low-vascular tissues. [41] Artificial dermis is beneficial for the reconstruction of these wounds because it promotes the early infiltration of mononuclear cells and fibroblasts and better growth of connective tissue strands and epithelium. [41-43]

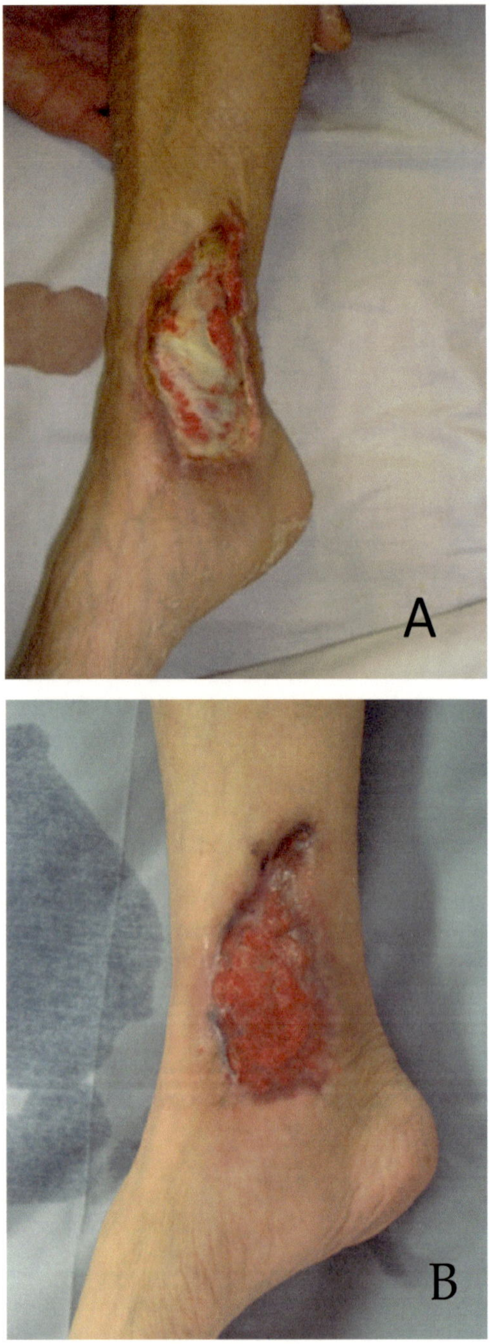

Fig. 18. (A) A 63-year-old female suffered from a tendon-exposed wound due to instillation into the subcutaneous tissue of the ankle. She had received hemodialysis because of chronic glomerulonephritis for 4 years. (B) Three weeks after wound bed preparation with basic fibroblast growth factor. Abundant granulation tissue suitable for free skin grafting was observed. The wound completely resurfaced after skin grafting.

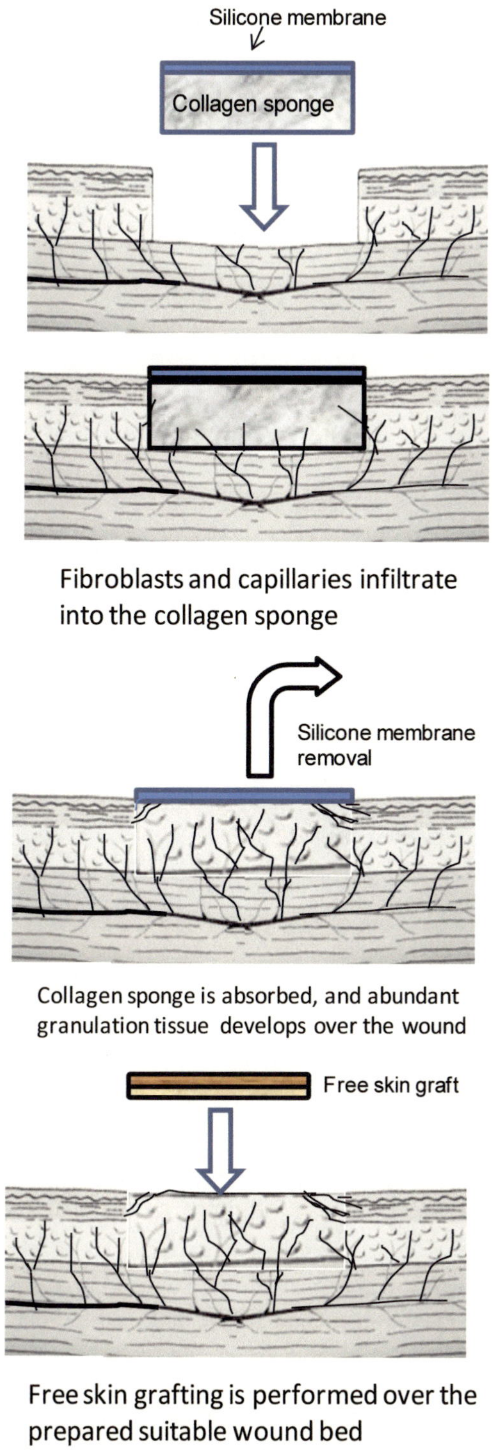

Fig. 19. Treatment of a full-thickness skin defect ulcer using artificial dermis.

Marks reported that dermal wounds treated with collagen sponge seeded with fibroblasts or coated with bFGF show an increased level of reepithelialization, indicating that this method facilitates early dermal and epidermal wound healing. [44 45] Consequently, this method improves complex wounds and quickly prepares a favorable wound bed (Figures 20, 21).

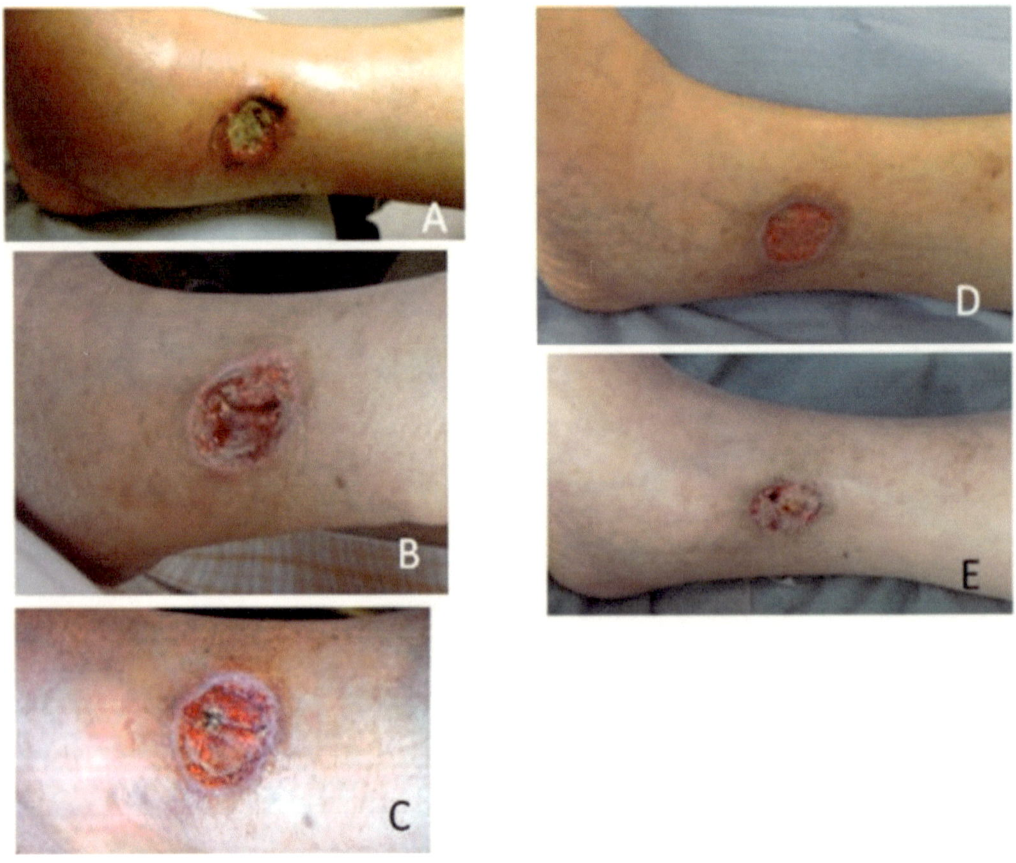

Fig. 20. (A) The photograph shows an unsatisfactory wound bed in a patient receiving HD because of DM at the initial examination. (B) A favorable wound bed did not develop, although cleansing and wet-to-dry dressing were continued for 2 weeks after debridement. (C) The wound became clean and a wound bed had developed 2 weeks after the start of combination treatment using bFGF and artificial dermis. (D) A favorable wound bed was prepared after 3 weeks of combination treatment. (E) The resurfaced wound 2 weeks after skin grafting.

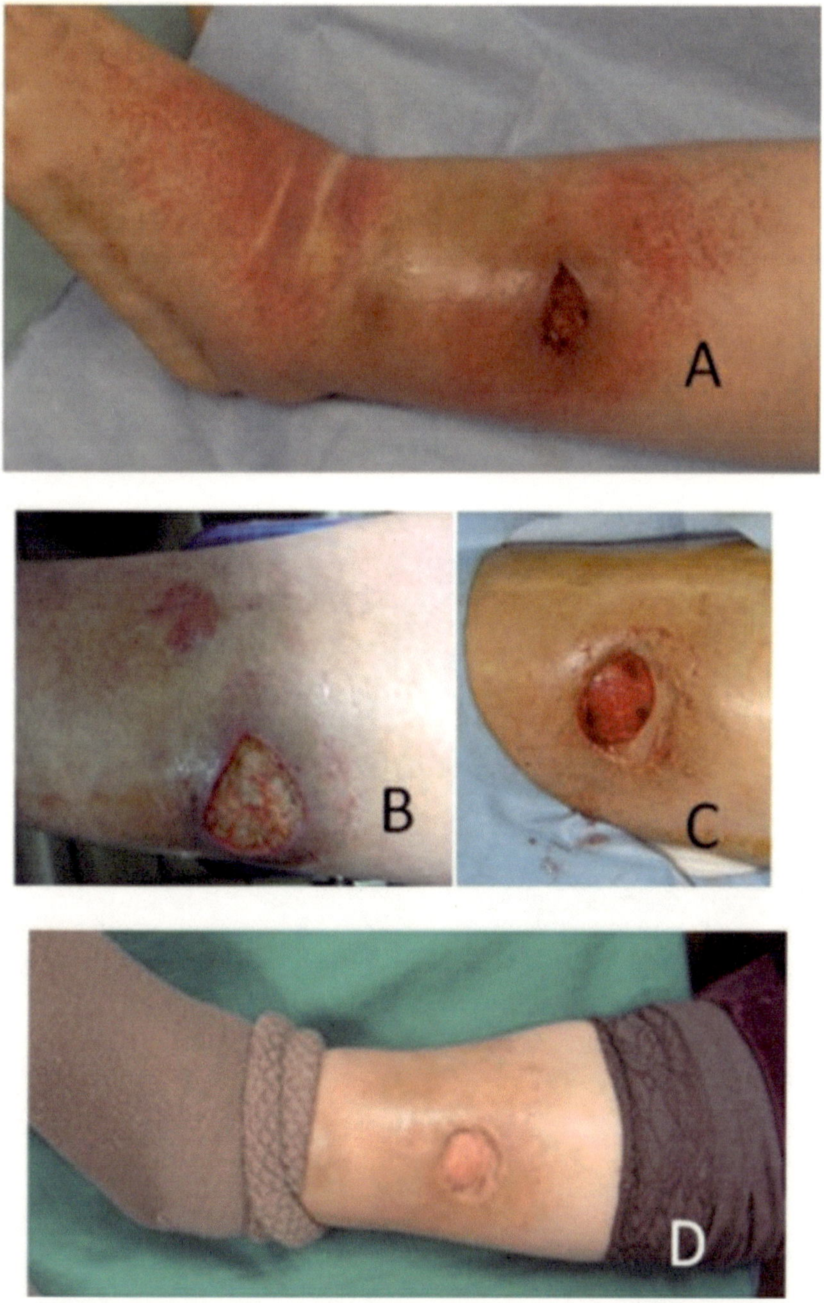

Fig. 21. (A) The photograph shows an infected wound in a patient receiving HD because of DM at the initial examination. (B) A favorable wound bed did not develop, although cleansing and wet-to-dry dressing were continued for 2 weeks after debridement. (C) The wound became clean and favorable for free skin grafting 2 weeks after the start of combination treatment using bFGF and artificial dermis. (D) The resurfaced wound 2 months after skin grafting.

Thirdly, negative pressure using a vacuum system has been proposed for speeding up treatment. A negative pressure wound therapy (NPWT) system is emerging as an acceptable option in patients with non-healing wounds of the foot, ankle, and lower limb[46]. Negative pressure wound therapy is a technique used to promote healing in acute or chronic wounds. A vacuum source is used to create sub-atmospheric pressure (125 mm Hg) in the local wound environment [47, 48]. A dressing, containing a drainage tube, is fitted to the contours of the wound and sealed with a transparent film. The tube is connected to a vacuum source, turning an open wound into a controlled, closed wound while removing excess fluid from the wound bed to enhance circulation and remove waste from the lymphatic system (Figure 22) [49]. It could be used effectively to prepare ulcers for closure via split-skin grafting or secondary closure in good time. We usually perform wound bed preparation with a combination of these therapies for improved clinical treatment of complex wounds (Figures 23), 24).

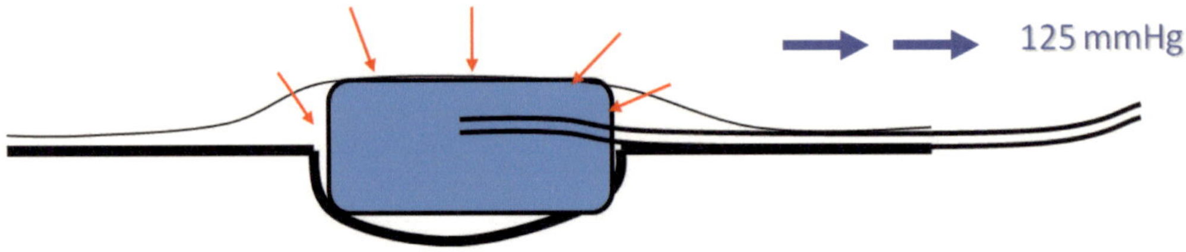

Fig. 22. Treatment of a full-thickness skin defect ulcer using artificial dermis.

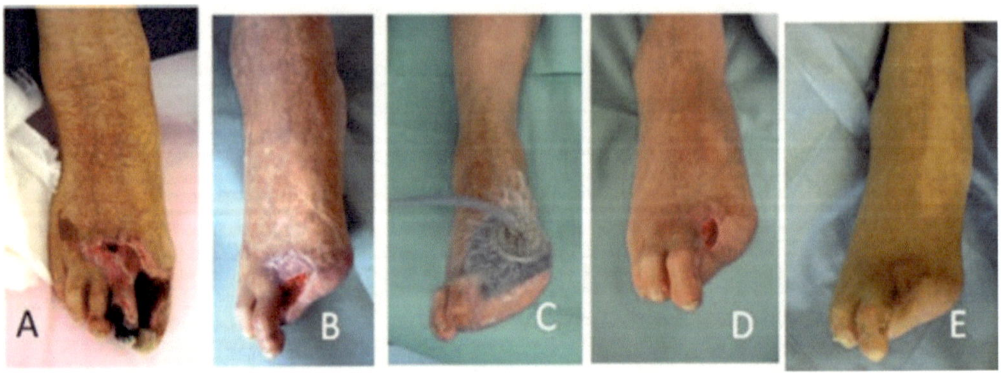

Fig. 23. (A) The photograph shows a necrotic wound of toes 1-3 in a patient receiving HD because of DM at the initial examination. He was also diagnosed ASO. He underwent amputation of toes 1-3, and the wound was sutured. (B) However, he developed a complex ulcer because of wound dehiscence. (C) Negative pressure wound therapy was performed. (D) Wound contraction was noted 2 weeks later. (E) The wound bed had closed completely 1 month later.

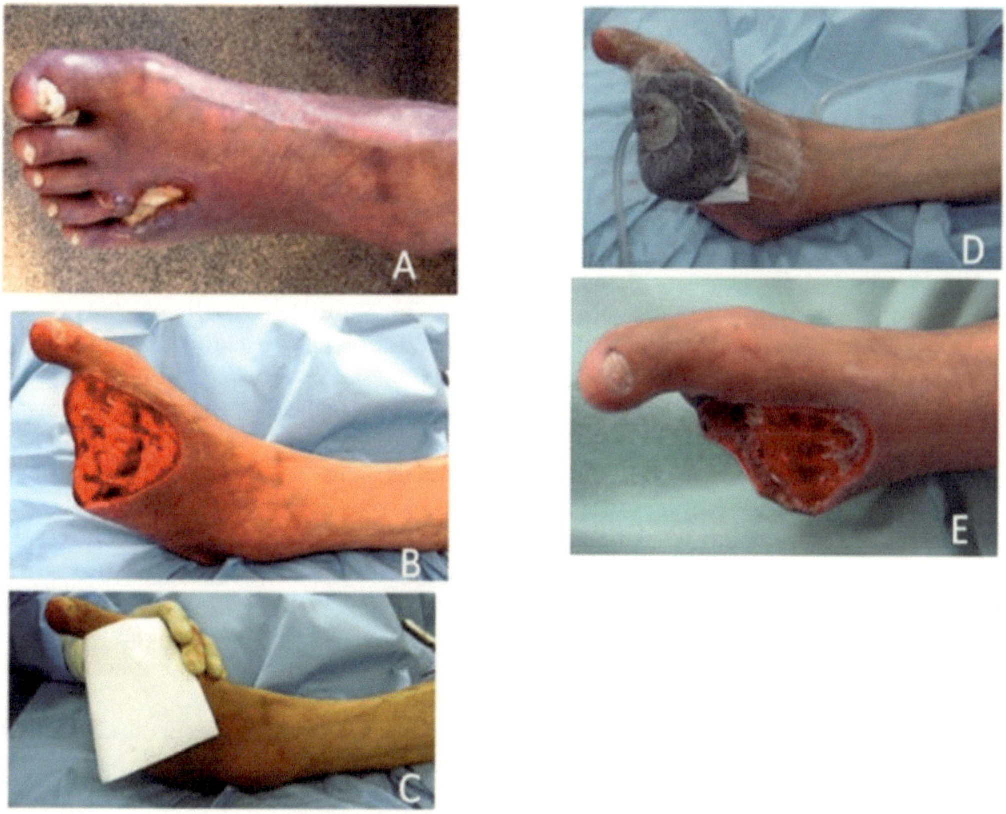

Fig. 24. (A) The photograph shows a complex wound in a patient receiving HD because of DM at the initial examination. He was also diagnosed with ASO. (B) He underwent amputation of toes 2-5, and the metacarpal bones were exposed. (C) Artificial dermis was applied on the wound. (D) Combined treatment of negative pressure wound therapy and artificial dermis was performed. (E) A favorable wound bed was prepared after 3 weeks of this combination treatment.

7. Conclusion

Patients receiving HD because of DM are likely to show more severe and rapidly developing complex wounds. They usually require immediate debridement before blood access shunts become infected.

8. References

[1] Akita S, Akino K, Imaizumi T, et al. The quality of pediatric burn scars is improved by early administration of basic fibroblast growth factor.J Burn Care Res. 2006;27:333-8.

[2] Attinger CE, Janis JE, Steinberg J, Schwartz J, Al-Attar A, Couch K.Clinical approach to wounds: débridement and wound bed preparation including the use of dressings and wound-healing adjuvants. Plast Reconstr Surg. 2006 Jun;117(7 Suppl):72S-109S.

[3] Bencini PL, Montagnino G, Citterio A, Graziani G, Crosti C, Ponticelli C. Cutaneous abnormalities in uremic patients. Nephron 1985;40:316-21.
[4] Bergesio F, Ciuti R, Salvadori M,et al.Are lipid abnormalities reliable cardiovascular risk factors in dialysis patients?Int J Artif Organs. 1989;12:677-682.
[5] Bird C.Managing malignant fungating wounds.Prof Nurse. 2000 ;15:253-256.
[6] Clare MP, Fitzgibbons TC, McMullen ST, Stice RC, Hayes DF, Henkel L. Experience with the vacuum assisted closure negative pressure technique in the treatment of non-healing diabetic and dysvascular wounds.
[7] Deery HG 2nd, Sangeorzan JA. Saving the diabetic foot with special reference to the patient with chronic renal failure. Infect Dis Clin North Am. 2001;15:953-981.
[8] Douglass J.Wound bed preparation: a systematic approach to chronic wounds. Br J Community Nurs 2003;8:26-34.
[9] Dowsett C, Ayello E.TIME principles of chronic wound bed preparation and treatment. Br J Nurs. 2004 Aug 12-Sep 8;13(15):S16-23.
[10] Dyachenko P, Shustak A, Rozenman D.Hemodialysis-related pruritus and associated cutaneous manifestations. Int J Dermatol 2006;45:664-667.
[11] Ferreira MC, Carvalho VF, Kamamoto F, Tuma P Jr, Paggiaro AO. Negative pressure therapy (vacuum) for wound bed preparation among diabetic patients: case series. Sao Paulo Med J. 2009;127(3):166-70.
[12] Fujioka M, Fujii T. Maxillary growth following atelocollagen implantation on mucoperiosteal denudation of the palatal process in young rabbits: implications for clinical cleft palate repair. Cleft Palate Craniofac J. 1997;34:297-308.
[13] Fujioka Masaki, Oka Kiyoshi, Kitamura Riko, Yakabe Aya. Complex wounds tend to develop more rapidly in patients receiving hemodialysis because of diabetes mellitus Hemodial Int. Apr;13(2):168-71. 2009
[14] Fujioka Masaki, Oka Kiyoshi, Kitamura Riko, Yakabe Aya. Complex wounds tend to develop more rapidly in patients receiving hemodialysis because of diabetes mellitus Hemodial Int. 2009.Apr;13(2):168-71.
[15] Fujioka Masaki. Combination treatment with basic fibroblast growth factor and artificial dermis improves complex wounds caused by collagen diseases with steroid use. Dermatologic Surgery2009;35(9):1422-5.
[16] Fujioka Masaki.Artificial dermis: A new material for wound treatment.JOURNAL OF WOUND TECHNOLOGY. No. 4 APRIL 13-19.2009
[17] Hajheydari Z, Makhlough A.Cutaneous and mucosal manifestations in patients on maintenance hemodialysis: a study of 101 patients in Sari, Iran.Iran J Kidney Dis. 2008 Apr;2(2):86-90
[18] Hajheydari Z, Makhlough A.Cutaneous and mucosal manifestations in patients on maintenance hemodialysis: a study of 101 patients in Sari, Iran.Iran J Kidney Dis. 2008 Apr;2(2):86-90)
[19] Ibels LS, Stewart JH, Mahony JF, Neale FC, Sheil AG.Occlusive arterial disease in uraemic and haemodialysis patients and renal transplant recipients. A study of the incidence of arterial disease and of the prevalence of risk factors implicated in the pathogenesis of arteriosclerosis.Q J Med. 1977;46:197-214.
[20] Iseki.K. Pharmacological control of secondary hyperparathyroidism in chronic hemodialysis patients: cinacalcet is coming to Japan.Expert Opin Pharmacother 2008;9:601-610.

[21] Jeanneret B, Magerl F. Treatment of osteomyelitis of the spine using percutaneous suction/irrigation and percutaneous external spinal fixation.J Spinal Disord. 1994 Jun;7(3):185-205.
[22] Kawamura A, Horie T, Tsuda I,et al.Clinical study of therapeutic angiogenesis by autologous peripheral blood stem cell (PBSC) transplantation in 92 patients with critically ischemic limbs.J Artif Organs. 2006;9:226-233.
[23] Lai MY, Lin YP, Yang WC.Fever with fulminant skin necrosis and digital gangrene in a uraemic woman.Nephrol Dial Transplant. 2007 May;22(5):1473-4.
[24] Lai MY, Lin YP, Yang WC.Fever with fulminant skin necrosis and digital gangrene in a uraemic woman.Nephrol Dial Transplant. 2007 May;22(5):1473-4.
[25] Marks MG, Doillon C, Silver FH. Effects of fibroblasts and basic fibroblast growth factor on facilitation of dermal wound healing by type I collagen matrices.J Biomed Mater Res. 1991 ;25:683-96.
[26] Mistik S, Utas S, Ferahbas A, et al An epidemiology study of patients with uremic pruritus. J Eur Acad Dermatol Venereol 2006;20:672-678
[27] Mistrík E, Dusilová-Sulková S, Bláha V, Sobotka L.Plasma albumin levels correlate with decreased microcirculation and the development of skin defects in hemodialyzed patients.Nutrition. 2010 Sep;26(9):880-5.
[28] Mistrík E, Dusilová-Sulková S, Bláha V, Sobotka L.Plasma albumin levels correlate with decreased microcirculation and the development of skin defects in hemodialyzed patients.Nutrition. 2010Sep;26(9):880-5.
[29] Nakase H, Matsuda R, Tamaki R, Tei R, Park YS, Sakaki T. Two-stage management for vertebral osteomyelitis and epidural abscess: technical note.Neurosurgery. 2006 Jun;58(6):1219.
[30] Nather A, Chionh SB, Han AY, Chan PP, Nambiar A. Foot Ankle Int. 2002 Oct;23(10):896-901.
[31] Nather A, Chionh SB, Han AY, Chan PP, Nambiar A.Effectiveness of vacuum-assisted closure (VAC) therapy in the healing of chronic diabetic foot ulcers. Ann Acad Med Singapore. 2010 May;39(5):353-8.
[32] Nease C. Using low pressure, NPWT for wound preparation & the management of split-thickness skin grafts in 3 patients with complex wound. Ostomy Wound Manage. 2009 Jun 1;55(6):32-42.
[33] Noordzij M, Boeschoten EW, Bos WJ, Dekker FW, Bossuyt PM, Krediet RT, Korevaar JC; for the NECOSAD Study Group.Disturbed mineral metabolism is associated with muscle and skin complaints in a prospective cohort of dialysis patients.Nephrol Dial Transplant. 2007 Oct;22(10):2944-9. Epub 2007 Jun 27.
[34] Palmer-Kazen U, Wariaro D, Luo F, et al. Vascular endothelial cell growth factor and fibroblast growth factor 2 expression in patients with critical limb ischemia. J Vasc Surg. 2004; 39: 621-8.
[35] Panuncialman J, Falanga V .The science of wound bed preparation.Surg Clin North Am. 2009 Jun;89(3):611-26.
[36] Patel MS, Malinoski DJ, Nguyen XM, Hoyt DB.The impact of select chronic diseases on outcomes after trauma: a study from the National Trauma Data Bank.J Am Coll Surg. 2011 Jan;212(1):96-104.
[37] Pico MR, Lugo-Somolinos A. Cutaneous alterations in patients with chronic renal failure. Int J Dermatol 1992;31:860-3.

[38] Pisoni RL, Wikstrom B, Elder SJ, Akizawa T, Asano Y, Keen ML, et al. Pruritus in haemodialysis patients: international results from the Dialysis Outcomes and Practice Patterns Study (DOPPS). Nephrol Dial Transplant 2006; 21: 3495–3505.

[39] Razeghi E, Omati H, Maziar S, Khashayar P, Mahdavi-Mazdeh M.Chronic inflammation increases risk in hemodialysis patients.Saudi J Kidney Dis Transpl. 2008 Sep;19(5):785-9.

[40] Robinson-Boston L, DiGiovanna JJ. Cutaneous Manifestations of end-stage renal descase. J Am Acad Dermatol. 2000;43:975-86.

[41] Schultz GS, Barillo DJ, Mozingo DW, Chin GA; Wound Bed Advisory Board Members. Wound bed preparation and a brief history of TIME.Int Wound J. 2004 Apr;1(1):19-32.

[42] Schultz GS, Sibbald RG, Falanga V, Ayello EA, Dowsett C, Harding K, Romanelli M, Stacey MC, Teot L, Vanscheidt W.Wound bed preparation: a systematic approach to wound management.Wound Repair Regen. 2003 Mar;11 Suppl 1:S1-28.

[43] Stein, A. A. and Wiersum, J.: The Role of Renal Dysfunction in Abdominal Wound Dehiscence.J. Urol., 82:271, 1959.

[44] Stojadinovic A, Carlson JW, Schultz GS, Davis TA, Elster EA. Topical advances in wound care. Gynecol Oncol. 2008 Nov;111(2 Suppl):70-80.

[45] Suzuki S, Kawai K, Ashoori F, et al. Long-term follow-up study of artificial dermis composed of outer silicone layer and inner collagen sponge. Br J Plast Surg. 2000; 53: 659-66.

[46] Udayakumar P, Balasubramanian S, Ramalingam KS, Lakshmi C, Srinivas CR, Mathew AC.Cutaneous manifestations in patients with chronic renal failure on hemodialysis.Indian J Dermatol Venereol Leprol. 2006 Mar-Apr;72(2):119-25.

[47] Wikström B. Itchy skin--a clinical problem for haemodialysis patients.Nephrol Dial Transplant. 2007 Jul;22 Suppl 5:v3-7.

[48] Yasuhara H, Naka S, Yanagie H, Nagawa H. Influence of diabetes on persistent nonhealing ischemic foot ulcer in end-stage renal disease.World J Surg. 2002;26:1360-1364.

[49] Yosipovitch G, Duque MI, Patel TS, Ishiuji Y, Guzman-Sanchez DA, Dawn AG, Freedman BI, Chan YH, Crumrine D, Elias PM.Skin barrier structure and function and their relationship to pruritus in end-stage renal disease.Nephrol Dial Transplant. 2007 Nov;22(11):3268-72.

9

Specifications of the Quality of Granulated Activated Charcoal Used in Water Systems Treatment in Hemodialysis Centers in Brazil

Eden Cavalcanti Albuquerque Júnior[1], Marcos Antonio de Souza Barros[1], Manoel O. Mendez[2], Aparecido R. Coutinho[2] and Telma T. Franco[3]
[1]*Professional Masters in Environmental Technology, Technology Institute of Pernambuco*
[2]*Energy and Environment Laboratory, Methodist University of Piracicaba*
[3]*School of Chemical Engineering, State University of Campinas*
Brazil

1. Introduction

According to the Brazilian Nephrology Society, in 2009, Brazil had approximately 600 Hemodialysis clinical centers. Currently, more than 77,000 Brazilians, who resort to specialized Hemodialysis services, are exposed to a volume of water of 18,000 to 36,000 L/year (Silva et al., 1996). Therefore, if the water used in these centers during the service is not duly treated, many chemical, toxic and bacteriological contaminants may be transferred to the patients, eliciting adverse effects, sometimes lethal (Buchanan et al., 1982; Arvanitidou et al., 2000).

The water used in these Hemodialysis centers come mainly from the public supply, and it is known that in many water reservoirs that are aimed for the population supply and consume, as the ones located in the Brazilian states like São Paulo, Paraná and Pernambuco, there is a propensity towards cyanobacteria toxic growing (Mendonça et al., 1999). The first report of human death from hepatotoxins of cyanobacteria, more specifically the microcystins -LR, -YR and -AR, happened in intravenous exposition in a Hemodialysis clinic in the city of Caruaru, Pernambuco, in 1996 (Carmichael et al., 2001).

In 2001, another incident involving Hemodialysis water contamination by microcystins was reported. Toxic growths of cyanobacteria with preponderance of the *Microcystis sp.* and *Anabaena sp.* were identified in the Funil reservoir and in the Guandu River, both used as water resources for the public supply in the city of Rio de Janeiro, RJ, Brazil. Thus, from that episode, microcystins concentration of the order of 4 μg/L and 0.32 μg/L, respectively were detected in the water and in the activated charcoal filter, used by the water treatment station of the Hemodialysis Center of the Clementino Fraga Filho Hospital of the Federal University of Rio de Janeiro, which is supplied by the water reservoir of Funil and the Guandu river.

As a consequence of this incident, a total of 44 uremic patients who had received care in this Hemodialysis Center, were believed to be exposed to the microcystins found in the water used in the preparation of the dialysate, being until the present time, monitored as to evaluate a possible chronic exposition to those toxins (Soares et al., 2006).

Considering thus the need to define the minimal criteria for the functioning and assessment of the public and private services which perform dialysis in outpatients, bearers of chronic renal insufficiency, as well as the mechanisms of their monitoring , moreover the need of risk reduction to which the dialysis patients are submitted , the ANVISA (The National Agency of Sanitary Surveillance) has established as resolution (RESOLUÇÃO-RDC nº 154, of June 15th, 2004, republished in May 31, 2006) which foresees the technical regulation for the functioning of these services in Brazil.

It was established from that resolution's publication, that the water used in the preparation of dialysate, must have its quality guaranteed in all phases of the treatment, storage and distribution through the monitoring of the microbiological and physic-chemical parameters, as well as the procedures for the treatment themselves. Therefore, the water provision of the dialysis services from the public supply, from wells and any other sources must have its drinking standard as provisioned in the Act MS Nr. 518 of March 25th, 2004, (Brazilian Health Ministry) or of any legal instrument which may replace that one. Regarding the cyanotoxins, according to the art. 14 of this regulation, it was established that the upper limit allowed of microcystins in water for public supply be of 1 μg/L, it was also recommended that the analysis for the cyanotoxins included the determination of cylindrospermopsin and saxitoxins (STX), taking into consideration, respectively, the value limits of 15.0 μg/L e 3.0 μg/L of STX/L equivalents.

A good example of cyanotoxins monitoring is being made in the systems of water collection which supply the city of São Paulo, Brazil (systems Rio Grande, Alto Tiête and Guarapiranga) by the Basic Sanitation Company and water treatment of São Paulo,- SABESP. It has been noticed that despite the mycrocystin levels are below the standard established by the MS 518/2004, many Hemodialysis clinics, in where this water is used, are at alert, as the water used by them for the Hemodialysis treatment needs to be with microcystins concentration equal to zero.

In Brazil, according to the Brazilian Society of Nephrology, in order to guarantee the water quality used for renal patients, more than 80% of the Hemodialysis centers have water treatment systems which use reverse osmoses, deionization, integrated system of reverse osmoses + deionization, besides activated charcoal.

The granulated activated charcoal (GAC) is an adsorbent used in processes of water treatment (activated charcoal filters) to remove micropollutants present in water, as pesticides, industrial chemical agents, cyanobacterial secondary metabolites such as geosmim and 2-methyl isoborneol (MIB) which give taste and odor to water, and toxins like hepatotoxins (microcystins) and neurotoxins (Newcombe, 1999).

The adsorption capacity of activated charcoals (AC) by compounds in the water is mainly influenced by the physical structure and chemical characteristics of the surface of these adsorbents, their previous material, and their preparation condition (Newcombe, 1999; Karanfil et al., 1999). Different research groups have shown that the ACs with pore volume developed in the regions of mesopores and secondary micropores can be very effective in the removal of microcystins (Falconer et al., 1989; Donati et al., 1994; Pendleton et al. 2001; Campinas & Rosas, 2010a, 2010b). Therefore, it is indispensable to estimate the distribution of pores in these regions, whether by means of adsorbing in liquid phase by using the methylene blue solution or in gaseous phase using N_2.

The Hemodialysis Centers are concerned with the correct quality parameters which would indicate from those parameters which is the best charcoal to be used in their water treatment, as the activated charcoal, associated with other technologies, is commonly used by water treatment stations in Hemodialysis Centers. Thus, in this Chapter, are discussed the adsorption techniques in liquid and gaseous phase which were used aiming to assess the adsorption capacity of the GAC commonly used by water treatment stations in the Brazilian Hemodialysis Centers, providing indicators which may be used as to purchase these adsorbents.

2. Sampling of activated charcoals

Activated charcoals used in two Brazilian Hemodialysis Centers, located in the city of Recife/Pernambuco, Brazil - Hemodialysis Center of the Clinical Hospital of the Federal University of Pernambuco, coordinates 08°03'15.40"S 34°52'52.52"W (termed A) - and in the city of Campinas/São Paulo, Brazil - Hemodialysis Center of the Clinical Hospital of the State University of Campinas, coordinates 22°54'25.58"S 47°03'47.66"W (termed B) - were used in this study. Besides that, sugarcane bagasse (CA-R-H) and dry coconut shell (CA-R-G) based-activated charcoal were specially produced for this work and used as reference charcoals (termed R) (Table 1). These charcoals were activated with water steam at temperature close to 900 °C. The raw material preparation conditions, the carbonization and activation, besides those charcoals full characteristics, in liquid and gaseous phase, are thoroughly described by Albuquerque Junior et al. (2005)*.

Reference	Origin	Precursor
AC-A-A	Unknown	Coconut Tree wood
AC-A-B	Calgon®, EUA	Coconut Shell
AC-A-C	Calgon®, EUA	Coconut Shell
AC-A-D	Criciúma, Brazil	Coal
AC-B-E	Carboleste, Brazil	Babaçu coconut endocarp
AC-B-F	Bahia Carbon®, Brazil	Coconut shell
AC-R-G	Author*	Coconut shell
AC-R-H	Author*	Sugar Cane Bagasse

Table 1. Assessed Activated Charcoals

2.1 Characterization of activated charcoals

For the characterization in liquid phase by means of use of methylene blue solution and in gaseous phase by N_2, the charcoals were marked in mortar and pestle, grinded in a sieve with nominal opening mesh of 0.075mm. Whereas the ones used in the experiments in fixed bed column were grinded in sieves with nominal opening mesh of 0.50mm and 0.35mm, being the obtained material in this last sieve collected for the referred experiment. The charcoals were then dried in greenhouse at 150 °C by 3 hours minimally, and then cooled in desiccators with silica gel until reached room temperature for its posterior use.

2.1.1 Adsorption in gaseous phase: Specific surface area and distribution of pores size

As the analysis procedures, all the ACs were degasified in vacuum at 150 °C for 24 h. A software in interface with a gas analyzer (model NOVA-1200, Quantachrome Corp.) was used in the measures of specific surface area and distribution of pores size. Equilibrium data obtained from the isothermal of adsorption /desorption of gaseous nitrogen at 196 °C were used to determine the specific surface area by means of application of the method developed by Brunauer, Emmet and Teller (BET). The micropores area was obtained by the "t-plot" method. The total volume of the pores was determined converting in liquid volume the nitrogen aborted volume in the saturation point ($P/P_0 \sim 0.99$). The micropores and primary micropores were calculated from the intercept point of the t-plot linear region after the saturation of the micropores and primary micropores respectively. The volume of the mesopores was calculated from the difference between the total volume of the pores and the volume of the micropores, also, the volume of the secondary micropores was calculated by the difference between the volume of the mesopores and the volume of the primary micropores. The distribution of the size of the pores in the micropore and mesopore regions in the ACs was obtained from the methods developed by Horvath-Kawazoe (HK) and Barrett-Joyner-Halenda (BJH), respectively (Webb & Orr, 1997).

2.1.2 Adsorption in liquid phase: Methylene blue index and [D-Leucine[1]]microcystin-LR

2.1.2.1 Batch experiments

An isotherm study of adsorption equilibrium is important as to describe an interaction between adsorbate and adsorbents, and it is critical in the optimization of these materials for both studies in continuous or in batch process. Information regarding the distribution of the sizes of the AC pores were obtained from comparison of the adsorption characteristic for three different adsorbates: methylene blue and [D-Leucine[1]]microcystin-LR ([D-Leu[1]]MCYST-LR). The choice of these molecules is justified by their properties, forms and polarities, being the first commonly used for foretelling the capacity of the activated charcoal in adsorbing micropollutants in industrial effluents (Hsieh & Teng, 2000; Lussier et al., 1994), besides providing an estimate of the volumes in secondary micropores + mesopores, as foretold in previous works by Albuquerque Junior et al. (2005).
The trihydrate methylene blue (99.95%, Merck, EUA) analytical grade was used in the solution preparation as to determine the Methylene Blue Index (MBI). The adsorption experiments were made in accordance with the norm JIS (Japanese Industrial Standard), JIS-K 1474 (1991). The methylene blue concentrations in the liquid phase after the equilibrium were determined indirectly from molecular adsorption spectrophotometry (spectrophotometer GBC UV/VIS - 911 A) in the wave length of 665 nm. The experimental data were adjusted to the Freundlich's model, and the quantity of the methylene blue adsorbed by the charcoals (q) was calculated according to the equation 1.

$$q = \frac{(C_0 - C)}{m} V \tag{1}$$

For the foretelling of the capacity and removal de microcystine in water by activated charcoal, an aqueous extract of [D-Leu[1]]MCYST-LR of concentration around to 6000 μg/L, prepared in drinkable water exempt of chloride, was used as adsorbate. This toxin has been already identified in growths in Lagoa dos Patos, Rio Grande do Sul, Brazil, (coordinates 31° 9'56.93"S 51°25'51.45"W) by Matthiensen et al. (2001) and in Lagoa de Jacarepaguá, Rio de Janeiro, Brasil (22°59'10.69"S 43°23'57.95"W) by Oliveira et al. (2004). The preparation of the respective extract, as in the quantification model of the referred toxin by High Performance Liquid Chromatography (HPLC) was fully discussed by Kuroda et al. (2005). The experimental data were adjusted to the Langmuir's model and the quantity of adsorbed toxin by the activated charcoals was measured from the equation 1.

2.1.2.2 Experiments in fixed bed columns: Adsorption of [D-leucine[1]]MCYST-LR

In order to evaluate the microcystin dynamics in experiments in fixed bed column, an acrylic column was used of 2.5 cm de d_i and height of up to 25 cm, adjusted by means of a piston. A distributor plate with five orifices of 1mm openings, made of stainless steel, was inserted in the base of this column. A net of 60 µm was used below the distributor and in the entrance of the piston through which the fluid that passed the column flowed, avoiding that possible loss of adsorbent by reflux (Fig. 1).

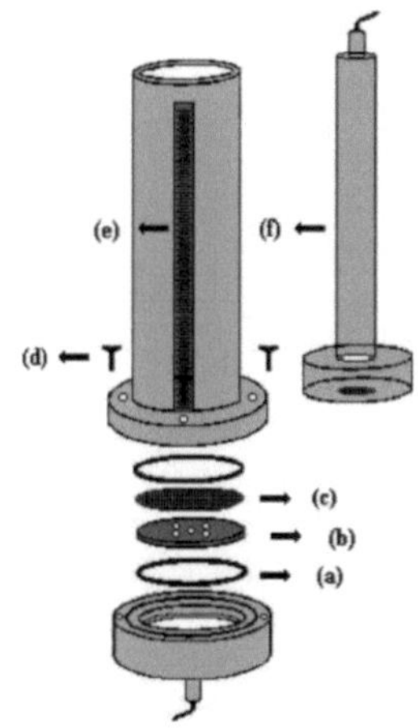

Fig. 1. The column scheme used in this work (a) *o*-ring, (b) distributor (perforated plate), (c) net (60 µm), (d) screw, (e) rule, (f) piston. Source: Santos et al., 2002.

The charcoal bed was continuously percolated by a solution having [D-Leu[1]]MCYST-LR of varied concentration, from which effluent samples were intermittently collected until the bed saturation. The toxin concentration in the liquid phase was determined by HPLC and the evaluation of the continuous process of adsorption was made by means of breakthrough curves sizing, which is the relation between the ration of the initial concentration by the toxin concentration in the column effluent (C/C_0) vs time (t).

3. Results

3.1 Textual characteristics of activated charcoals

The activated charcoals are formed by an interconnected net of pores, which according to IUPAC (International Union of Pure and Applied Chemistry) may be classified according to its diameters in different categories: macropores (di > 50 nm), mesopores (2 nm < di < 50 nm), primary micropores (di < 0,8 nm) and secondary micropores(0,8 nm < di < 2nm) (Everett, 1988).

The activated charcoal porosity may be estimated from the form of the isotherm of Nitrogen adsorption according to the Brunauer, Deming, Deming and Teller (BDDT) (Gregg & Sing, 1982) classification. Therefore, from that classification, it was observed that the AC-B-F, AC has presented an isotherm characteristic of the type I, typical of micropores material, with relatively small external surface area. Nevertheless, loops characteristic from hysteresis in partial pressures (P/P_0) above 0,4 in other ACs, which indicate that these charcoals must present a small band of pores in the secondary micropore region and mesopores. Thus, these other charcoals have presented a combination between the isotherms I and II, the same observed for charcoals taken as reference (fig. 2).

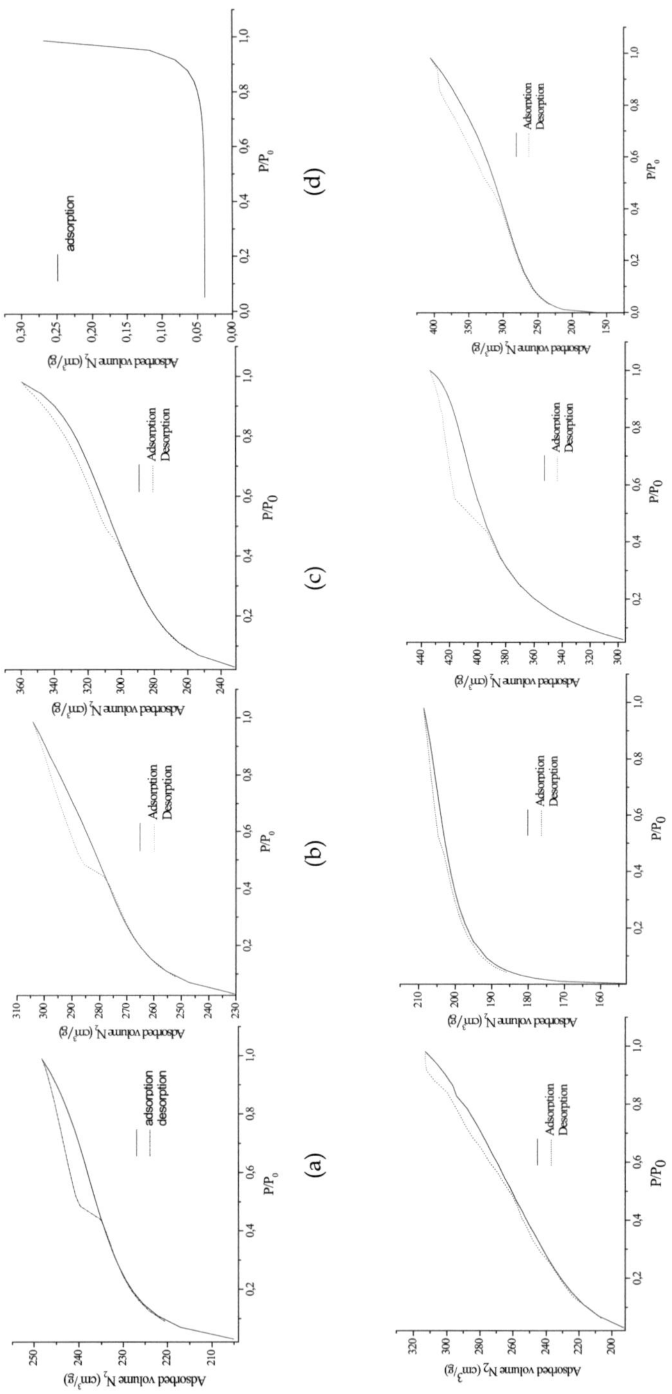

Fig. 2. Nitrogen adsorption/desorption Isothermes at -196°C. (a) AC-A-A, (b) AC-A-B, (c) AC-A-C, (d) AC-A-D, (e) AC-B-E, (f) AC-B-F, (g) AC-R-G and (h) AC-R-H

The adsorption isotherms could also be analyzed from the hysteresis loop format according to the standard classification, which contains 4 types: H1–H4 (Girgis & Hendawy, 2002). The hysteresis loops appear in multilayer regions of isothermal of physiosorption, and are considered as being associated to capillary condensation. The hysteresis loop style found for the analyzed charcoals was of the H4 type, which was originated from the influence, even small, of the existing secondary micropores and mesopores in these materials.
The charcoal sample AC-A-D has presented an unusual behavior from the obtained isothermal data of N_2 adsorption/desorption, as it has shown a very low Nitrogen adsorpted volume, around 0.27 cm^3/g, when compared with those obtained by other sampled charcoals, which then Nitrogen adsorpted volumes were above 248 cm^3/g (Figure 2d). By the adsorption behavior of that charcoal, it is assumed that the same is an activated charcoal and, thus, could not be used in the water treatment station in the Hemodialysis Centers A (HC Campinas) for the removal of contaminants.
The used ACs in the water treatment station of the Hemodialysis Center A have presented BET area (S_{BET}) between 764.9 m^2/g e 1,017.4 m^2/g, whereas the ones used in the Hemodialysis Center B have presented S_{BET} between 632.8 m^2/g and 789.5 m^2/g (Table 2).

	Surface area (m^2/g)			Pore Volume (cm^3/g)			
REF.	BET	Micro	Meso	Primary micropore (%)	*Secondary micropore (%)	Mesopore (%)	Total
AC-A-A	764.9	756.2	8.7	0.16 (44.7)	0.21 (55.3)	0.01 (2.6)	0.38
AC-A-B	871.2	857.6	13.6	0.12 (31.9)	0.32 (68.1)	0.03 (6.4)	0.47
AC-A-C	1017.4	967.9	49.5	0.08 (31.9)	0.38 (69.1)	0.09 (16.4)	0.55
*AC-A-D	4.6	4.5	0.015	-	-	-	0.003
AC-B-E	632.8	610.2	22.6	0.17 (55.9)	0.15 (44.1)	0.02 (5.9)	0.34
AC-B-F	789.5	772.0	17.5	0.14 (37.5)	0.30 (62.5)	0.04 (8.3)	0.48
AC-R-G	1079.5	1014.2	65.3	0.08 (50.0)	0.29 (50.0)	0.20 (34.5)	0.58
AC-R-H	1174.3	1097.3	77.3	0.10 (22.3)	0.35 (77.7)	0.39 (41.8)	0.76

* The very low adsorption capacity has not allowed the calculation of these parameters.

Table 2. Activated Charcoals textural properties.

A first observation of these results would imply in the choice of charcoals of any of the two centers, however, according to Quinlivan et al. (2005), the BET area (SBET) is a poor indicator of the adsorption capacity of activated charcoals, hence, the sampled charcoals quality cannot be assessed only by their BET (SBET) area data, so, other effectiveness parameters must be taken into consideration in order to choose a charcoal for a determined aim. Thus, beyond that parameter, the secondary micropores and mesopores volumetric fractions must also be considered in the choice of an activated charcoal for the use in water treatment, as these pores are significantly important in the adsorption of organic micropollutants like the microcystins by the activated charcoals according to Donati et al. (1994) and Pendleton et al. (2001). According to Donati et al. (1994), there is no correlation between the adsorption capacity of activated charcoals by microcystins and the BET area, the micropores volume and the number of Iodine. However, the mesopores presence in these adsorbents may favor the adsorption of the cyanobacterium toxin. Moreover, Pendleton et al. (2001), have shown that besides the mesopores volume, the adsorption capacity of that toxin, was also influenced by the volumetric fraction correspondent to the secondary micropores. In these charcoals, the secondary micropores and mesopores volumetric fractions have exceeded 37% e 28%, respectively, favoring the adsorption of microcystin in 200.0 μg/mg.

The activated charcoals of the water treatment in the hemodialysis Center (A and B) have presented secondary micropores and mesopores volumetric portions of 0.15 to 0.38 cm^3/g (44.1 to 69.1%) and of 0.01 to 0.09 cm^3/g (2.6 to 16.4%), respectively. These charcoals have presented secondary micropores portions higher than those found by Pendleton et al. (2001), however, they have also presented very low mesopores volumetric fractions, around 8% in average, which characterizes microporous charcoals. Nevertheless, those commercial activated charcoals obtained as reference by the authors, have presented secondary micropores volumetric fractions and mesopores of 59.2 to 63.6% and of 34.5 to 41.8%, respectively, which can be characterized as a good indicator for the AC for the treatment water use.

A visualization of the pores size distribution can be obtained from the distribution function calculated by the HK and BJH (Figure 3) methods. The (A), (B) and (C) charcoals have shown a distribution function HK/BJH, with dW/dLo of 0.04; 0.07 and 0.06 $cm^3/nm/g$ consisting of pores average diameters of 3.81, 3.80 and 3.28 nm, respectively. Due to the low adsorption capacity of the D charcoal, it was not possible to obtain its distribution of the pores sizes. For the E charcoal, the distribution function dW/dLo has presented two peaks with 0.02 and 0.01 $cm^3/nm/g$ a 2.53 and 4.15 nm in pores average diameter; while the AC-B-F has presented dW/dLo ≈ 0.06 $cm^3/nm/g$ to an average pore diameter of 2.7 nm. In contrast with these results, the standards AC-R-G and AC-R-H have shown a distribution function a little higher: (AC-R-G) dW/dLo ≈ 0.3 $cm^3/nm/g$ with 1.61 nm of pore average diameter, and AC-R-H has presented two peaks with dW/dLo ≈ 0.17 and 0.08 $cm^3/nm/g$ with pore average diameter of approximately 1.71 and 3.00 nm, respectively.

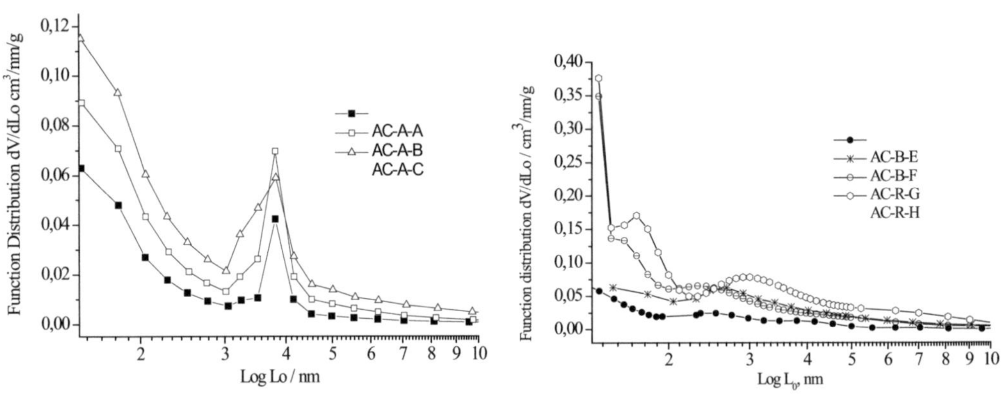

(a) (b)

Fig. 3. Function distribution HK/BJH: (■) AC-A-A; (□) AC-A-B; (Δ) AC-A-C; (●) AC-B-E; (✱) AC-B-F; (Θ) AC-R-G; (O) AC-R-H.

According to Lanaras et al. (1991) the MCYST-LR when dissolved in water, has a solvated volume of 2.63 nm, length of 1.9nm, height of 1.5nm, thickness of 1.1nm, and solvated area of 1.8 nm^2. The [D-Leu[1]]MCYST-LR has an amino acid residue, D-Leucine, which has replaced the amino acid residue, D-Alanine, of MCYST-LR, that confers the [D-Leu[1]]MCYST-LR more hydrophobicity than the MCYST-LR. But, these differences between their chemical structures are not so significant regarding their heights, solvated volume and transversal section area, enabling that approximate dimensions of the first MCYST-LR might be taken as referential of the latter. Thus, taken the approximate dimensions of the MCYST-LR it is presumed that the [D-Leu[1]]MCYST-LR is adsorbed in the activated charcoal pores with an internal diameter close to 2-3 nm.

The distribution of the pores size (Figure 3) estimated from the HK/BJK has allowed to observe that the sampled charcoals have a pores average diameter between 2.5-4 nm, which would make these charcoals potential adsorbents for their use in the removal of the water microcystin, but the low volume of the pores observed in this 2.5-4 nm band is smaller than 0.07 cm^3/g, which makes these charcoals adsorbents of low adsorption capacity for such aim.

3.2 Adsorption on liquid phase

3.2.1 Batch experiments

Knowing the adsorption equilibrium represents the first step in investigating the possibilities for using an adsorbent in a determined separation process. Besides, additional information regarding the distribution of the sizes of the activated charcoal pores can be obtained by comparing the adsorption characteristics of adsorbate by taking those obtained from adsorption data in gaseous phase.

Methylene blue (MB) has been widely used as an adsorbate to estimate the adsorption capacity of CA from continuous in fixed bed or batch experiments (Kumar & Sivanesan, 2006; Macedo et al., 2006; Zhang et al., 2006). Studies on MB adsorption equilibrium in activated charcoal can provide important information about the selectivity of these adsorbents regarding this molecule, given that the MB is accessible to the charcoal pores with an inner diameter greater than 1.5 nm, being important for the characterization of the secondary micropores ($0.8 < di < 2.0$ nm) and mesopores (2 nm $< di <$ 50 nm) mainly, besides being a model compost used for predicting the adsorption of organic contaminants found in industrial effluents such as textile dye and microcystines (Barton, 1987; Baçaoui et al., 2001).

According to the JIS norm (1994), the Methylene Blue Index is operationally defined as the adsorbed amount of that molecule when its residual concentration in liquid phase after equilibrium is of 0.24 mg/L. This adsorption capacity was obtained from an equilibrium isotherm where the experimental data were adjusted to Freundlich's adsorption model. The correlation coefficients for linear regression from the adjustment of the experimental data to the respective linearized model along with its empirical parameters, K and 1/n, besides the charcoals' Methylene Blue Index (MBI), are displayed on Table 3.

	Freundlich's model parameters			
	Methylene Blue Index			
Reference	K (L/mg)	1/n	r^2	MBI (mg/g)
AC-A-A	9.2	0.13	0.91	7.6
AC-A-B	40.7	0.07	0.98	36.6
AC-A-C	43.4	0.02	0.95	42.1
* AC-A-D	-	-	-	-
AC-A-E	35.4	0.1	0.97	32.5
AC-A-F	85.6	0.05	0.99	79.2
AC-A-G	104.5	0.08	0.94	92.6
AC-A-H	271.4	0.16	0.99	217.5

*This charcoal has a very low adsorption capacity (close to zero) for methylene blue, which makes it impossible to calculate the MBI.

Table 3. Freundlich's model adsorption parameters.

Standard international and national norms regarding the quality of activated charcoal for water treatment bring specifications primarily concerning the minimal iodine adsorption limit (iodine number), 600 mg/g (ABNT - EB-2133, 1991 and AWWA – B600-05) and 900 mg/g (ASTM - D 4607-96), making no mention to the minimal limits of methylene blue adsorption. It is known that iodine is a small molecule of approximately 0.8 nm and being thus associated with micropore adsorption. Therefore, the iodine number cannot be the sole specification of quality standard adopted for an activated charcoal destined for water treatment, because it is a well-applied parameter for microporous charcoals.

In Marroco, the activated charcoals destined for water treatment have in their specifications the minimal limits established for the methylene blue adsorption capacity of 180.0mg/g (Baçaoui et al., 2001). Thus, if we consider this minimal limit as a specification for the activated charcoal sampled in both the Hemodialysis Centers, we would see that none of these charcoals could be used for water treatment, because they are specifically microporous activated charcoals.

3.2.1.1 Adsorption of [D-Leucine[1]]MCYST-LR

From results obtained in the characterization of the hemodialysis centers AC regarding the pore volume and methylene blue adsorption, it was possible to choose the best AC in each center and use it in the adsorption studies with the cyanobacteria toxin. The adsorption kinetics of the [D-Leucine[1]]MCYST-LR on the charcoals was studied, from which we could estimate the efficiency of the removal of this cyanobateria toxin by those adsorbents. Other two activated charcoals produced by Albuquerque et al. (2005) (AC-R-G and AC-R-H, originating from the sugarcane bagasse and coconut tree endocarp) were also studied regarding their removal efficiencies for [D-Leu[1]]MCYST-LR on water.

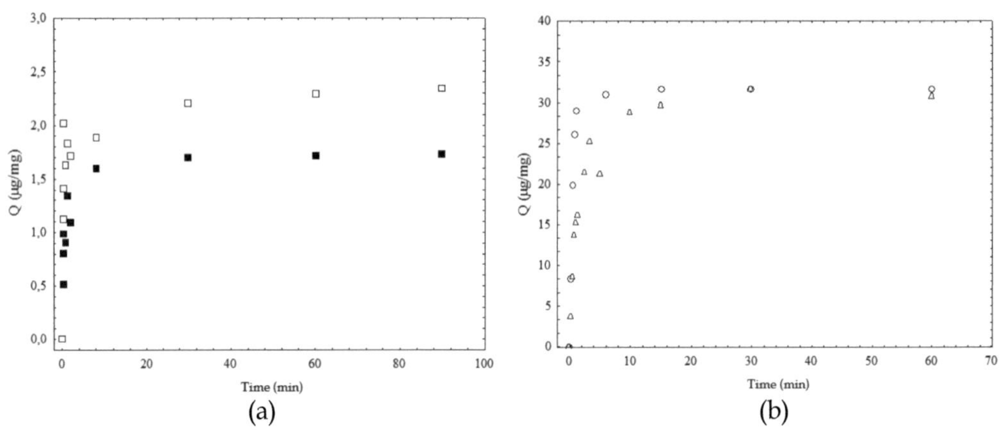

Fig. 4. Adsorption kinetics of [D-Leucine[1]]MCYST-LR on the activated charcoals: (a) □ AC-B-F, ■ AC-A-B, and (b) ○ AC-R-G and Δ AC- CS – F.

After 15 seconds of contact between the [D-Leu[1]]MCYST-LR and the charcoals, removal efficiencies of 7.40% (AC-R-G) and 26.47% (AC-R-H) were observed, compared to the very low results obtained by the AC-A-B and AC-B-F with removal efficiency of 1.96 and 2.26%, respectively. The adsorption kinetics evolved gradually with time until the adsorption balance was reached in around 30 minutes for the AC-R-G and AC-R-H, and of 60 minutes for the AC-A-B and AC-B-F (Figure 4). The removal efficiencies by these AC in the respective equilibrium times were of 62.31% (AC-R-G), 98.73% (AC-R-H), 4.3% (AC-B-F) and 3.7% (AC-A-B). Still in the equilibrium, toxin adsorption in the charcoals of 30 μg/mg (AC-R-G), 32 μg/mg (AC-R-H), 1.4 μg/mg (AC-A-B) and 1.7 μg/mg (AC-B- F) were observed. The low removal efficiency of the two last charcoals (from hemodialysis centers) can be explained by their low mesopore volumes, around 0.04 cm^3/g in average, when compared to those of other charcoals taken as standards, AC-R-G and AC-R-H (0.20-0.39 cm^3/g).

3.2.2 Experiments in fixed bed column

In the dinamic adsorption dynamic of the [D-Leu[1]]MCYST-LR in a fixed bed of activated charcoal, the latter removed that toxin from a solution until the saturation of the bed, wherein the performance of this continuous adsorption process is affected, among other parameters, by the concentration of the entry solution (Gomes et al., 2001) and by operational conditionals such as particle size and fluid flow in the column (Inglezakis et al., 2002). According to Sag & Aktay (2001) and Barros et al. (2001), the solutions which are more concentrated saturate the bed faster, and small particles diminish the resistance to mass transfer. It is also known that an increase in the flow of the solution on the bed reduced its adsorption capacity, increasing the lenght of the mass transfer zone, because the phenomenon of mass transfer necessary for adsorption of [D-Leu[1]]MCYST-LR might not be able to continue in higher mass transfer rates, brought forth by an increase in the flow of the fluid (Watson, 1999). Besides, the bed flow can be deviated from the ideal because of the flow channeling due to insufficient material wettability. Those problems can reduce the adsorption process efficiency, because it is important that the column operates as close as possible to the flow/runoff conditions as the one observed for a tubular-type "plug flow" reactor. Hence, in order to correctely plan and operate the continuous adsorption process of that toxin in a AC fixed bed, as the one found in many water treatment stations of hemodialysis centers, it is necessary to study the kinetics and adsorption equilibrium for that toxin, besides knowing its adsorption dynamics in a fixed bed through the sizing of the breakthrough curves. The first step in a adsorption project for [D-Leu[1]]MCYST-LR in fixed bed column is the establishment of optimal conditions for preparing the process, that is, those that minimize the diffusional resistances both in the film and in the interior of adsorbent particles, thus favoring a greater interaction between the charcoals' active sites, accessible to adsorption, and the adsorbate.

In this experiment, the previous studies of methylene blue adsorption in activated charcoal fixed bed have shown flows between approximately 8 and 12 mL/min and average particle size of 0.425 mm would be conditions that could reduce to minimum those mass transfer resistances without significant increase in charge loss on the bed, and thus be taken as a starting point for the planning of a continuous adsorption process for that toxin. Under these conditions, one should expect that the breakthrough curves come closer to a perfect degree, which is desirable (Mccabe et al., 2001). Thus, taking such conditions like particle size, flow and height of the bed, new experiments with solutions [D-Leu[1]]MCYST-LR were carried out aiming to evaluate the removal of this toxin from the treated water using fixed bed columns of AC-A-B charcoals and AC-B-F, besides the AC taken as standards AC-R-G and AC-R-H (Table 4).

Aiming to recover the solution initially containing [D-Leu[1]]MCYST-LR kept in contact in a continuous fashion with an activated charcoal bed initially free from it, the concentration of this toxin in the exit of the bed was monitored, in function of the time, producing curves as shown in Figure 5 denominated breakthrough curves.

REF.	C_0 (µg/L)	Flow (mL/min)	Hbed (cm)	mZ (g)
AC-A-B	12,779.6	11.1	2.4	8.3
AC-B-F	12,460.6	8.5	2.3	8.1
AC-R-G	13,496.4	10.5	2.4	9.2
AC-R-H	19,153.5	12.2	2.3	7.0

Table 4. Experimental conditions and adsorption results in continuous regime

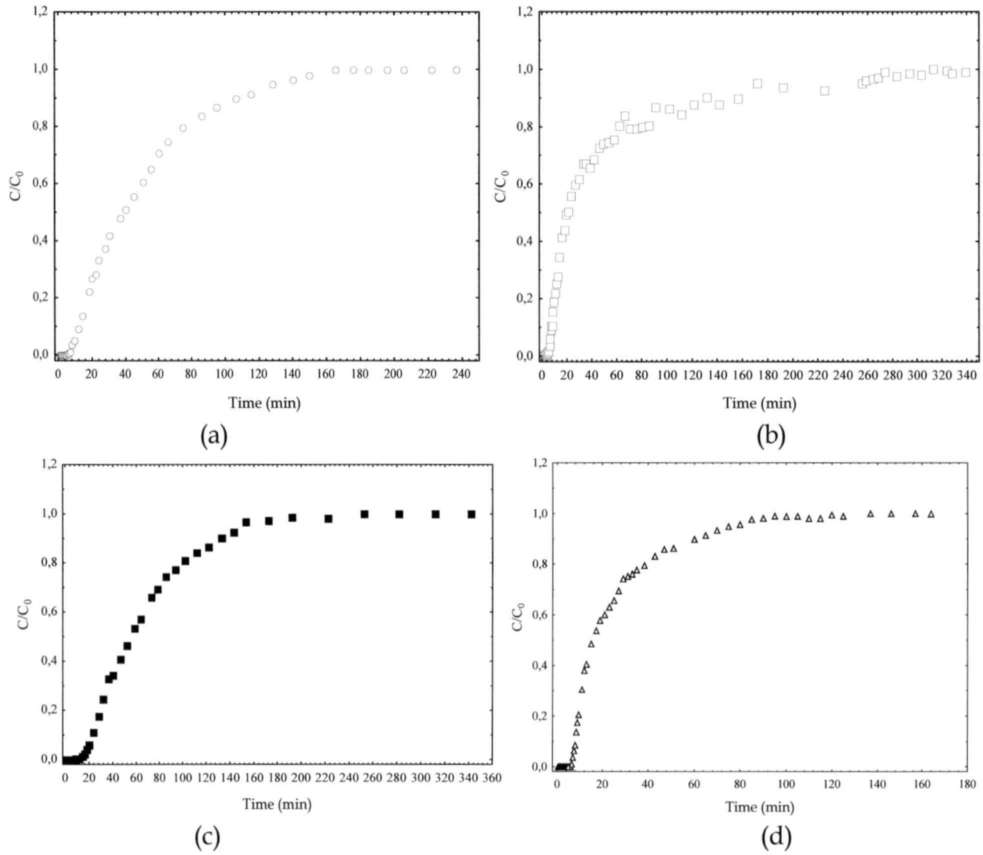

Fig. 5. Breakthrough curves of activated charcoals (C/C_0 versus time): (a) AC-R-H, (b) AC-A- B, (c) AC-B- F, (d) AC-R-G.

Initially, the adsorbent layer located in the inferior part of the bed adsorbs the solution quickly and effectively thus reducing the concentration of that toxin in the exit of the column. The effluent on the top of the bed is practically free of solute. In this situation, the inferior layer of the bed is practically saturated and the adsorption occurs in an adsorption zone (Zad) that is relativelly narrow and the concentration changes rapidly. Continuing with the solution flow, the Adsorption Zone flow (Zad) moves in an ascendant way like a wave, at an ordinarily much slower rate than the linear fluid velocity through the bed. In a certain time, practically half of the bed is saturated with the solute, but the concentration in the effluent is still substantially zero. When the adsorption zone (Zad) has reached the top of the bed, and the solute concentration in the effluent increases sensibly, the system is said to initiate rupture, so the solute concentration in the effluent increases rapidly when the adsorption zone (Zad) passes through the bed bottom and the solute concentration is substantially equated to the concentration value in the initial solution (C_0).

Based on the data obtained from the Breakthrough curves, it was possible to estimate the needed time for the C/C_0 = 0.05 ratio to be reached in the exit of the column, which denominated breakthrough time (t_b). Hence, for the AC fixed beds composed by the samples from the Recife (AC-B-F) and Campinas (AC-A-B) Hemodialysis Centers, this time was of 24 and 3 min. This results indicated that each charcoal bed composed by 8.12g (AC-B-F) and 8.26g (AC-A-B) of activated charcoal displayed an adsorbed mass of [D-Leu^1]MCYST-LR of around 2541.9 μg (24 min × 0.0085 L/min = 0.204 L; 0.240 L × 12460.6 μg/L = 2541.9 μg) and 424.8 μg (3 min × 0.01108 L/min = 0.03324 L; 0.03324 L × 12779.6 μg/L = 424.8 μg), corresponding to 0.31 μg/mg and 0.05 μg/mg, respectively.

With the continuous adsorption process until the exhaustion of each bed in 282 min (AC-B-F) and 310 min (AC-A-B), when the C/C_0 = 1 ration was achieved in the column exit, it was possible to estimate the [D-Leu^1]MCYST-LR mass adsorbed by the bed in those times. Under this conditions, each bed showed an adsorbed mass of [D-Leu^1]MCYST-LR of 29,868.05 μg (282 min × 0.0085 L/min = 2.237 L; 2.237 L × 12,460.6 μg/L) (AC-B-F) and 43,895.37 μg (310 min × 0.01108 L/min = 3.435 L; 3.435 L × 12,779.6 μg/L) (AC-A-B), this corresponded to about 3.678μg/mg and 5.314μg/mg, respectively.

Comparing the performance of the beds above with those composed by the activated charcoals AC-R-G and AC-B-F, adsorbed masses of [D-Leu^1]MCYST-LR of 1,017.29 μg (7.5 min × 0.01005 L/min = 0.0754L; 0.0754L × 13,496.4μg/L) and 2,072.02 μg (9 min × 0.01202 L/min = 0.1082 L; 0.0754 L × 19,153.5 μg/L) were observed, which corresponds to 0.113 μg/mg and 0.296 μg/mg, respectively. These beds displayed an exhaustion time of 132 and 165 min. In those times, the beds presented adsorbed masses of 18,706.01 μg (132 min × 0.01005 L/min = 1.326 L; 1.326 L × 13,496.4 μg/L) and 37,987.13 μg (165 min × 0.01202 L/min = 1.9833 L; 1.9833 L × 19,153.5 μg/L), which corresponded to 2.07 and 5.43 μg/mg, respectively.

REF.	*t_b (min)	t_e (min)	t_u (min)	t_t (min)
AC-A-B	7.0	320	45.7	593.2
AC-B-F	24	282	153.5	615.6
AC-R-G	7.5	132	59.2	276.1
AC-R-H	9.0	165	56.6	384.9

*t_b is the breakthrough time, t_e exhaustion time, t_u utile time and t_t stoichiometry time.

Table 5. Properties of the activated charcoal beds.

Comparing the results obtained from the activated charcoals AC-R-G and AC-R-H with the Bernezeau (1994) data (50 μg microcystin-LR/12 mg Powdered Activated Charcoal - PAC), the sugarcane bagasse based-activated charcoal showed an adsorption capacity 1.3 times bigger than the PAC studied by the aforementioned researcher, remembering that in our studies we have used an extract with four microcystins.

According to Zambon (2002), qualitative information regarding the resistance to mass transfer can be obtained from the form of breakthrough. If the mass transfer zone is narrow, the breakthrough curve will be more inclined, whereas if the zone is wider, the curve will be more elongated. From Figure 6, it is possible to see that such zones differed from charcoal to charcoal according to the operational parameters established in each experiment such as initial concentration, flow and bed height. Hence, in the case of the Breakthrough curves obtained for the AC-R-G, AC-A-B and AC-R-H beds, a narrower S-shaped curved indicating a narrower mass transfer zone and, therefore, with mass transfer resistance to be considered. Nonetheless, the breakthrough curve obtained from the bed packaged with charcoal AC-B-F (Hemodialysis Center B) displayed a more elongated S-shaped curved, as seen on Figure 5, indicating a broader mass transfer zone and, therefore, little resistance to mass transfer. The supposition of the adsorption zone provides the basis for a method for a much simpler project, which makes it possible to scale up the experiments from a small laboratory scale. However, besides the Mass Transfer Zone (MTZ) concept, the estimative of parameters such as average residence time and dimensionless variance can help in the design of an adsorption column (activated charcoal filter).

4. Conclusion

Granulated Activated charcoals are largely used in adsorption continuous processes in fixed bed for the water treatment in Hemodialysis Centers. The quality of the water used in these centers is intrinsically associated with the quality of these charcoals. As in Brazil, there are no norms, and neither, entities which control the quality of these adsorbents; it is each day more important to find the correct parameters indicators of quality. Activated charcoals used in two water treatment stations in hemodialysis centers were sampled as to assess their qualities. The Specific Surface Area (S_{BET}) of the charcoal sampled in the water treatment stations in the two centers have presented values between 600 and 1000 m^2/g approximately. S_{BET} values around 800 m^2/g are usually taken as reference value, for those who acquire such adsorbents, mainly those destined to the water treatment. From that principle, it is verified that the sampled charcoals of both Hemodialysis Centers are in accordance with this parameter, however, it was also observed, that the same charcoals have mesopores volume of (0.01-0.09 cm^3/g), which are significantly below from those specified in the literature (0.40 cm^3/g), thus, the charcoals from both centers must be rejected for such aim or used with caution. The blue methylene adsorption was proposed as adsorption capacity measure of activated charcoals, as this molecule has been used as to estimate the charcoal mesopores volume. It was observed that the activated charcoals which have presented higher mesopores+ secondary micropores volume have more adsorption capacity to that molecule, and, hence, may be taken as a model to estimate the referred pores region, which is important for the charcoals used in the water treatment.

Regarding the first estimate of the adsorption capacity in batch of the activated charcoal in both hemodialysis centers for the cyanobacterium toxin [D-Leu[1]]MCYST-LR, low removal efficiencies for that toxin were observed (close to 4%), compared with the activated charcoal from sugarcane bagasse (close 99%). The behavior in the adsorption of the sampled charcoals in the hemodialysis centers is associated with its low mesopores volumes, smaller than 0.04 cm^3/g, contrary to the sugarcane bagasse based-activated charcoal whose mesopores volume is around 0.40 cm^3/g.

Preliminary studies regarding the dynamic adsorption of the [D-Leu[1]]MCYST-LR in fixed beds of the activated charcoals in the Hemodialysis Centers have shown low adsorption capacity between 3.67 and 5.31 $\mu g/mg$. Regarding the coconut shell and the sugarcane bagasse based-activated charcoals it was observed a 2.07 and 5.43 μg/mg adsorption capacity of the respective beds.

5. Acknowledgment

The authors acknowledge the financial support (02-11529-8) received from the Fundação de Amparo à Pesquisa do Estado de São Paulo (FAPESP) and fellowship from the Conselho Nacional de Desenvolvimento Científico e Tecnológico (CNPq) for development this work.

6. References

Albuquerque Junior, EC.; Mendez, M.O.; Coutinho, A.R. & Franco, T.T. (2005). Production and characterization of physically activated carbon from Brazilian agricultural and industrial residues. In: *Proceedings of III Brazilian Congress of Carbon.* Rio de Janeiro, RJ, Brazil, p. 401-410.

American Society for Testing and Materials. ASTM, D 4607-96; Standard Test Method for Determination of Iodine Number of Activated Carbon. PA, EUA, 1999. 2p.

American Water Works Assosiation Standards, Denver, CO. AWWA B600-05; Powdered Activated Carbon. Denver, CO, EUA, 2005. 24p.

Arvanitidou, M.; Spaia, S.; Tsoubaris, P.; Katsinas, C.; Askepidis, N.; Pagidis, P.; Kanetidis, D.; Pazarloglou, M.; Bersos, G.; Digenis, P.; Katsouyannopoulos, V. & Vayonas, G. (1999). Chemical Quality of Hemodialysis Water in Greece: A Multicenter Study. *Dialysis & transplantation*, Vol.29, No.9, pp.519-525, ISSN 0090-2934.

Associação Brasileira de Normas Técnicas. Rio de Janeiro. EB 2133; Carvão ativado pulverizado: especificação. Rio de Janeiro, 1991. 54p.

Baçaoui, A.; Yaacoubi, A.; Dahbi, A.; Bennouna, C.; Phan Tan Luu, R.; Maldonado-Hodar, F. J.; Rivera-Utrilla, J. & Moreno-Castilla, C. (2001). Optimization of conditions for the preparation of activated carbons olive-waste cakes. Carbon, Vol.39, No. 3, pp.425-432, ISSN 0008-6223.

Barros, M.A.S.D.; Arroyo, P. A. Métodos de remoção de cromo de águas residuais - troca iônica. IN: Maria Angélica Simões D. De Barros; Pedro Augusto Arroyo; Eduardo Falabella Sousa-Aguiar; Pedro Avila García. (Org.). Problemas Ambientais com soluções analíticas. Vol. I. O Cromo no processamento de peles. Madri: CYTED, 2001, v. 1, p. 84-98.

Barton, S. S. (1987). The adsorption of methylene blue by active carbon. *Carbon*, Vol.25, No. 3, pp.343-350, ISSN 0008-6223.

Buchanan, M.; Stevens, B.; Marshal, A.; Plomley, R.; d'Apice, A. & Kincaid-Smith, P. (1982). Aluminium associated bone disease: clinic-pathologic correlations. *American Journal of Kidney Disease*, Vol. 2, No. , pp. 255-263, ISSN 0272-6386.

Brazilian Society of Nephrology. Available from: <http://www.sbn.org.br>. Accessed in February, 2011.

Campinas, M. & Rosa, M.J. (2010a). The ionic strength effect on microcystin and natural organic matter surrogate adsorption onto PAC. *Journal of Colloid and Interface Science*, Vol.299, No.2, pp. 520-529, ISSN 0021-9797.

Campinas, M. & Rosa, M.J. (2010b). Removal of microcystins by PAC/UF. *Separation and Purification Technology*, Vol. 71, No. 1, p. 114-120, ISSN 1383-5866.

Carmichael, W.W.; Azevedo, S.M.F.O., A.N.J.; Molica, R.J.R.; Jochimsen, E.M.; Lau, S.; Rinehart, K.L.; Shaw, G.R.; Eaglesham, G.K. (2001). Human fatalities from cyanobacteria: chemical and biological evidence for cyanotoxins. *Environmental Health Perspective*, Vol. 109, No. 7, pp. 663– 668, ISSN 0091-6765.

Donati, C., Drikas, M., Hayes, R., Newcombe, G. (1994). Microcystin-LR adsorption by powdered activated carbon. *Water Research*, Vol. 28, No. 8, pp. 1735-1742, ISSN 0043-1354.

Everett, D.H. (1987). Pore Systems and Their Characteristics. In: *Characterization of Porous Solids*, K.K. Unger, J. Rouquerol, K.S.W. Sing and H. Kral, (Ed.), 1-21, Elsevier, ISBN 9780-4444-2953-7, Amsterdam, The Netherlands.

Falconer, I.R., Runnegar, M.T.C., Buckley, T., Huyn, V.L. & Bradshaw, P. (1989). Using activated carbon to remove toxicity from drinking water containing cyanobacteria blooms. *Journal American of Water Works Association*, Vol.81, No. 2, pp. 102-105, ISSN 1551-8833.

Girgis, B.S. & El-Hendawy, A.N.A. (2002). Porosity development in activated carbons obtained from date pits under chemical activation with phosphoric acid. *Microporous and mesoporous materials*, Vol. 52, No. 2, pp. 105-117, ISSN 1387-1811.

Gregg, S.J. & Sing, K.S.W. (1982). *Adsorption, Surface Area and Porosity*, Academic Press, 303p., 0123-0095-61, ISBN 0123009561 , London.

Gomes, C.P.; Almeida, M.F. & Loureiro, J.M. (2001). Gold recovery with ion exchange used resins. *Separation and Purification Technology*, Vol.24, No. 1-2, pp.35-57, ISSN 1383-5866.

Hsieh, C. & Teng, H. (2000). Influence of mesopore volume and adsorbate size on adsorption capacities of activated carbons in aqueous solutions. *Carbon*, Vol. 38, No. 6, pp. 863-869, ISSN 0008-6223.

Inglezakis, V.J.; Loizidou, M.D. & Grigoropoulou, H.P. (2002). Equilibrium and kinetic ion exchange studies of Pb^{2+}, Cr^{3+}, Fe^{3+} and Cu^{2+} on natural clinoptilolite. *Water Research.*, Vol. 36, No. 11, pp. 2784-2792, ISSN 0043-1354.

Japanese Industrial Standard. JIS K 1474. (1991). Test methods for activated carbon. Japanese Standards Association, Tokyo.

Kumar, K.V. & Sivanesan, S. (2006). Equilibrium data, isotherm parameters and process design for partial and complete isotherm of methylene blue onto activated carbon. *Journal of Hazardous Materials*, Vol. 134, No. 1-3, pp. 237–244, ISSN 0304-3894.

Kuroda, E.K.; Albuquerque Júnior, E.C.; Di Bernardo, L. & Trofino, J.C. Characterization and choice kind of activated charcoal to be employed in water treatment with microcystins. In: *Proceedings of XXIII Brazilian Congress of Sanitation and Environmental Engineering*. Campo Grande, MS, Brazil.

Lanaras, T.; Cook, C.M.; Eriksoon, J.E.; Meriluoto, J.A.O.; Hotokka, M. (1991). Computer modeling of the 3-dimensional structures of the cyanobacterial hepatotoxins microcystin-LR and nodularin. Toxicon, Vol. 29, pp. 901–907.

Lussier, M. G.; Shull, J. C. & Miller, D. J. (1991). Activated carbon from cherry stones. *Carbon*, Vol.29, pp.613-619.

Mccabe, W. L.; Smith, J. C.; Harriot, P. Unit Operations of Chemical Engineering. New York, USA: McGraw-Hill International Ed., 6th ed., 2001.

Macedo, J. S.; Costa Júnior, N. B.; Almeida, L. E.; Vieira, E. F. S.; Cestari, A. R.; Gimenez, I. F.; Carreño, N. L. V.; Barreto, L. S. Kinetic and calorimetric study of the adsorption of dyes on mesoporous activated carbon prepared from coconut coir dust. *Journal of Colloid and Interface Science*, Vol. 298, pp. 515–522, 2006.

Matthiensen, A.; Beattie, K.A.; Yunes, J.S.; Kaya, K.; Codd, G.A. (2000). [D-Leu[1]]Microcystin-LR, from the cyanobacterium Microcystis RST 9501 and from a Microcystis bloom in the Patos Lagoon estuary, Brazil. *Phytochemistry*, Vol. 55, pp. 383-387.

Mendonça, D. F. P.; Bouvy, M.; Marinho, M. E.; Moura, A. N. (1999). Microfitoplâncton e condições limnológicas em reservatórios de cinco bacias hidrográficas do Estado de Pernambuco: ênfase ao gênero Cylindrospermopsis. In: *VIII Brazilian Meeting of Phicology*. Porto de Galinhas-PE, Brazil, p. 120.

Newcombe, G. (1999). Charge vs. porosity - some influences on the adsorption of natural organic matter (NOM) by activated carbon. *Water Science and Technology*, Vol.40, pp.191–198.

Oliveira, A.C.R.; Magalhães, S.V.F.; Soares, R.M. & Azevedo, S.M.F.O. (2005). Influence of drinking water composition on quantitation and biological activity of dissolved microcystin (cyanotoxin). *Environmental toxicology*, Vol. 20, No. 2, pp. 126-130.

Act GM/MS No. 518, March 25th, 2004. Available from: <http://www.saude.ba.gov.br/divisa/arquivos/legislacao/Portaria_MS_518-04.pd>. Accessed in August 30th, 2005.

Pendleton, P.; Schumann, R.; Wong, S.H. (2001). Microcystin-LR adsorption by activated carbon. *Journal of Colloid and Interface Science*, Vol.240, pp.1-8.

Quinlivan, P.A.; Li, L. & Knappe, D.R.U. (2005). Effects of activated carbon characteristics on the simultaneous adsorption of aqueous organic micropollutants and natural organic matter. *Water Research*, Vol.39, pp.1663–1673.

Resolução-RDC N° 154, June 15th, 2004. Available from: <http://www.sbn.org.br/portarias/RDC154.doc>. Accessed in July 10th, 2006.

Sağ, Y. & Aktay, Y. (2001). Application of Equilibrium and mass transfer models to dynamic removal of Cr (VI) ions by Chitin in packed column reactor. Process Biochem., Vol. 36, pp. 1187-1197.

Santos, E. S.; Guirardello, R & Franco, T. T. (2002). Preparative chromatography of xylanase using expanded bed adsorption. *Journal of Chromatography A*, Vol.944, No.1-2, pp.217-224.

Silva, A.M.M.; Martins, C.T.B.; Raboli, R.F.; Getti, V.J. & Romão Junior, J.E. (2006). Review/Updating in dialysis: Water for hemodialysis. *Journal of Brazilian Nefrology*, Vol. 18, No. 2, pp. 180-188.

Soares, R.M.; Yuan, M.; Servaites, J.C.; Delgado, A.; Magalhães, V.F.; Hilborn, E.D.; Carmichael, W.W & Azevedo, S.M.F.O. (2006). Sublethal exposure from microcystins to renal insufficiency patients in Rio de Janeiro, Brazil. *Environmental Toxicology*, Vol.21, pp.95–103.

Sridhar, P.; Sastri, N.V.S.; Modak, J.M. & Mukherjee, A.K. (1994). Mathematical simulation of bioseparation in an affinity packed column. *Chemical and Engineering Technology*, Vol.17, No.6, pp. 422-429.

Watson, J.S. (1999). Separation methods for waste and environmental applications. ISBN 0824799437, New York: Marcel Dekker Inc.

Webb, P.A. & Orr Jr, C. (1997). *Analytical methods in fine particle technology*. Micromeritics Instrument Corp., Norcross, ISBN 978-096-567-830-8.

Zambon, G. A. (2002). Removal of Lead (Pb^{2+}) using natural zeolite Clinoptilolita. State University of Campinas, 102p. Master's Disseratation.

Zhang, C.; Wang, Y. & Yan, X. (2006). Liquid-phase adsorption: Characterization and use of activated carbon prepared from diosgenin production residue. *Colloids and Surfaces. A, Physicochemical and Engineering Aspects*, Vol.280, No.1-3, pp. 9–16, ISSN 0927-7757.

10

Bioimpedance Measurement in the Kidney Disease Patient

Joëlle Cridlig, Mustapha Nadi and Michèle Kessler
Université Henri Poincaré Nancy 1
France

1. Introduction

1.1 The problematic of hydration status in the kidney disease patient

Dry weight corresponds to the body weight of a person with normal extracellular fluid volume [1]. In the context of hemodialysis, dry weight is the weight reached at the end of the dialysis session by patients who will remain free of orthostatic hypotension or hypertension until the next session. Clinicians are thus obliged to estimate the appropriate dry weight each individual patient should reach at the end of a dialysis session. If this weight is underestimated, the patients are at risk of various incidents ranging from simple yawning to death. Low dry weight also carries a permanent risk of hypotension, cramps, nausea, vomiting or ischemia. If this weight is overestimated, chronic hyperhydration can cause acute events including pulmonary edema, or hypertension, but also long-term consequences affecting cardiovascular morbidity and mortality [2]. This important notion of dry weight is however quite problematic because it corresponds to a transient state, making it necessary to anticipate weight gain between two dialysis sessions and thus to reach a certain degree of dehydration at the end of each hemodialysis session.

The many methods proposed for measuring dry weight and body composition are still under investigation. The difficulty encountered in establishing a reliable comparative tool for measuring these parameters arises from inevitable physiological, anatomical and physical variability. Most approaches remain empirical, relying on feedback from trial and error [3].

In practice, dry weight is estimated clinically [4]. Physical examination is a classic but limited tool. Solid evidence-based analysis of specific physical findings such as systolic blood pressure, orthostatic blood pressure, or the presence or not of edema is lacking. Such clinical symptoms can also be related to conditions other than a dry weight or body composition problem. Several tests have been proposed to assess the dry weight of hemodialysis patients [5]. Echocardiographic inferior vena cava diameter and biochemical markers are available but results exhibit high variability and poor correlation with extra-cellular volume; there are also unserviceable in detecting volume depletion.

Bioimpedance spectroscopy measurement has been demonstrated as a potentially useful method to determine the physiological status of living tissues [6]. Disease-related alterations are associated with variations in essential tissue parameters such as physical structure or ionic composition that can be detected as changes in passive electrical properties.

Bioimpedance spectroscopy can be used as a diagnostic tool reflecting the overall status of a patient or of an individual organ. The range of applications derived from this method is wide making this non-destructive and non-invasive approach a promising technique for the characterization of the physiological status of the human body.

This chapter presents the use of bioimpedance spectroscopy as a tool for measuring the dry weight of the hemodialysis patient. The first part summarizes the basic fundamentals of the method, describing the underlying electrical and biological principles and the potential interest for applications in hemodialysis. Techniques and models are presented and discussed. The second part discusses clinical results obtained at the hemodialysis center of the Nancy University Hospital, with focus on patient-related parameters influencing or limiting measurements and their interpretation.

1.2 Basic principles of bioimpedance spectroscopy

1.2.1 Physical principles

The bioelectrical properties of the human body depend on the nature of the biological tissues composing it and their relative conductivities. These properties lead to the notion of impedance of a biological medium which varies as a function of the frequency of an electrical current applied across it. This in turn leads to the notion of bioimpedance spectroscopy.

Impedance is a complex quantity $(\underline{Z})$ describing, in compliance with Ohm's law (assuming sinusoidal voltage), the relationship between the voltage difference across the medium and the amplitude of the electrical current. Because of the capacitive nature of biological media, all impedance measurements of the human body involve a phase shift between the voltage and the current, yielding complex values. Biological media are weak conductors due to the dissipation (or loss) of energy in the media and can be considered as energy-loosing dielectrics. The quantities of interest can thus be defined using a schematic representation of a biological suspension placed between two electrodes (Fig. 1).

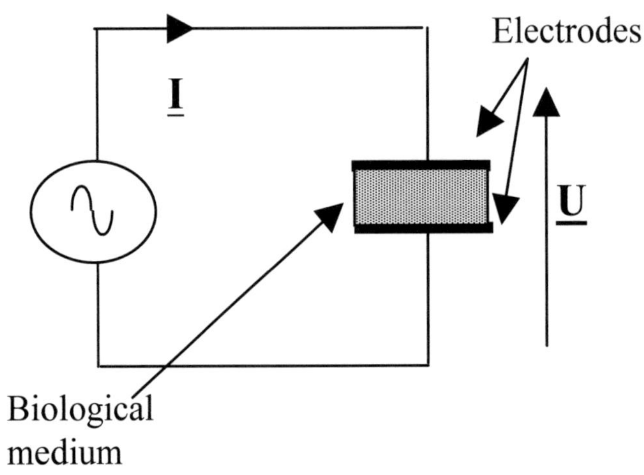

Fig. 1. Basic principle of bioimpedance spectroscopy

$\underline{U}$ and $\underline{I}$ are sinusoidal quantities with phase shift ϕ

$$\underline{U} = Uo\, e^{j\omega t} ; \underline{I} = Io\, e^{j(\omega t + \phi)} \quad (1)$$

The impedance of a biological medium is thus the relationship between the voltage difference across the medium and the current amplitude as described by Ohm's law:
$\underline{U} = \underline{Z}\,\underline{I}$ where $\underline{Z}$ is the complex impedance expressed in Ohms (Ω). In Cartesian form this gives $\underline{Z} = R + jX$ where R is the resistance, X is the reactance, both expressed in Ohms, and j the imaginary unit, $j = \sqrt{-1}$
Setting $Z = \sqrt{R^2 + X^2}$ and $\phi = \text{arctg}\,(X/R)$ gives the polar form $\underline{Z} = Z\,e^{j\,\phi}$
The bioelectric impedance $\underline{Z}$ describes the inertia of a biological medium opposing passage of a sinusoidal current with intensity $\underline{I}$ and pulsation ω (rad/s). Along the lines of the electrical current, this impedance generates a difference of potential $\underline{U}$. Bioelectrical impedance can be represented in a complex plane. It is perfectly defined by knowledge of either its real and imaginary components (R and X), or by its module and its argument, $\underline{Z}$ and ϕ.
For an isotropic, homogeneous, linear medium, impedance is a function of the medium's electrical properties, conductivity and permitivity, but also depends on the geometric features of the measurement cell. This so-called bioimpedance is a well-known tool for characterizing different physiological water compartments [7]. Because of the complexity and highly heterogeneous nature of living tissues, a global approach is used, considering the whole body as a suspension of cells in water and electrolytes [8].

1.2.2 Biological basis

Biological tissues cannot be considered as ideal conductors. They are ionic conductors with heterogeneous structures. If we limit our considerations to the sole electrical aspect of interest here, biological tissues can very schematically be considered as a combination of two components: *i*) a free water medium called the extracellular fluid, within which are suspended *ii*) cells surrounded by a membrane containing and thus limiting a volume of intracellular fluid (Fig. 2). The cell concentration can vary greatly, depending on the nature of the tissue.
The fluid components (extracellular fluid, plasma and intracellular fluid) can be considered as electrolytic suspensions of ions whose concentration, electrical charge and mobility, taking into account the viscosity of the medium, will essentially determine the impedance of the suspension, mainly arising from resistive type resistance. Cell membranes however constitute a more complex component. Cole demonstrated that cell membranes can be likened to capacitors [9, 10, 11]. This divides biological media into two basic components, resistors (R) and capacitors (C), which when connected in parallel produce an electrical equivalent model as described by Fricke [13] (Fig. 2). This simplified model (R_e, R_i and C are not ideal) enables an interpretation of observed biophysical phenomena.
Theoretically, tissue impedance, like any electric impedance, can be measured. The mass of tissue to study simply has to be delimited and linked to a measurement device via a system of electrodes. In practice however, measuring the electrical characteristics of biological tissues raise many specific problems. It is useful to recognize the electrical properties of

biological tissues and their components because of their interest both in medicine, where many diagnostic methods are based on electrical principles, and in fundamental physiology, where these same properties contribute to the structural analysis of cell organization, the study of cell excitation mechanisms, or to the analysis of protein molecules. Debye, Cole-Cole and Maxwell-Wagner models have been developed to represent the theoretical interpretations of these phenomena. These models can be used to demonstrate important factors characterizing biological tissues [12].

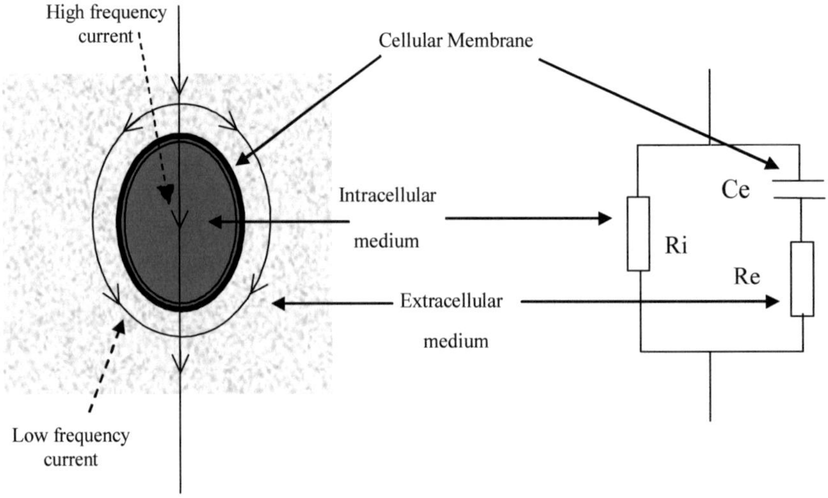

Fig. 2. Electrical equivalent model (Fricke's model) of a biological cell in suspension in the extracellular fluid. Ri : intra-cellular resistance, Re : extra-cellular resistance, Ce : capacitance

Capacitance and resistance can be combined either in series or in parallel, leading to several variants of the Fricke model. Resistivity (charge accumulation) and conductivity (conduction of electrical current) are however two independent processes for which the parallel model has been found to be more representative. Formulas used for biological tissues are thus all based on the Fricke model [13]. Applying these models to bioimpedance spectroscopy curves allows a quantification of value differences corresponding to the intracellular fluid and the extracellular fluid and thus their corresponding masses. The interest for hemodialysis is obvious.

1.3 Usefulness of bioimpedance for the kidney disease patient

Much research has been devoted to the determination of body hydration status and fluid compartments, particularly in hemodialysis patients [14]. Work has focused on various physiological parameters with different modalities to study individual segments of the body or the whole body [15, 16, 17] using multiple or unique frequencies [18]. One of the goals is to improve predictive equations and to identify the effect of different parameters on the measures obtained [19, 20]. In dialysis for example, it has been shown that fluid is removed predominantly from the extracellular and peripheral (arms, legs) compartments [21]. Thus, different biofluid models have been proposed to describe the whole body or individual organs. Basically, applying the bioimpedance method to determine body composition consists in placing electrodes conveniently on the arms and legs in order to impose an electrical current and measure the voltage it induces across the body. For a reasonable current density, the behavior is linear so that Ohm's law remains valid. Intra- and extra-cellular fluids are mainly resistive, whereas cell membranes act as an insulator between these two compartments. Rare bioimpedance spectroscopy studies conducted in kidney graft recipients have shown a trend towards improved hydration after transplantation. We have been unable to find any study evaluating hydration changes in patients with acute kidney disease.

2. Theoretical and experimental models

2.1 Principles of bioimpédance in hemodialysis

Many different instruments have been marketed using algorithms based on different equations predicting body composition from impedance measurements [22, 23, 24, 25]. The validity of these different equations remains a question of debate since most have been established empirically. Moreover, the equations actually used by the algorithms of commercial microcomputers are not readily accessible, making it rather difficult to discuss their validity or make necessary corrections. The voltage produced by the current is measured to calculate the impedance. The relationships between impedance and other variables such as body water volume have been established using statistical correlations observed in specific populations rather than on a real biophysical basis. Actually, the theoretical basis can be summarized by the following statement: the human body is a complex conductive volume composed of heterogeneous tissues and intra- and extra-cellular compartments in perpetual movement.

Basically, the algorithms applied are based on regression laws used as a tool predictive of the relationship between two or more body variables constituting a database. Thus for total body water (TBW) the regression equation is written as [26](with H: Height):

$$TBW = a \,.\, H^2 / R + b \,.\, weight + c \,.\, Age + d \qquad (2)$$

TBW is measured in a large population using a gold standard, e.g. isotopic dilution (Fig. 3). The statistical software then uses regression analysis to establish the best fitting equation describing the relationship between TBW and the different measurements, e.g. height, weight, age, gender, resistance... For subsequent resistance measurements, a software inserts the recorded data into the accepted formula and delivers the results as TBW (Fig. 4).

2.1.1 Prediction of total body water

2.1.1.1 Historical background

One of the most commonly cited relationship is the cylinder model where the volume of a conductive cylinder is function of its length (L) and its resistance (R). High frequency current penetrates into the cell and runs across body fluids. A TBW value can thus be obtained by modeling the human body as a sum of cylinders. Devices applying this method are calibrated by dilution techniques. These devices rely on the following relationship:

$$TBW = \left(a.H^2\right) / R + c \qquad (3)$$

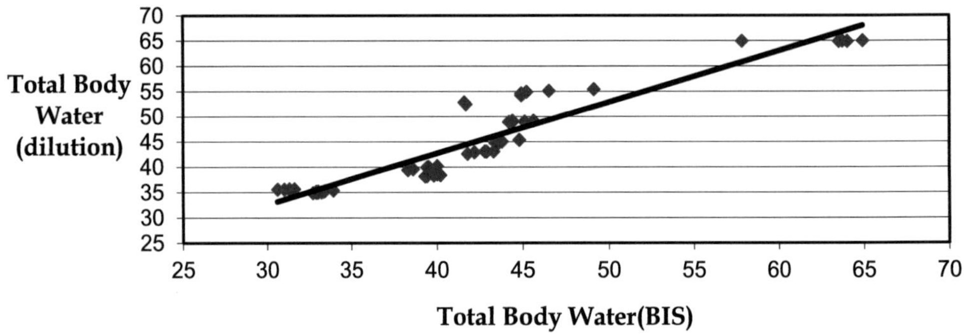

Fig. 3. Correlation between isotopic dilution and bioimpedance (BIS)

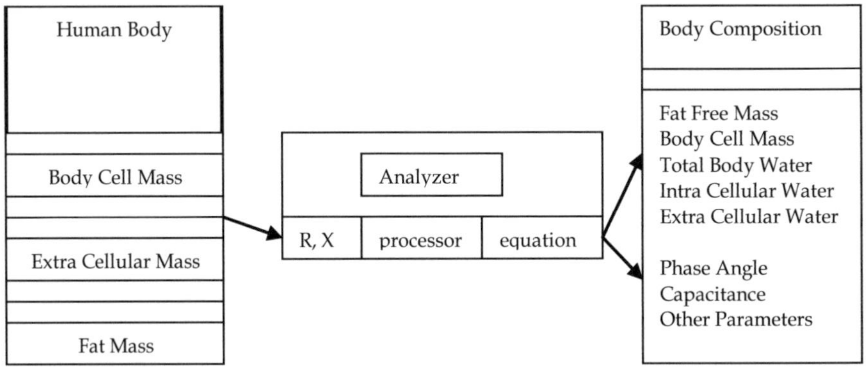

Fig. 4. Exemple of bioimpedance analysis block diagram [23] (R : resistance, X : Reactance)

Thomasset [27, 28] was the first, in 1963, to use two frequencies (1 et 100 kHz), to measure extracellular and total water respectively using the Cole-Cole model (Fig.5). Subsequently, several different formulas have been proposed based on regression equations.

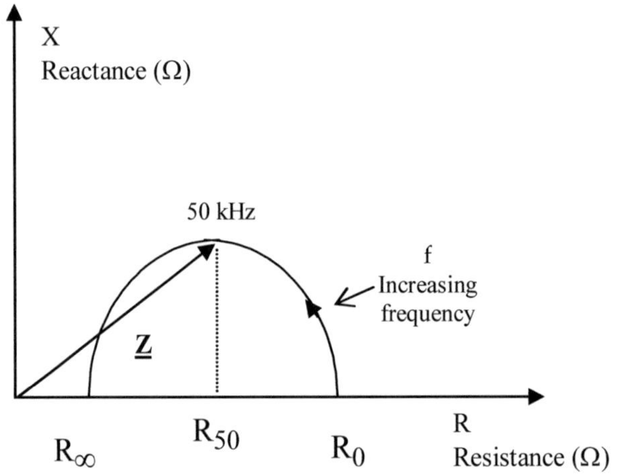

Fig. 5. Cole-Cole model

2.1.1.2 Theories used

Three techniques are generally described, using multiple frequencies, high and low frequencies, and a unique 50 kHz frequency.

The multifrequency mode is the most widely studied. It is based on the Cole-Cole model and allows differentiation between intra- and extra-cellular volumes. But the relationship between resistance and water volume is not linear, so that the multifrequency mode is associated with Hanaï theory, which takes into account the non-conductive element, connected in a parallel, to distinguish the different compartments. The parallel model described by Fricke takes into account the conductive elements exhibiting a certain degree of resistance connected in parallel and isolated by a cell membrane. This method has been validated by Van Loan [29, 30, 31]. At high and low frequencies, the Hanaï theory takes into account the presence of non-conductive elements connected in parallel. The measurement improvement mainly concerns the extracellular compartment [32, 33]. At the unique 50 kHz frequency, the theory enables a measurement of TBW (and lean body mass) [28]. Many different formulas have been published, using the term: H^2/R_{50}, where H is the subject's height in cm and R_{50} the wrist-ankle resistance. These methods have not been validated and generally cannot detect small volume changes. This limitation may be related to the relative uniformity of tissue elements considered in the formulas which do not take into consideration changes in tissue composition. Simple calculations allow extrapolations for extracellular water [34].

These different theories can then be applied to measure body segments or the whole body [35, 36, 37, 38]. For segmental measures, the mathematical models remain empirical and actual measures remain dependent on electrode position. Differences appear in comparison with whole body measures with a trend to underestimate water loss during a dialysis session compared with a segmental measurement, particularly in the event of hypotension [39]. One advantage is that the segmental technique would be less sensitive to changes in patient position from one measure to the next [40].

2.1.1.3 From theory to measure

The problem is then to transform a resistance measurement into a calculation of body composition. Geometry plays an important role. As seen in Figure 6, three objects with a constant height exhibit the same resistance from top to bottom, despite their different volumes [41].

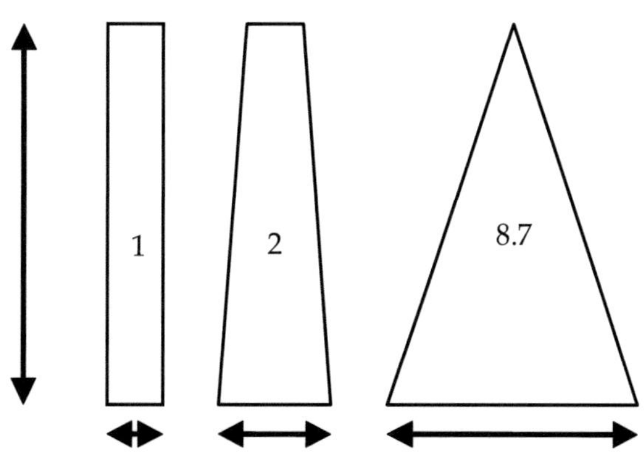

Fig. 6. Complexity of the body geometry-measurement relationship

Thus in many models, the human body is considered to be the sum of five compartments (Fig. 7) (the four limbs and the trunk), with a dimension homogeneity factor K_b.

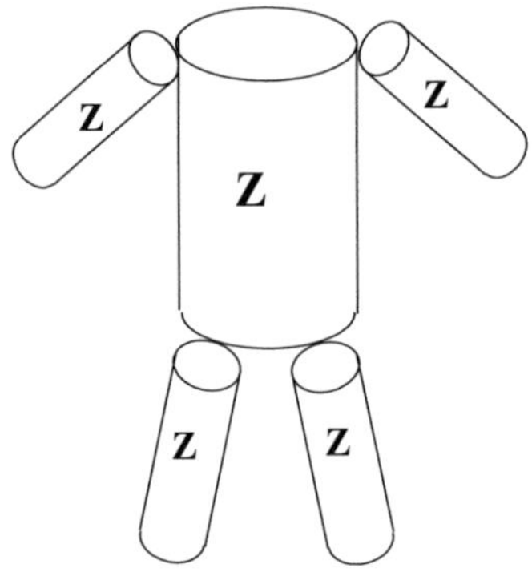

Fig. 7. The 5-compartment human body model

The homogeneity factor is calculated from the resistance of a cylinder (R) which is function of its resistivity (ρ), its length (L) and its cross-section (A) [42]

$$R = \rho \frac{L}{A} \tag{4}$$

Then, by calculating the volume of the cylinder, and separating, arms, legs and trunk, the following formula is established with *l* for leg, *t* for trunk and *a* for arm:

$$R = \rho 4\pi . \left(\frac{L_l}{C_l^2} + \frac{L_t}{C_t^2} + \frac{L_a}{C_a^2} \right) \tag{5}$$

This formula, together with the classical formula for the volume of a cylinder, yields the dimension homogeneity constant, K_B, which represents a characteristic anthropometric parameter independent of the electrical parameters.

$$V = K_B \rho \frac{L^2}{A} \tag{6}$$

$$K_b = \frac{1}{L^2} . \left(\frac{L_l}{C_l^2} + \frac{L_t}{C_t^2} + \frac{L_a}{C_a^2} \right) (2L_a C_a^2 + 2L_l C_l^2 + L_t C_t^2) \tag{7}$$

2.1.1.4 Formula validity and limitations

When these formulas are applied to measure body composition, the result is always significantly different from gold standard measurements. Thus Fenech [43] and Jaffrin [44] proposed a direct calculation of TBW using the same method as for extracellular water, assuming that TBW is a homogeneous quantity of fluid. The mean resistivity of this TBW was validated by comparison with body composition data obtained using the DEXA method. Jaffrin then raised the question of extrapolating total body resistance from the resistance value measured at 50 kHz [45], using a proportional intermediary multiplier.

Finally, the superiority of multifrequency impedance over the monofrequency impedance has not been demonstrated. Similarly no one formula has been found superior to the others.

2.2 Available clinical applications

Several studies have been conducted in hemodialysis patients. Three approaches have been particularly fruitful, the nomovolemia/hypervolemia curves established by Chamney [46, 47, 48, 49], the resistance/reactance curves by Piccoli [50, 51, 52] and Zhu's continuous curves [53, 54]. Although essential, these approaches will not be detailed here. Readers may usefully refer to the cited references.

2.2.1 Problems and solutions

2.2.1.1 Changes of body position

It has been shown that resistance/reactance curves are modified reversibly by changes in body position (reclining, sitting, upright position). Physical studies have demonstrated a modification in the lines of current passing through the body with changes in body position. In addition, length and resistance measures vary [55]. In the healthy subject, comparison of whole body and segmental measures shows an increase in resistance in all sectors (peripheral and central compartments) when moving from the upright to the reclining position [56, 57]. This is logical for the peripheral sector, related to the decrease in water in this sector which is redistributed to the central sector by cancelation of the gravity effect. However, surprisingly, resistance increases in the trunk, despite the increase in water. One explanation is that impedancemetry poorly evaluates the central sector. In the dialysis patient, and using the segmental mode, resistances vary with electrode position. The volumes calculated using the segmental mode are much higher than with the whole body mode and than with the anthropometric formulas [58]. In conclusion, segmental measures are insufficient to eliminate artifacts related to changes in body position.

2.2.1.2 Underestimation of extracellular volume variations in dialysis patients

These calculations are made from variations in plasma sodium content, accepting the hypothesis of zero sodium exchange between intra- and extra-cellular compartments or with the dialysis solute (obviously a false assumption). These results show that the contribution of the extracellular volume is superior to that measured by impedancemetry, with certain aberrant results [59, 60]. Conductivity variability is well known in dialysis and is most likely responsible for these problems of fluctuating resistivity for different compartments during dialysis.

3. Experimental materials and methods

3.1 Tanita (TBF-300)

Tanita (TBF-300) is a device for measuring body impedance between the two legs. It is simple to use and does not require electrodes. Manufactured in Japan, the devise presents as a weight scale with a built-in body composition analyzer which calculates TBW, total body fat and fat-free body mass [61]. The National Institute of Health has not validated the results. For these measurements, the person stands barefoot on a four-point platform. Impedance measurements are made using a high frequency (50kHz) and low intensity (500 μA) current between the feet. (formula are not known)

3.2 Body composition monitor

The body composition monitor (BCM) was developed by Fresenius® Medical Care. BCM is a rapid non-invasive 4-electrodes method for monitoring body composition by measuring the electrical impedance response to a multifrequency signal (50 frequencies from 5 kHz to 1 MHz). The Cole-Cole model is applied, with Hanaï mixture theory, to distinguish extracellular water (ECW), intracellular water (ICW) and total body water. Integrated software can also display over-hydration status. The device has been validated in healthy people, in comparison with reference methods (isotopic dilution).

The advantage of this device is to provide a quantitative diagnosis of over-hydration. The model is based on tissue hydration constants observed in the healthy individual which can then be applied to quantify excess water in kidney disease patients. The validation study, based on gold standard methods (bromide dilution for the extracellular compartment, deuterium dilution for TBW, potassium dilution for intracellular compartment and DEXA for fat mass), included 500 healthy subjects. The measures were then compared with the hemodialysis patient, before and after dialysis. This technique assumes that intracellular water, fat-free mass, and fat mass remain unchanged during the course of the dialysis session despite the ultrafiltration [62].

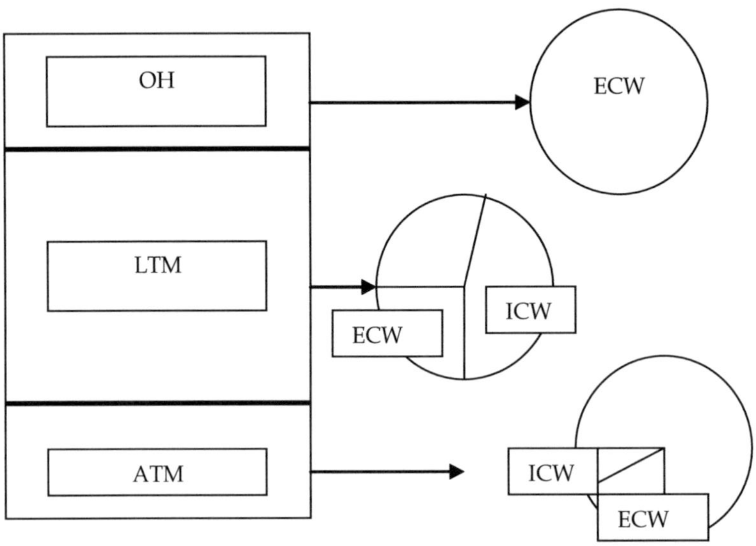

Fig. 8. Physiological model used by the body composition monitor (BCM) to determine the hydration constant of tissues and thus overhydration (OH). ATM: adipocyte tissue mass; LTM: lean tissue mass

The novel aspect of this model is the introduction of a third compartment corresponding to the excess fluid (Fig. 8) or over-hydration (OH) in comparison with the healthy individual. This over-hydration is considered to concern the extracellular compartment exclusively. Lean body mass contains exactly 73.2% water and includes the intra- and extra-cellular compartments, the intracellular compartment predominating. Lean body mass includes protein (muscles) and mineral (bone) matter. The sum of the intracellular compartment plus the protein mass defines the cell mass. Adipose tissue mass, or fat mass, contains 26.8% water, the extracellular compartment predominates. The notion of a third compartment avoids the problems related to the fact that the ratio between the extracellular and

intracellular water is not constant. Comparing total and extracellular water measurements obtained in the healthy population and in the dialysis population defines the notion of over-hydration. Time-course curves of the different compartments provide a picture of the evolving state of hydration.
In Figure 9, the notion of hydration status in the dialysis patient is combined with systolic blood pressure. Four sectors are defined. I: over-hydration and hypertension, II: normo-hydration and hypertension, III: normo-hydration and normo-tension IV: over-hydration and normo- or hypo-tension. Trends can be plotted.

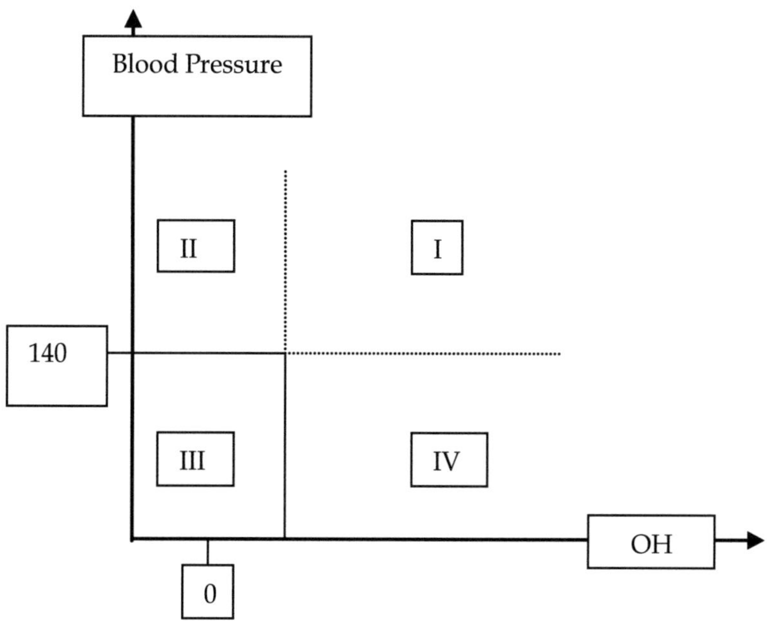

Fig. 9. Hydration reference

3.3 Experimental works and results
3.3.1 Hemodialysis patients

3.3.1.1 Elaborating a dry-weight index using Tanita

We first used the Tanita TBF-300 analyzer to obtain bioimpedance measures in 238 hemodialysis sessions. The mean total body water (TBW) was 41.9±7.9 kg before sessions and 39.6±7.3 kg after sessions. Mean body weight was 76.6±18.2 kg before and 74.2±17.1 kg after. Statistically, body weight remained stable during this study and was thus valid for assessing reliability. This enabled the definition of patient populations used to hypothesize the pathophysiology of hyperhydration, dehydration and normohydration state based on a body-weight index (Fig.10). Change in weight (ΔW) and TBW (ΔTBW) was noted and compared with ultrafiltration. In theory, these three variables should be similar, because during dialysis sessions, the ultrafiltration applied corresponds to a subtraction of water, and consequently to the change in w or TBW before and after the water depletion. But net ultrafiltration and ΔW correlated poorly (c=0.62) with ΔTBW. This led to the definition of a dry-weight index, I. It was hypothesized that this Index would be 0 when patients reach their dry weight: **I = ΔW– ΔTBW**

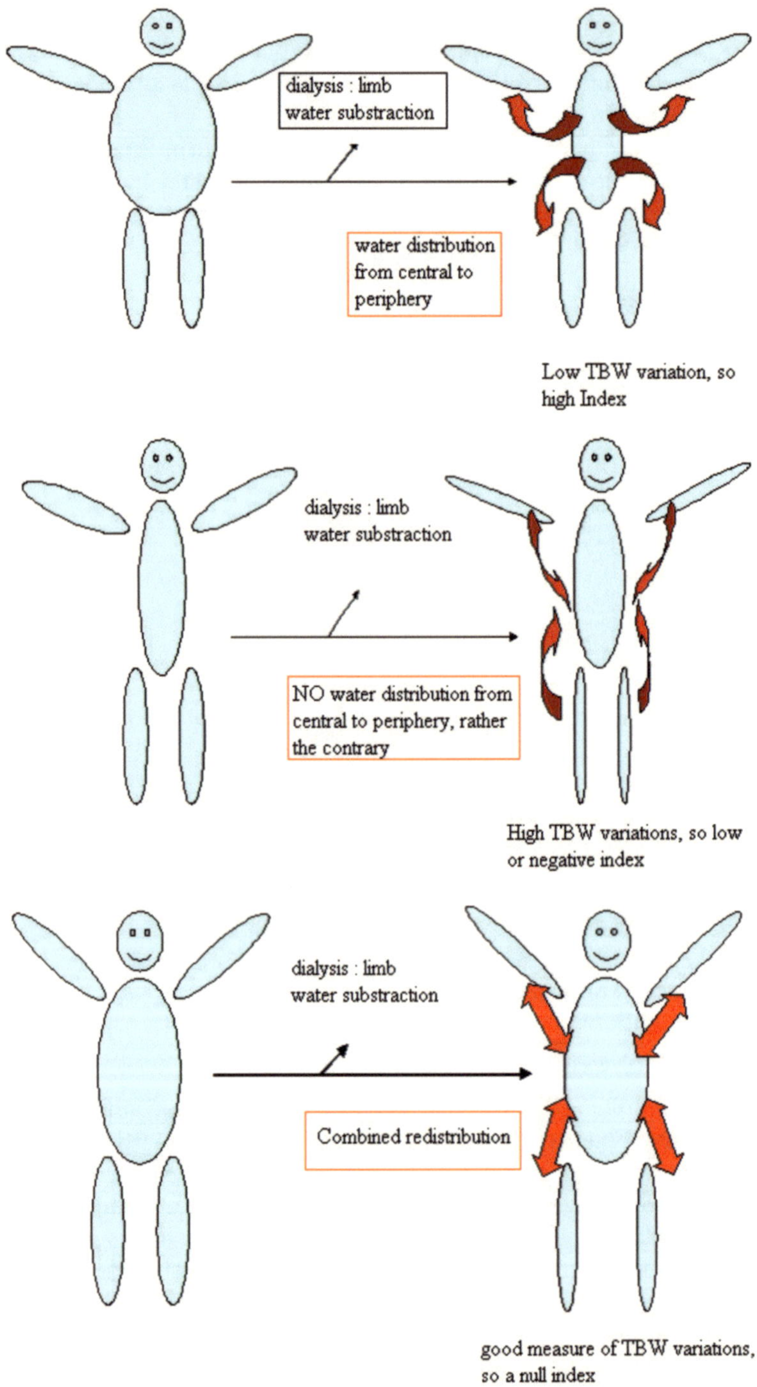

Fig. 10. Pathophysiology of hydration state. **upper panel:** hyperhydration; **middle panel**: dehydration; **lower panel**: normo-hydration. TBW = total body water, W = body weight. Dry-weight index : $\mathbf{I = \Delta W - \Delta TBW}$

3.3.1.2 Body composition monitoring of the elderly hemodialysis patients

Body composition was monitored for a 1.5-month period under standardized conditions in 10 hemodialysis patients aged over 80 years with the BCM. The data collected (Table 1) showed that these elderly patients exhibited a different water distribution pattern during ultrafiltration and also different refilling behavior. Thus ultrafiltration did not fully reflect changes in over-hydration. The only valid and clearly coherent measures were those recorded before the dialysis session. While the Cole-Cole model remained valid, implanted devices or specific clinical situations such as heart failure affected the impedance results. Pacemaker behavior (patient n° 8) was unaffected by the very small current used, but the presence of conductive metal (orthopedic prosthesis in patient 10) modified the bioimpedance measures. In such patients, change in weight and ultrafiltration followed a similar pattern, but TBW recordings were obviously incorrect in light of the weight loss (Table 1) and the over-hydration diagnosis (Table 2).

	Δ Weight (kg)		**UF (l)**		**Δ TBW (l)**		**Δ ECW (l)**		**Δ ICW (l)**	
	mean	***SD***	**mean**	***SD***	**mean**	***SD***	**mean**	***SD***	**mean**	***SD***
patient 1	2,03	*0,36*	2,1	*0,59*	2,5	*0,96*	2,07	*0,47*	0,47	*0,47*
patient 2	1,22	*0,2*	1,22	*0,32*	1,26	*0,41*	1,12	*0,19*	0,16	*0,29*
patient 9	1,43	*0,68*	1,76	*0,72*	1,53	*0,46*	1,2	*0,62*	0,3	*0,82*
patient 3	1,58	*0,3*	1,3	*0,23*	0,78	*0,43*	0,55	*0,06*	0,23	*0,46*
patient 5	1,52	*0,51*	1,28	*0,31*	0,46	*1,46*	0,82	*0,48*	-0,3	*0,17*
patient 6	2,9	*0,29*	2,8	*0,15*	1	*0,71*	1,85	*0,35*	-0,95	*1,06*
patient 10	1,3	*0,99*	1,52	*0,55*	0,77	*0,75*	0,6	*0,36*	0,17	*0,42*
patient 4	1,33	*0,22*	1,18	*0,16*	2,7	*0*	1,7	*0,17*	0,97	*0,15*
patient 8	2,63	*0,43*	2,34	*0,34*	6,83	*2,48*	1,5	*0,53*	5,43	*2,94*
patient 7	1,53	*2,19*	0,72	*0,19*	0,78	*0,57*	1	*0,68*	-0,25	*0,17*

Table 1. Participation of fluid compartments during ultrafiltration (UF)

Four patient profiles could be identified from the data presented in Table 1.

- Patients 1, 2 and 9 exhibited good correlation between weight loss, applied ultrafiltration, and TBW variation during dialysis sessions.
- Patients 3, 5, 6 and 10 exhibited a different type of behavior. The decline in TBW from the beginning to the end of the dialysis session was underestimated as compared with the variation in weight or applied ultrafiltration.
- Inversely, for patients 4 and 8, the decline in TBW during dialysis was overestimated, compared with the very similar variations in weight or ultrafiltration.
- In one patient (n° 7), ultrafiltration and TBW correlated well with each other, but not with weight loss.

As expected, dialysis-related water depletion mainly involved a reduction of the extracellular compartment compared with the intracellular compartment. This well-known phenomenon is called refilling. In three patients (n° 5, 6 and 7), the bioimpedance measures predicted fluid overload in the intracellular compartment, with a smaller fall in TBW than in extracellular water. This might be related to a "reverse refilling" phenomenon. For patient n° 8 who had a pacemaker, fluid removal seemed to occur exclusively from the intracellular compartment.

	OH before (l)		OH after (l)	
	mean	*SD*	**mean**	*SD*
patient 1	0,1	*0,49*	-1,77	*0,55*
patient 2	1,7	*0,21*	0,72	*0,13*
patient 3	0,78	*0,11*	0,53	*0,21*
patient 4	0,98	*0,29*	-0,17	*0,12*
patient 5	0,72	*0,33*	-0,1	*0,39*
patient 6	2,6	*0,71*	0,57	*0,15*
patient 7	0,62	*0,63*	-0,15	*0,77*
patient 8	0,5	*1,59*	1,63	*0,8*
patient 9	0,84	*0,65*	-0,2	*0,26*
patient 10	-0,6	*0,12*	-0,97	*0,21*

Table 2. Body composition monitoring (BCM) diagnosis of over-hydration (OH) status

The over-hydration data presented in Table 2 show that, according to the BCM findings, all patients except two (n° 8 and 10), were over-hydrated at dialysis onset and underhydrated at dialysis end. Comparing the clinical diagnosis of over-hydration established by the nephrologist programming the ultrafiltration at the beginning of the session (Table 1) with the over-hydration status diagnosis established by BCM before dialysis (Table 2) revealed different trends. The nephrologist tended to overestimate over-hydration before dialysis while the BCM tended towards an underestimation. At the end of the ultrafiltration six of the patients were dehydrated, but not far from their dry weight, with a difference of ≤0.5 liters from normo-hydration.

3.3.2 Body composition monitoring in living-donor transplant recipients

We prospectively studied five transplanted patients who had received a living-donor graft after a period of hemodialysis. These five patients had exhibited particularly rapid recovery of normal renal function after transplantation. We took bioimpedance measures before surgery and several times during a mean 2-months period after transplantation. Our findings produced a bell-shaped curve showing weight gain with increasing over-hydration followed by weight loss with normo-hydration, in correlation with the normalization of kidney graft function (Table 3).

BCM diagnosis	Day 1 post-transplantation	Day 50 post-transplantation
Over-hydration	1.04±0.7 liters	0.56±0.3 liters

Table 3. Over-hydration after kidney transplantation

Clinically, the patients' blood pressure improved and edema disappeared. For example, one patient weighed 48.4 kg on day 4 post-transplantation and 47.3 kg on day 10. There was a reduction of the hyperhydration, the Cole-Cole curves shifting to the right (Fig. 11), and an increase in maximal reactance (X) (from 50.6 to 62.5 Ohm). The frequency at which this reactance reached its maximum also declined from 60 kHz to 50 kHz, a frequency which is commonly observed in normo-hydration subjects.

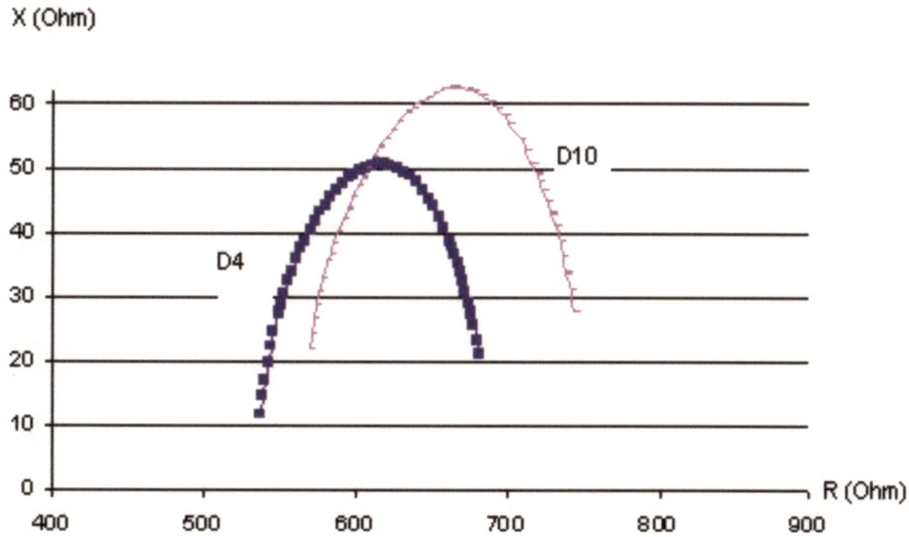

Fig. 11. Cole-Cole time curves after kidney transplantation. In blue at Day 4 post transplantation (OH +0.5), in red at Day 10 post transplantation (OH +0.6)

3.3.3 Body composition monitoring in acute kidney failure

We studied three patients with acute reversible kidney disease. Body composition monitoring was started at the time of the acute disease and continued to the recovery period. Results (impedance, reactance, phase shift, Cole-Cole curve) showed an over-hydration period that disappeared with the normalization of kidney function. The time course of improved hydration status in this patient is represented in Figure 12. Over-hydration and weight variations followed the same pattern, rising and declining in parallel.

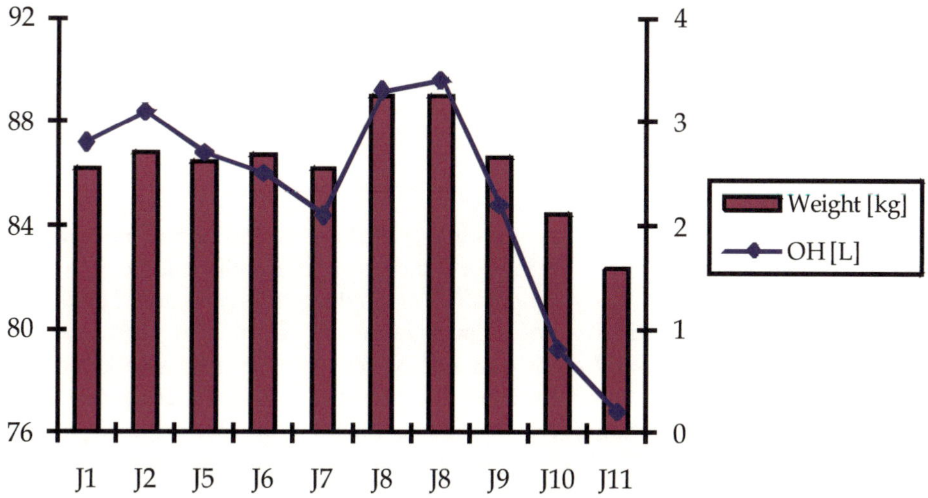

Fig. 12. Hydration status time course in a patient recovering normal kidney function.

	Day 1	Day 11
weight (kg)	86.2	82.3
Over-hydration (Kg)	2.8	0.2
Maximal reactance	25	37.7
Resistance (Ohm)	410	540
Frequency (kHz)	67	5O

Table 4. Resistance and frequency values at maximal reactance

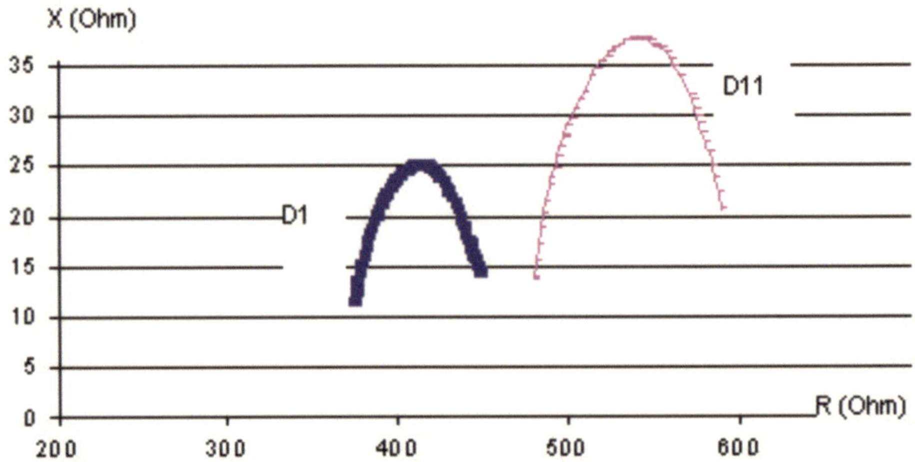

Fig. 13. Cole-Cole curves with recovery of kidney function from Day 1 (blue) to Day 11 (red)

Figure 13 also shows that the Cole-Cole curves shifted to the right as hydration status returned to normal. This right shift being the expression of lesser hyperhydration. On day 1, the resistance levels at 0 and ∞ frequency went from 450 to 370 Ohms with a maximum reactance of 26 for a resistance of 410. By day 11, the curves had shifted to the right, corresponding to lesser hyperhydration, weight loss, and a diagnosis of lower over-hydration. These values ranged from 590 to 480 Ohms and maximal reactance of 37.7 with a corresponding resistance at 540 (Table 4). These physical elements also corresponded to clinical reality since blood pressure levels returned to normal with involution of lower limbs edema.

4. Conclusion

Bioimpedance is an easy-to-use tool providing a useful evaluation of patients' dry weight. The method remains limited due to the lack of standards of normality. Moreover, changes in electrolytes, red cells, protein, body temperature or implanted devices affect bioimpedance measures, further compromising use of bioimpedance for determining the dry weight or normal hydration level of hemodialysis patients. Nevertheless, measurable values such as impedance, reactance, or phase shift enable the identification of patient groups and the description of trends. Impedance, reactance and phase shift can be used to identify population groups with similar behavior patterns useful for determining dry weight or detecting hydration disorders. Analysis of correlations between physical data and clinical findings is another point of interest discussed in this chapter.

5. References

[1] Charra, B. (1998). "Dry weight in dialysis": the history of a concept. Nephrol Dial Transplant, Vol 7, pp.1882-1885

[2] Wabel, P.; Moissl, U.; Chamney, P.; Jirka, T.; Machek, P.; Ponce, P. & Wizemann, V. (2008). Towards improved cardiovascular management: the necessity of combining blood pressure and fluid overload. Nephrol Dial Transplant, Vol 23, pp.2965-2971

[3] Kooman, J.; Van des Sande, F. & Leunissen, K. (2009). *Wet or dry in dialysis-Can new technologies help*. Seminars in Dialysis, Vol 22, No.1, (January 2009), pp.9-12, Maastricht, The Netherlands

[4] McGee, S.; Abernethy, Wb. & Simel, DL. (1999). The rational clinical examination. Is this patient hypovolemic? JAMA, Vol 281, pp.1022-1029

[5] Ishibe, S.; Peixoto, A. (2004). Methods of assessment of volume status and intercompartmental fluid shifts in hemodialysis patients: implications in clinical practise. Seminars in Dialysis, Vol 17, No.1, (January 2004), pp.37-43

[6] Kraemer, M. (2006). A new model for the determination of fluid status and body composition from bioimpedance measurements. Physiol Measurement, Vol 27, pp.901-919

[7] Jaffrin, M.Y, Fenech, M., de Fremont, J.F. & Tolani, M. (2002). Continuous monitoring of plasma, interstitial and intracellular fluid volumes in dialyzed patients by bio-impedance and hematocrit measurements. ASAIO J, Vol, 48, pp.326-333

[8] Morucci, JP.; Chauveau, N. ; Rigaud, B. ; Felice, C. & Marcili, P. (1996). Bioelectrical impedance techniques in medicine. Crit Rev Biomed Eng, Vol 24, pp.257-677

[9] Cole, K. (1928). Electrical impedance of suspension of spheres. J Gen Physiol, Vol 12, pp. 29-36

[10] Cole, K. (1934). Alternating current conductance and direct current excitation of nerve. Science, Vol 79, pp.164-165

[11] Cole, K. (1940). Permeability and impermeability of cell membranes for ions. Cold Spring Harbor Symp. Quant. Biol Vol 8, pp. 110-122

[12] Foster, K.R. & Schwan, H.P. (1994). Dielectric properties of tissues. In C Polk, E Postow (eds), Handbook of Biological Effects of Electromagnetic Fields, 2d ed

[13] Fricke, H. (1925). A mathematical treatment of the electrical conductivity and capacity of disperse system. II. The capacity of a suspension of conducting speroids surrounded by a nonconducting membrane for a current of low frequency. Phys Rev, Vol 26, pp. 678-681

[14] Ho, LT.; Kushner, RF.; Schoeller, DA.; Gudivaka, R. & Spiegel, DM. (1994). Bioimpedance analysis of total body water in hemodialysis patients. Kidney, Vol 46, pp.1438-1442

[15] Zhu, F.; Schneditz, D. & Levin NW. (1999). Sum of segmental bioimpedance analysis during ultrafiltration and hemodialysis reduces sensitivity to changes in body position. Kidney Int, Vol 56, pp.692-699

[16] Zhu, F.; Schneditz, D.; Wang, E.; Martin, K.; Morris, AT. & Levin, NW. (1998).Validation of changes in extracellular volume measured during hemodialysis using a segmental bioimpedance technique. ASAIO J, Vol 44, pp541-545

[17] Chanchairujira, T. & Mehta, RL.(2001) Assessing fluid change in hemodialysis: whole body versus sum of segmental bioimpedance spectroscopy. Kidney Int, Vol 60, pp.2337-2342

[18] Gudivaka, R.; Schoeller, D.; Kushner, R. & Bolt, M. (1999). Single- and multifrequency models for bioelectrical impedance analysis of body water compartments. J Appl Physiol, Vol 87, pp.1087-1096

[19] Chertow, G.; Lazarus, J.; Lew, N.; Ma, L. & Lowrie E. (1997). Bioimpedance norms for the hemodialysis population. Kidney Int, Vol 52, pp.1617-1621

[20] Buchholz, A.; Bartok, C. & Schoeller, D. (2004). The validity of bioelectrical impedance models in clinical populations. Nutr Clin Pract, Vol 19, p.433-446

[21] Shulman, T., Heidenheim, A., Kianfar, C., Shulman, S. & Lindsay, R. (2001). Preserving central blood volume changes in body fluid compartments during hemodialysis. ASAIO J, Vol 47, pp. 615-618

[22] Lafargue, L.A., Cabrales, L.B. & Larramendi, R.M. (2002). Bioelectrical parameters of the whole human body obtained through bioelectrical impedance analysis. Bioeelectromagnetics, Vol 23, pp.450-454

[23] Aloia, J.F., Vaswabi, A., Flaster, E. & Ma, R. (1998). Relationship of body water compartments to age, race, and fat-free mass. J Lab Clin Med, Vol 132, pp.483-490

[24] Basile, C., Vernaglione, L., Di Lorio, B., Bellizzi, V., Chimienti, D., Lomonte, C., Rubino, A. & D'Ambrosino, N. (2007). Development and validation of bioimpedance analysis prediction equation for dry weight in hemodialysis patients. Clin J Am Soc Nephrol, Vol 2, pp.675-680

[25] Lukaski, H.C. (1996). Biological indexes considered in the derivation of the bioelectrical impednce analysis. Am J Clin Nutr, Vol 64, pp.397-404

[26] Kushner, R.F. & Schoeller, D.A. (1986). Estimation of total body water by bioelectrical impedance analysis. Am J Clin Nutr, Vol 44, pp.417-424

[27] Thomasset, A. (1963). Bio-electrical properties of tissue impedance measurements. Lyon Med, Vol 209, pp.1325-1352

[28] Hoffer, E.C., Meador, C.K. & Simpson, D.C. (1969). Correlation of whole-body impedance with total body water volume. J Appl Physiol, Vol 27, pp.531-534

[29] Van Loan, M.D., Withers, P., Matthie, J. & Mayclin, P.L. (1993). Use of bioimpedance spectroscopy to determine extracellular fluid (ECF), intracellular fluid (ICF), total body water (TBW), and fat free mass (FFM). In: human body composition: in vivo methods, models and assessment , edited by Ellis, K.J. & Eastman, J.D., pp.67-70, New York: Plenum

[30] Van Marken Lichtenbelt, W.D., Westerterp, K.R., Wouters, L. & Luijendijk, S. (1994). Validation of bioelectrical impedance measurements as a method to estimate body-water compartments. Am J Clin Nutr, Vol 60, pp.159-166

[31] Ho, L.T., Kushner, R., Schoeller, A., Gudivaka, R. & Spiegel, D.M. (1994). Bioimpedance analysis of total body water in hemodialysis patients. Kidney Int, Vol 46, pp.1438-1442

[32] Deurenberg, P., Andreoli, A. & De Lorenzo, A. (1996). Multifrequency bioelectrical impedance: a comparison between the Cole-Cole modeling and Hanaï equations with the classical impedance index approach. Ann Hum Biol, Vol 6, pp.31-40

[33] Segal, K.R., Burastero, S., Chun, A., Coronel, P., Pierson, R.N. Jr, & Wang, J. (1991). Estimation of extracellular and total body water by multiple-frequency bioelectrical -impedance measurement. Am J Clin nutr, Vol 54, pp.26-29

[34] Lukaski, H.C. & Bolonchuk, W.W. (1988). Estimation of body fluid volumes using tetrapolar bioelectrical impedance measurements. Aviat Space Environ Med, Vol 59, pp.1163-1169

[35] Park, J. Yang, W.S., Kim, S.B., Paark, S.K., Lee, S.K., Park, J.S. & Chang, J.W. (2008). Usefulness of segmental bioimpedance ration to determine dry body weight in new hemodialysis patients: a pilot study. Am J of Nephrol, Vol 29, pp.25-30

[36] Levin, N.W., Zhu, F., Seibert, E., Ronco, C. & Kuhlmann, M.K. (2005). Use of segmental multifrequency spectroscopy in hemeodialysis. Contrib to Nephrol, Vol 149, pp.162-167

[37] Chanchairujira, T. & Mehta, R.L. (2001). Assessing fluid change in hemodialysis : whole body versus sum of segmental bioimpedance spectroscopy. Kidney Int, Vol 60, pp.2337-2342

[38] Zhu, F., Ronco, C., Schneditz, D., De Simone, L. & Levin, N.W. (2000). Estimation of dry body weight by segmental bioimpedance analysis during hemodialysis. ASAIO J; Vol 46, pp.221

[39] Zaluska, W.T., Schneditz, D. & Kaufman, A.M. (1998). Relative underestimation of fluid removal during hemodialysis hypotension measured by whole body bioimpedance. ASAIO J, Vol 44, pp.823-827

[40] Zhu, F., Schneditz, D. & Levin, N.W. (1999). Sum of segmental bioimpednce analysis during ultrafiltration and hemodialysis reduces sensitivity to changes in body position. Kidney Int, Vol 56, pp.692-699

[41] Foster, K.R. & Lukeaski, H.C. (1996). Whole-body impedance-what does it measure? Am J Clin Nutr, Vol 64, pp.388-396

[42] De Lorenzo, A., Andreoli, A., Matthie, J. & Withers, P. (1997). Predicting body cell mass with bioimpedance by using theoretical methods : a technological review. J Appl Physiol, Vol 82, pp.1542-1558

[43] Jaffrin, M.Y. & Morel, H. (2008). Body fluid volumes measurements by impedance: a review of bioimpedance spectroscopy (BIS) and bioimpedance analysis (BIA) methods. Med Eng Phys, doi: 10.1016/j.medengphy.2008.06.009

[44] Jaffrin, M.Y., Fenech, M., Moreno, M.V. & Kieffer, R. (2006). Total body water measurement by a modification of the bioimpedance spectroscopy method. Med Biol Eng Comput, Vol 44, PP.873-882

[45] Morel, H. & Jaffrin, M.Y. (2008). A bridge from bioimpedance spectroscopy to 50 kHz bioimpedance analysis: application to total body water measurements. Physiol Meas, Vol 29, pp.465-478

[46] Matthie, J.R. (2005). Second generaation mixture theory equation for estimating intracellular water using bioimpedance spectroscopy. J Appl Physiol, Vol 99, 780-781

[47] Matthie, J.R., Zaroutz, B. &De Lorenzo, A. (1998). Analytic assessment of various bioimpedance methods used to estimate body water. J Appl Physiol, Vol 84, PP.1801-1816

[48] Moissl, U.M., Wabel, P., Chamney, P.W., Bosaeus, I. & Levin, N.W. (2006). Body fluid volume determination via body composition spectroscopy in health and disease. Physiol Meas, Vol 27, pp.921-933

[49] Chamney, P.W., Krämer, M, Rode, C., Kleinekofort, W. & Wizemann, V. (2002). A new technique for establisching dry weight in hemodialysis patients via whole body bioimpedance. Kidney Int, Vol 61, pp.2250-2258
[50] Piccoli, A. (1998). Identification of opèrational clues to dry weight prescription in hemodialysis using bioimpedance vector analysis. Kidney Int, Vol 53, pp.1036-1043
[51] Epstein, B.R. & Foster K.R. (1983). Anisotropy in the dielectric properties of skeletal muscle. Med Biol Eng Comp, Vol 21, pp.51-55
[52] Piccoli, A., Pastori, G. & Guizzo, M. (2005). Equivalence of information from single versus multiple frequency bioimpedance vector analysis in hemodialysis. Kidney Int, Vol 67, pp.301-313
[53] Zhu, F., Kuhlmann, M.K. & Sarkars, S. (2004). Adjustment of dry weight in hemodialysis patients using intradialytic continuous multifrequency bioimpedance of the calf. Int J Artif Organs, Vol 27, pp.104-109
[54] Zhu, F., Leonard, E.F. & Levin, N.W. (2005). Body composition modeling in the calf using an equivalent circuit model of multi-frequency bioimpedance analysis. Physiol Meas, Vol 26, pp.133-143
[55] Zhu, F.; Schneditz, D., Wang, E. & Levin NW. (1998). Dynamics of segmental extracellular volumes during changes in body position by bioimpedance analysis. J Appl Physiol, Vol 85, pp.497-504
[56] Zhu, F., Kuhlmann, M.K., Kaysen, G.A., Sarkar, S., Kaitwatcharachai, C., Khilnani, R., Stevens, L., Leonard, E.F., Wang, J., Heymsfield, S. & Levin N.W. (2006). Segment-specific resistivity improves body fluid volume estimates from bioimpedance spectroscopy in hemodialysis patients. J Appl Physiol, Vol 100, pp.717-724
[57] Scharfetter, H., Monif, M., Laszlo, Z., Lambauer, T., Hutten, H. & Hinghofer-Szalkay, H. (1997). Effect of postural changes on the reliability of volumes estimations from bioimpedance spectroscopy data. Kidney Int, Vol 51, pp.1078-1087
[58] Chertow, G.M., Lazarus, J.M., Lew, N.L., Ma, L. & Lowrir E.G. (1997). Bioimpedance norms for the hemodialysis population. Kidney Int, Vol 52, pp.1617-1621
[59] Kyle, U.G., Bosaeus, I, De Lorenzo, A;, Deurenberg, P., Elia, M;, Gomez, J.F., Heitmann, B.L., Kent-Smith, L., Malchior, J.C., Pirlich, M., Scharfetter, H., Schols, A. & Pichard, C. (2004). Bioelectrical impedance analysis-part I: review of principles and methods. Clin Nutr, Vol 23, pp.1226-1243
[60] Kyle, U.G., Bosaeus, I, De Lorenzo, A;, Deurenberg, P., Elia, M;, Gomez, J.F., Heitmann, B.L., Kent-Smith, L., Malchior, J.C., Pirlich, M., Scharfetter, H., Schols, A. & Pichard, C. (2004). Bioelectrical impedance analysis-part II: utilization in clinical practise. Clin Nutr, Vol 23, pp.1430-1453
[61] Jebb, S.A., Cole, T.J., Doman, D., Murgatroyd, P.R. & Prentice, A.M. (2000). Evaluation of the novel Tanita body-fat analyser to measure body composition by comparision with a four-compartment model. British J of Nutr, Vol 83, pp.115-122
[62] Chamney P.W., Wabel, P., Moissl, U.M., Müller, M.J., Bosy-Westphal, A., Korth, O. & Fuller, N.J. (2007). A whole-body model to distinguish excess fluid from the hydration of major body tissues. Am J Clin Nutr, Vol 85, pp.80-89

11

Management of Fluid Status in Haemodialysis Patients: The Roles of Technology and Dietary Advice

Elizabeth Lindley, Lynne Aspinall, Claire Gardiner and Elizabeth Garthwaite
Department of Renal Medicine, Leeds Teaching Hospitals NHS Trust
United Kingdom

1. Introduction

The kidneys play a vital role in maintaining normal tissue hydration and serum sodium level. In haemodialysis patients, with impaired or absent kidney function, fluid status is managed by removing excess fluid using ultrafiltration and by restricting dietary sodium intake. Ideally, haemodialysis patients should remain close to normal hydration throughout the interdialytic period, with minimal periods of excessive dehydration or fluid overload and with no fluid-related co-morbidity.

Optimal fluid management is achieved by adjusting the post-dialysis 'target' weight and, where necessary, limiting the fluid gained between dialysis sessions. While clinical history and examination remain the basis for prescribing the target weight, technology can provide useful objective information especially where the clinical indications are ambiguous. A simple non-invasive test can now be carried out when a patient attends for dialysis enabling staff to pick up changes in body composition so that their target weight can be adjusted to maintain optimal fluid status.

In most patients, interdialytic fluid gain (IDFG) is directly related to sodium intake. Acceptable fluid gains can usually be achieved by limiting salt intake to the recommended daily allowance for the general population and avoiding unnecessary sodium loading during dialysis. Low pre-dialysis serum sodium levels can help identify patients with other causes of high IDFG, such as high blood sugar or social drinking, who need additional counselling. For the patients, lowering sodium intake may also improve blood pressure control and reduce requirements for antihypertensive medication. Staff education, and preferably participation, is vital when implementing salt restriction in a haemodialysis unit.

2. Optimisation of the target weight

2.1 What is meant by target weight?

A typical definition found on patient-focussed websites is 'the weight your doctor thinks you would be when all the extra fluid is removed from your body'(DaVita, n.d.). This actually defines the 'normally hydrated' weight which is a very useful concept but not necessarily the weight the patient should achieve post-dialysis.

Most publications aimed at professionals define the target weight as the lowest weight a patient can tolerate without the development of symptoms or hypotension (Henderson, 1980). Variations of this definition have appeared in publications for over 30 years though it is unhelpful in those patients who are hypotensive when clearly fluid overloaded based on other clinical assessments. It also suggests that patients should be dehydrated to the point at which they become symptomatic regardless of the effect on residual renal function (RRF).

The importance of preserving RRF is undisputed in peritoneal dialysis (Marrón et al, 2008) but, until recently, it has been widely assumed that RRF is of no significance once a patient has started haemodialysis. Bioincompatible membranes and contaminated dialysis fluid probably did contribute to accelerated loss of RRF in haemodialysis. However with modern technology both single centre (Vilar et al, 2009) and national (van der Wal et al, 2011) studies have shown that RRF can be preserved in haemodialysis, and that loss of RRF is a powerful a predictor of mortality (Brener et al, 2010).

A more holistic definition of target weight is the post-dialysis weight that enables the patient to remain close to normal hydration throughout the interdialytic period, without experiencing discomfort or compromising residual function.

2.2 Clinical indicators of hydration status

Regular clinical assessments are an essential element in the overall management of haemodialysis patients. Table 1 lists the parameters that are typically used to assess fluid status and which should be reviewed regularly whether or not there are concerns about the patient's fluid status.

Parameter	Fluid overload	Fluid depletion
Trend in body weight	Recent weight loss Anorexia, hospital admission Nausea, vomiting, diarrhoea	Recent weight gain Improved appetite Nutritional support started
Residual renal function	Usually minimal or absent	May be significant
Blood pressure	May be elevated	May be low
Neck veins	Full	Usually flat
Breathing	May be breathless May be unable to lie flat	Usually breathing normally
Oedema	May have facial oedema May have ankle/hand oedema	No generalised oedema
Intradialytic problems	May have intradialytic hypotension	May be unable to achieve target weight May have cramps, dizziness
Post-dialysis problems	Usually recovers quickly May have headaches	Usually feels washed out May be thirsty, have croaky voice
Chest X-ray (if available)	May show enlarged heart	Usually shows normal heart

Table 1. Parameters used in a typical clinical assessment of fluid status

Unfortunately haemodialysis patients often have co-morbidity that can make the signs of fluid status ambiguous. Heart failure can lead to low blood pressure in a patient with severe fluid overload while an inadequately blocked renin-angiotensin system can lead to high blood pressure in a patient who is dehydrated. Many patients with fluid overload show no obvious signs of oedema and have no breathing difficulties, while chest infections or anaemia can cause breathlessness in fluid depleted patients.

Where the clinical assessment is not straightforward, as in the patient who is hypotensive but clearly oedematous, technology can provide objective information to help inform the appropriate adjustment of target weight (Charra, 2007; Jaeger and Metha, 1999). This chapter covers the technology that is commercially available and intended for routine use in the out-patient haemodialysis setting.

2.3 Continuous blood volume monitoring

Blood volume monitoring (BVM) was introduced in the 1990's. The monitors used ultrasonic or optical sensors to measure changes in haematocrit in the arterial blood line. An increase in haematocrit during dialysis indicates a decrease in blood volume. BVM was intended to alert staff (or automatically adjust the machine) when poor refilling of the intravascular space from the tissues led to an excessive drop in blood volume as fluid was removed by ultrafiltration. However, on introducing BVM, many units found a significant proportion of the patients appeared to be chronically fluid overloaded.

When fluid accumulates in the body, most of the excess is contained in the extracellular space. Figure 1 shows how the blood volume changes as the extracellular fluid volume increases. Initially there is a steady increase in blood volume, but at about 7 litres the intravascular space is unable to accommodate any more fluid and the blood volume remains constant and all additional fluid is stored in the tissues. If the BVM shows no change in blood volume while a significant amount of fluid is removed, this gives a clear diagnosis of severe fluid overload. When BVM was introduced in St James's Hospital in Leeds, approximately 20% of patients were found to be overloaded on the first measurement. They were usually asymptomatic with blood pressure controlled using medication. In most cases the patient's target weight was successfully decreased.

The 'flat-line' BVM when removing fluid gives an unequivocal indication of fluid overload. A falling BVM trace has to be interpreted with caution for a number of reasons. At best, the BVM can only tell you how easily the patient is refilling as fluid is removed. A patient may be overloaded but not refilling adequately which could lead staff to believe they are normally hydrated or dry. Redistribution of blood from the central to the micro-circulation (e.g. to the splanchnic circulation when eating) can look like a rapid drop in blood volume. This is because the lower haematocrit in capillaries causes haemoconcentration in the central vessels (Mitra et al, 2004) from which the blood is taken to the dialysis machine. Patients may become symptomatic as a result of redistribution of blood, but the solution is not to increase target weight.

Other problems that can occur when using BVM to assess fluid status are interpretation of overhydration in patients with good residual function who have minimal change in blood volume because they required little fluid removal, and confusing dehydration with normal hydration. The latter occurs because, as shown in figure 1, the rate of change in blood volume with extracellular fluid removal is the same above and below normal hydration.

Misinterpretation of BVM traces may have contributed to the higher mortality observed in patients randomised to receive optional BVM measurements in the CLIMB study (Reddan et al, 2005). With adequate training, BVM can help in the assessment of fluid status but it is best used to identify and implement fluid removal strategies that minimise symptoms.

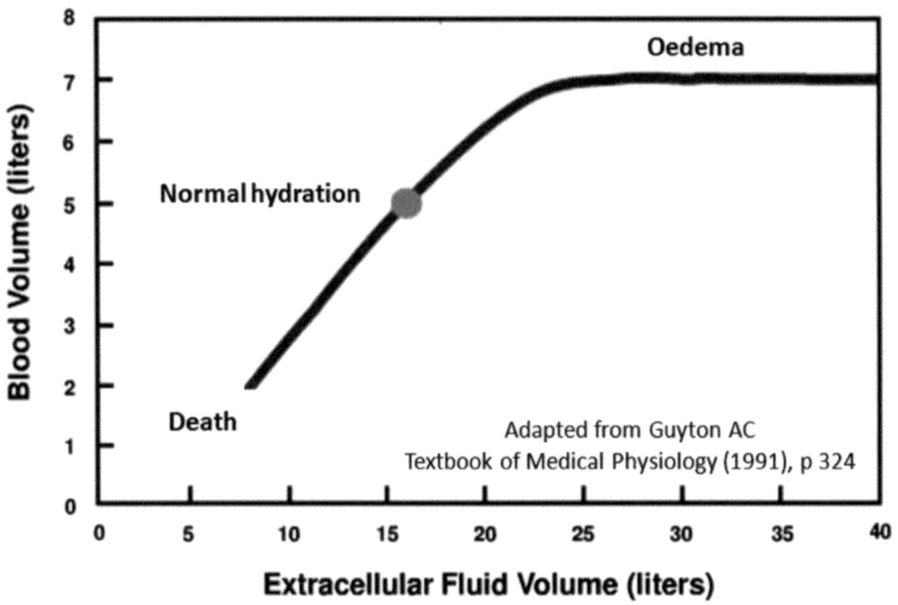

Fig. 1. Variation in blood volume with extracellular volume

2.4 Bioimpedance and body composition monitoring

Bioimpedance monitors can provide quick, cheap, non-invasive bedside measurements of fluid status with good reproducibility. However, until recently the use of bioimpedance has been restricted to a relatively small number of centres with both a clinical and an academic interest in the technology.

In 'single frequency' bioimpedance monitors, a tiny 50 kHz alternating current is passed between a pair of electrodes, usually placed on the hand and foot. Sensing electrodes, placed just inside the current carrying electrodes, measure 'resistance' and 'reactance' to the passage of the current. Resistance and reactance combine to give the overall 'impedance'. An increase in body water makes it easier for current to pass through the body so that resistance decreases. Reactance, which is due to the capacitance of cell membranes, decreases as the number and/or integrity of the membranes decreases.

Single frequency bioimpedance monitors are widely used in health clubs as they can give an estimate of body fat and muscle mass. The technology is also built into bathroom scales where the current is passed between the feet. In dialysis patients, the equations used to derive body composition from the impedance at 50 kHz are unreliable if the patient has an abnormal fluid status.

Prof Antonio Piccoli and co-workers recognised this and developed bioimpedance vector analysis (BIVA) which simply looks at the hydration of the body tissues between electrodes placed on the hand and foot. The resistance and reactance measurements are normalised to height and interpreted using gender-specific nomograms derived from large studies of normal subjects and of populations with altered body composition (Piccoli 1994, 1995). As shown in figure 2, fluid overload is associated with movement of the vector downward and to the left whilst dehydration moves the vector up and to the right.

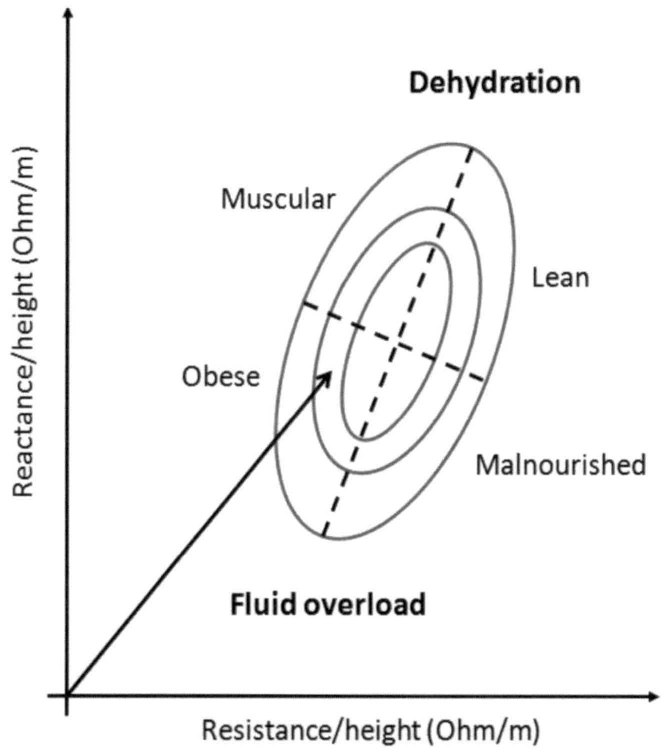

Fig. 2. Nomogram used for interpreting single frequency bioimpedance measurements. The outer ellipse encloses 95% of readings for normal subjects.

BIVA could provide practical information on changes in fluid status using very simple equipment that would cost little more than a set of bathroom scales if the market was larger. The reason BIVA cannot give an accurate indication of the patient's normally hydrated weight is clear when you examine Figure 2. The vector shown could be obtained from a slightly overweight subject with normal hydration, from a muscular subject with fluid overload or from an obese subject who is dehydrated. The confusion arises because adipose tissue contains very little intracellular water as fat cells are filled with triglycerides, but does have water in the extracellular space. So, like overhydration, an increase in body fat leads to an increase in the proportion of fluid in the extracellular space leading to a shorter vector.

In whole body bioimpedance spectroscopy (BIS), the electrodes are placed as for BIVA and resistance and reactance is measured over a range of frequencies. The results, together with the height, weight and gender of the subject, are used to compute the intracellular and extracellular water volumes (ECW and ICW). Fluid overload is associated with an increase in the proportion of water in the extracellular space but until recently, it was necessary for the user to decide what this proportion should be at normal hydration. There are a number of published methods for doing this (for example Lindley et al, 2005; Lopot et al, 2002) but they involve comparing dialysis patients with normal controls. As with BIVA, this makes it difficult to assess fluid status in patients with abnormal body composition.

Body composition monitoring (BCM) is the most recent commercially available development in bioimpedance monitoring. It uses the same electronic measurements as BIS to determine ECW and ICW but incorporates additional modelling (Moissl et al, 2006; Chamney et al, 2007) to take account of the amount of body fat the patient actually has, rather than assuming they have the average amount for a person of their age and gender. Essentially, the BCM model assumes that the body is composed of normally hydrated lean tissue, normally hydrated adipose tissue and excess fluid (or missing fluid if the patient is dehydrated). For any combination of ECW, ICW and weight, there is only one matching combination of lean tissue, fat and excess/missing fluid.

With BCM, we can get an estimate of normal hydration and, for the first time, select a target weight that minimises the unwanted effects of dehydration as well as those of overhydration. Just as the introduction of BVM revealed a cohort of chronically overloaded patients, introducing BCM as part of the assessment of fluid status identified a group who were excessively dehydrated. In some of the cases identified in this way, an increase in target weight led to a reduction in interdialytic fluid gain as the patient's kidneys were able to produce more urine.

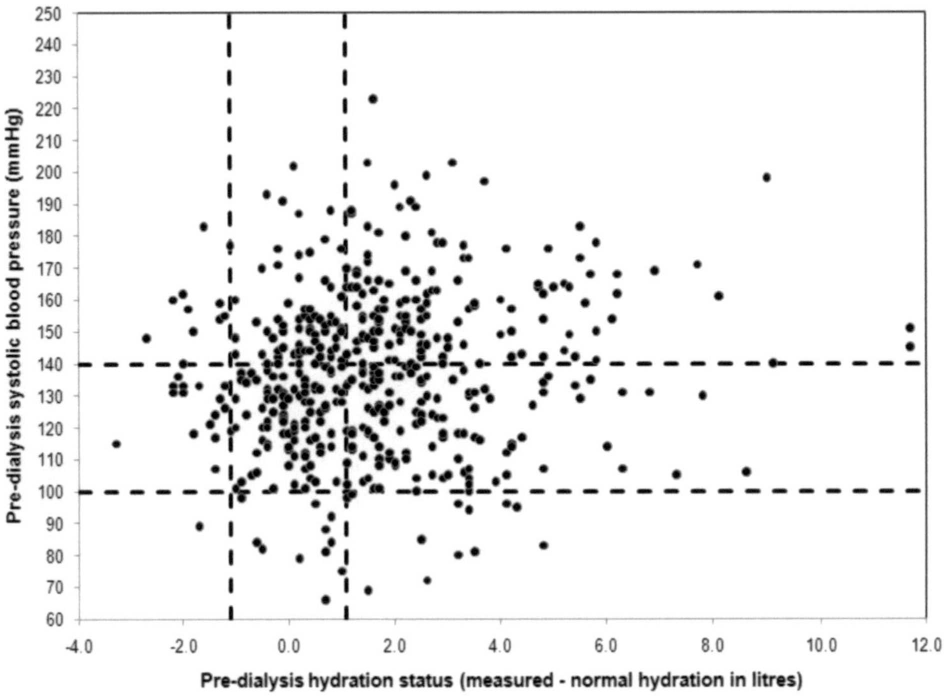

Fig. 3. Pre-dialysis systolic blood pressure vs hydration status

Users of BCM soon become aware that blood pressure can be misleading when evaluating fluid status. The scatter plot in Figure 3 shows the relationship between pre-dialysis systolic blood pressure and hydration status (the difference between measured and normal hydration in litres), for the first BCM measurement made in 474 haemodialysis patients under the care of Leeds Teaching Hospitals. A very similar plot was obtained in a cross-sectional study of 639 PD patients (Van Biesen et al, 2010). The expected increase in blood pressure with fluid overload is present, but only as a trend for the population. For an individual patient, a single high or low blood pressure measurement is a rather poor predictor of fluid status, though a trend to higher or lower blood pressures in the same patient does provide important clinical information.

A significant number of patients who are normally hydrated, or even dehydrated, pre-dialysis have high blood pressure. The traditional method for treating these patients by systematically decreasing their target weight could compromise their residual renal function, cause cramps and leave them feeling exhausted for hours after dialysis.

When the BCM measurement is combined with the clinical indicators in Table 1, and knowledge of the patient's usual IDFG, it is possible to customise the target weight as described in 2.1. Introducing BCM has been shown to improve blood pressure control and reduce intradialytic adverse events (Machek, 2010). Ideally BCM should be carried out at least quarterly, though more frequent measurements will be needed for patients who are unwell (especially if admitted to hospital) or who are trying to gain or lose weight. As well as ensuring timely adjustments to the prescribed target weight, BCM gives valuable information on changes in body fat and lean tissue and provides an accurate urea distribution volume for use in on-line measurements of dialysis adequacy.

3. Control of interdialytic fluid gain (IDFG)

3.1 Salt and fluid balance: Osmometric thirst and the sodium 'set-point'

The patient's hydration status during the interdialytic period depends on both the weight achieved after dialysis and the fluid gained by the patient before the next session. Very high IDFG can make it impossible for the patient to remain close to normal hydration and to control pre-dialysis blood pressure. Another problem, particularly in elderly and malnourished patients, is the inability to tolerate the ultrafiltration rates required to remove a moderate volume of accumulated fluid. Whether the patient is gaining excessive volumes or failing to transfer fluid from the tissues into the circulation sufficiently rapidly, the solution is to try and reduce their IDFG.

A typical haemodialysis patient in the UK accumulates about 2 litres of excess fluid in the intervals between sessions. When they attend for dialysis the machine is programmed to remove the excess fluid by ultrafiltration. Every litre removed in this way will carry with it about 137 mmol of sodium ions, though the actual amount will depend on the serum sodium level at the time the fluid was removed. As 137 mmol is the amount of sodium in 8 g of salt, the typical UK patient loses sodium equivalent to about 16 g of salt at each dialysis session. The body does have 'non-osmotic' sodium stores in tissues such as the skin and connective tissues (Titze, 2008) and it is possible that sodium can be recruited into or removed from these stores to buffer short term fluctuations in serum sodium. However, if the patient is assumed to be in steady state on the timescale of the interdialytic period, they must be making up for the sodium lost by taking in the equivalent of 16 g of salt between sessions. Sodium does come in other forms other than salt, such as sodium bicarbonate, but it is usually combined with chloride.

If retained in the body, the salt taken in will cause 'osmometric' thirst. Osmometric thirst is triggered when increased osmolarity of the extracellular fluid causes osmoreceptor cells in the hypothalamus to shrink. Volumetric thirst, which occurs when the body loses both water and salt, is triggered when baroreceptors in the atria sense low cardiac return volume. Haemodialysis patients may experience volumetric thirst immediately after dialysis if they are dehydrated, but at other times their thirst is primarily osmometric. Fluid drunk in response to post-dialysis dehydration does not usually lead to increased IDFG as it simply delays osmometric thirst until the patient has consumed enough salt. An important exception to this occurs if a patient with good residual renal function is dehydrated, as they will need to take in enough fluid to normalise their hydration before diuresis starts.

Osmometric thirst is part of the body's system for maintaining electrolyte balance. If our typical haemodialysis patient is anuric (unable to lose sodium via the kidneys), they will need to take in about one litre of water to dilute every 8g salt consumed to a normal physiological level. The patient will consume fluid with their food, when taking medications and in beverages taken socially. They may not even be aware of feeling thirsty, although many haemodialysis patients do find thirst a problem, but if salt consumption gets ahead of fluid intake, osmometric thirst will force the patient to drink enough to restore their serum sodium to an acceptable level. This level varies between patients and has been called the sodium 'set-point' or the 'osmostat' (Keen & Gotch, 2007).

Patients who take in no more fluid than is needed to avoid (or satisfy) salt-induced thirst will present for dialysis with a relatively constant serum sodium. Figure 4 shows pre-dialysis serum sodium averaged over 12 months for 375 haemodialysis patients in the care of the Leeds Teaching Hospitals (Gardiner et al, 2006). The majority of patients appear to have a well defined sodium set point that lies within the normal range of 135 to 145 mmol/l. The patients with relatively high pre-dialysis sodium levels could have a high set-point, but they could also be overriding their thirst to limit fluid gain or be unable to drink freely.

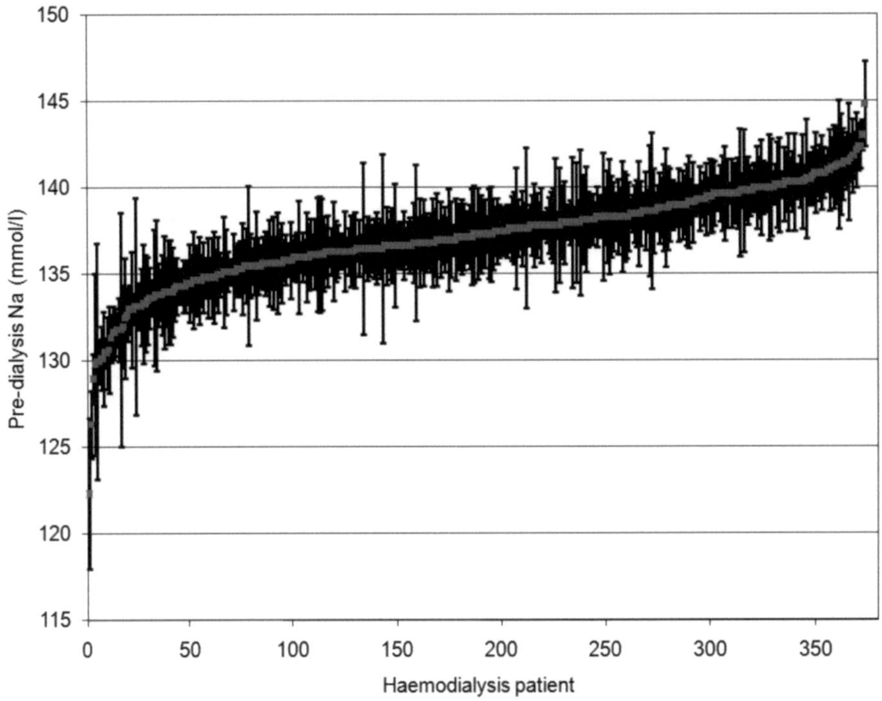

Fig. 4. Pre-dialysis serum sodium level for 375 HD patients. Each bar represents the distribution (mean and standard deviation) of 6 monthly measurements in a single patient.

Low pre-dialysis serum sodium may be due to urinary losses, but this will normally be associated with low IDFG. In patients with low sodium and high IDFG, elevated blood sugar may be responsible. In the group shown in Figure 4, the 28 poorly controlled diabetics (glycosylated haemoglobin >7%) had lower serum sodium (136 vs. 137 mmol/l, p=0.03) and higher fluid gain (2.3 vs. 1.7 kg, p=0.01) compared to well controlled diabetics and non-diabetics. However, the lowest pre-dialysis sodium levels occurred in non-diabetic patients with relatively high IDFG. These patients are taking in excess free water for various reasons including xerostomia (dry mouth, often due to medications), and comfort or social drinking. While patients with high IDFG and low pre-dialysis sodium will benefit from dietary salt restriction, other factors leading to fluid intake should be investigated and resolved if possible.

3.2 Minimising sodium loading during dialysis

During dialysis, sodium diffuses between the dialysate and the plasma water across the dialyser membrane until equilibrium is achieved. The plasma contains negatively charged proteins that are too large to pass through the dialyser membrane. This leads to retention of positively charged ions like sodium in the plasma water to maintain electric neutrality. This trapping of positively charged ions by negatively charged proteins leads to a higher concentration of sodium in the plasma water than in the dialysate at equilibrium (this is called the Gibbs-Donnan effect). Most labs measure the sodium concentration in the total plasma (the serum sodium), rather than the plasma water. Electrolytes in the total plasma are diluted by about 6% because of the volume taken up by the proteins and lipids. In most patients, this dilution more-or-less cancels out the Gibbs Donnan effect so that the measured serum sodium post-dialysis is usually close to the dialysate sodium level.

Through the plasma water, the sodium level in the patient's extracellular water equilibrates with the dialysate sodium during dialysis. Patients treated with dialysate sodium that is higher than their pre-dialysis serum level will receive an infusion of sodium during dialysis. Consider an anuric 70 kg male patient whose set point leads him to come for dialysis with a serum sodium of around 137 mmol/l. If he is treated with dialysate sodium of 140 mmol/l, there will be a net transfer of between 45 and 100 mmol of sodium from the dialysate to the patient during the session. The actual amount will depend on the movement of water out of the intracellular space to achieve osmotic equilibrium and transfers of other solutes. Although this sodium transfer is much smaller than the typical loss through ultrafiltration (about 275 mmol for 2 litres removed), reducing the dialysate sodium by 3 mmol/l should lead to a decrease in IDFG of at least 0.3 kg in this patient.

To eliminate unnecessary intradialytic sodium loading, and avoid the associated fluid gain, individualisation of the dialysate sodium based on the patient's pre-dialysis serum or plasma water sodium level has been recommended (de Paula et al, 2004; Santos & Peixoto, 2008). A simpler approach, which will achieve similar benefits in terms of reduced IDFG and blood pressure control, is to standardise the dialysate sodium levels towards the lower end of the normal range. Patients who normally have high serum sodium levels may experience osmotic disequilibrium (headache, nausea and hypertension) if treated with dialysate sodium of 135-137 mmol/l, but many will have no symptoms. Patients who have very low pre-dialysis sodium levels will gain sodium during dialysis, but this will not necessarily increase IDFG if their fluid intake is not controlled by osmometric thirst. Resetting of the sodium set-point, or 'osmostat', to very low levels has been reported (for example, as a complication of spinal cord injury) but it is rare and would lead to unbearable thirst after dialysis with dialysate sodium in the normal range.

3.3 Recommended salt consumption

Control of interdialytic fluid gains is important both in the maintenance of near-normal hydration and the minimisation of intradialytic hypotension and discomfort. Patients who consume less than 6 g of salt per day should accumulate no more than 0.8 l of fluid per day (it takes 750 ml of water to dilute 6 g salt to 137 mmol/l). Most patients are able to tolerate the ultrafiltration rates required to remove this amount of fluid. Smaller patients and those with impaired autonomic function may need a tighter salt restriction, especially when they have three days between dialysis sessions.

Unlike most of the dietary restrictions placed on dialysis patients, the recommendation to limit salt intake applies to the whole population, including healthcare professionals! The World Health Organisation recommends a maximum salt intake of 5 g/day and regularly convenes meetings to discuss reducing salt consumption at population level (WHO, 2010).

The USA, Canada, UK, Australia and New Zealand are among the countries that consider a recommended daily allowance (RDA) of 6 g/day to be achievable and sustainable. A salt intake of 6 g/day is equivalent to a sodium intake of 2.3 g/day or 100 mmol/day.

The RDA for patients with kidney failure, as with all patients at high risk of cardiovascular disease, should probably be lower than for the general population. However, the practical and psychological benefit of having the same dietary restriction as family and carers, as well as the risk of malnutrition due to an unappetising diet, makes the national RDA a more realistic target for most patients.

3.4 Dietary advice for patients

Before counselling patients with problematic fluid gains, it is essential to review their serum sodium. Patients with high IDFG who have normal pre-dialysis sodium levels are drinking in response to osmometric thirst and **must** be given advice on reducing their salt intake. Simply telling these patients to restrict fluid intake, as is common in many dialysis units (Lindley et al, 2005), will not succeed in reducing IDFG (Tomson, 2001).

Patients with high IDFG and low pre-dialysis sodium should be assessed for other reasons for fluid intake, such as high blood glucose or social drinking. These patients will probably benefit from salt restriction but they will also require individualised interventions.

The first step in reducing salt intake is to understand where the salt is coming from. In industrialized countries, 75-80% of salt consumed comes from manufactured foods including butter, cheese, biscuits, pastry, cereals, snacks, processed meats, sauces and ready-made soups and meals. In Canada, bread is reported to account for 14% of total dietary salt intake (WHO, 2010). Mhurchu et al report that bread purchased in the UK contain over 1 g of salt per 100g on average (Mhurchu et al, 2011). Restaurant meals and fast foods are frequently high in salt. In more rural populations, salt used as a preservative and added in cooking (usually in sauces) is the major source of salt in the diet. Fresh foods (meat, fish, vegetables) contribute 10% or less to salt intake.

Tips to reduce salt (sodium)

- Use fresh or frozen vegetables (if canned, look for low-sodium or no-salt-added on the label). If using food canned with salt, rinse the contents to remove as much as possible. Don't add salt to the water used for cooking.
- Try to use fresh poultry, fish and meat, rather than canned, smoked or processed products. Cheap processed meat often has salt added to make it absorb water and increase in weight.
- Cook rice, pasta and noodles without salt and avoid instant or flavoured products as they usually have added salt.
- Use ketchup, barbeque, soy and other sauces very sparingly.
- Make salad dressings and cooking sauces instead of buying them ready-made. Using other flavours (herbs, spices, lemon etc) may mean salt can be eliminated completely.
- Check nutrition labels on breakfast cereals, ready meals, soup and sauces to find products with lower salt/sodium. Food labelled as low in salt should contain less than 0.3 g of salt per serving, medium should mean 0.3 to 1.5 g per serving.

  Greater awareness of the need to reduce salt intake should increase the availability of low-salt products in the coming years, but always check that product labelled as low-salt do not contain potassium-based salt substitutes.

Fig. 5. Tips on reducing salt intake based on the DASH brochure (US NHBLI, 2006).

The importance of salt restriction for the whole population means that advice on lowering salt intake and recipes for low salt meals are widely available on the internet. The only modification required in dialysis patients is the need to be very careful of salt substitutes as they often contain potassium. Unfortunately the potassium content of processed food is often not clearly labelled. Figure 5 shows the tips for lowering salt intake from the 'Dietary Approaches to Stop Hypertension' brochure (US NHBLI, 2006) adapted for dialysis patients by a renal dietitian.

Patients who can tolerate only very limited fluid removal, and those who are hypertensive in the absence of fluid overload, may need to take further steps to reduce their salt consumption. This will include switching to unsalted butter and bread. If salt-free bread is not available, ways to substitute unsalted rice or pasta for bread should be sought. As these more stringent restrictions are difficult to implement, it is essential to prevent sodium loading during dialysis in these patients. Consideration should be given to lowering the dialysate sodium to 133-135 mmol/l and minimising infusion of normal saline (which contains 154 mmol/l sodium) at the end of dialysis (Penne et al, 2010).

Dialysis patients may have impaired taste sensitivity (Middleton 1999). If salt restriction leads to weight loss because the patient finds their food unappetising, they should be referred to a dietitian to look into the use of acceptable alternative flavourings. The need to check for weight loss and provide individual dietetic counselling is especially important in patients who need a very restricted salt intake as described above.

3.5 Implementing salt restriction: Staff education

There is a sound physiological basis for restricting intake of salt rather than fluids to control IDFG in most patients, though there are few published comparisons of the different approaches. Rupp et al compared patients on a traditional sodium and fluid restricted diet with those given a diet that just restricted sodium and found a significant decrease in IDFG only in the group on the simpler low-sodium diet (Rupp et al, 1978). Kayikcioglu et al compared cardiac function and blood pressure control in two units, one of which practiced a salt restriction strategy while the other relied on the use of anti-hypertensives (Kayikcioglu et al, 2009). The use of salt restriction not only reduced the requirement for antihypertensive medication (7% vs. 42%), but led to significantly lower IDFG (2.29 vs. 3.31 kg) and fewer episodes of intradialytic hypotension (11% vs. 27%).

With such clear benefits, it is surprising that there is not more emphasis on salt restriction in haemodialysis units. Patient information currently available via the internet tends to focus on fluid restriction, with advice such as using smaller cups, sipping slowly, sucking ice cubes or lemon wedges and keeping a fluid journal. The popularity of fluid restriction may be because fluid intake is relatively easy to monitor, while salt is hidden in manufactured foods and cutting out the 'visible' added salt has a disappointing impact on IDFG.

Dialysis staff can change the focus from fluid to salt restriction and establish a culture of sharing advice for reducing salt intake within the unit. With pressure from the World Health Organisation and national food safety bodies, we should see more low-salt products and increased disclosure of salt content. Tables of salt content in foods that can be used in educational material and quizzes are available from organisations such as the US Department of Agriculture (USDA, n.d.) and the Australian Healthy Eating Club (Healthy Eating Club, n.d.). Staff aiming to reduce their own salt intake to < 6 g/day will be able to swap tips rather than impose rules. How long does it take to get used to unsalted butter? Which breakfast cereals have the lowest salt content? How easy is it to make low salt bread?

Haemodialysis patients with little or no residual renal function can get feedback on the impact of any dietary modification simply by monitoring their fluid gains. As a rough guide, every kilogram gained between dialysis sessions corresponds to an intake of 8 g of salt. So a 0.5 kg decrease in IDWG over the short break shows they have managed to reduce their salt intake by 4 g (2 g/day). Staff will need to carry out 24 hour urine collections to check their own salt consumption.

The link between low IDFG and poor survival is well established (Sezer et al, 2002) and haemodialysis patients are often at risk of malnutrition, so it is essential to ensure that what appears to be a successful intervention to reduce salt intake does not lead to undiagnosed weight loss and fluid overload.

4. Conclusion

The implementation of bioimpedance measurements to assist in the optimisation of the patient's target weight, and the use of salt restriction to avoid excessive fluid gains, should enable most haemodialysis patients to stay close to normal hydration throughout the interdialytic period.

Future research in the use of bioimpedance will include verification of the BCM models in patients at the extremes of body composition and with conditions leading to very abnormal fluid distribution and the effect of transcellular fluid shifts caused by changes in electrolyte levels. Simple, inexpensive devices to allow patients to track changes in their fluid status should be developed. The effect of varying the target time-averaged hydration status on morbidity and mortality should be studied so that volume control can become a measure of dialysis adequacy as suggested by Ok and Mees (Ok & Mees, 2010).

For the majority of patients, interdialytic fluid gain can be controlled by using a standard low-normal dialysate sodium and keeping salt consumption to no more than 6 g/day. Staff will also benefit from keeping to this recommended salt intake. Patients who tolerate ultrafiltration very poorly will need careful management of sodium loading on dialysis together with a customised low-salt diet. An individualised approach, including improved diabetic control and motivational interviewing will also be required for patients with very low pre-dialysis serum sodium levels whose fluid intake does not depend on salt.

5. References

Brener ZZ, Kotanko P, Thijssen S, Winchester JF & Bergman M. (2010) Clinical benefit of preserving residual renal function in dialysis patients: an update for clinicians. *Am J Med Sci.*, Vol. 339 (2010), pp. 453-6.

Chamney PW, Wabel P, Moissl UM, Müller MJ, Bosy-Westphal A, Korth O, Fuller NJ. (2007) A whole-body model to distinguish excess fluid from the hydration of major body tissues. *Am J Clin Nutr* Vol. 85 (2007), pp. 80–89.

Charra B. (2007) Fluid balance, dry weight, and blood pressure in dialysis. *Hemodial Int*, Vol. 11 (2007), 21-31.

Davita. The hemodialysis diet. http://www.davita.com/kidney-disease/diet-and-nutrition/diet-basics/the-hemodialysis-diet/e/5314 (accessed May 2011).

de Paula FM, Peixoto AJ, Pinto LV, Dorigo D, Patricio PJ & Santos SF. (2004) Clinical consequences of an individualized dialysate sodium prescription in hemodialysis patients. *Kidney Int*, Vol. 66 (2004), pp. 1232-1238.

Gardiner C, Scott H, Wright M, Greaves E & Lindley E. (2006) IDWG, salt and water – an audit of dialysis staff. British Journal of Renal Medicine, Vol. 11 No. 3 (2006), pp. 12-14.

Healthy Eating Club. Sodium Food Charts. http://www.healthyeatingclub.org/info/books-phds/books/foodfacts/html/data/data5a.html (accessed May 2011).

Henderson LW. (1980). Symptomatic hypotension during hemodialysis. *Kidney Int*, Vol. 17 (1980), pp. 571-576.

Jaeger JQ, Mehta RL. (1999) Assessment of dry weight in hemodialysis: an overview. *J Am Soc Nephrol,* Vol. 10 (1999), pp. 392-403.

Keen ML & Gotch FA. (2007) The association of the sodium 'setpoint' to interdialytic fluid gain and blood pressure in hemodialysis patients. *Int J Artif Organs,* Vol. 30 (2007), pp. 971-9.

Kayikcioglu M, Tumuklu M, Ozkahya M, Ozdogan O, Asci G, Duman S, Toz H, Can LH, Basci A & Ok E. (2009) The benefit of salt restriction in the treatment of end-stage renal disease by haemodialysis. *Nephrol Dial Transplant,* Vol. 24 (2009), pp. 956-962.

Lindley E, Devine Y, Hall L, Cullen M, Cuthbert S, Woodrow G & Lopot F. (2005) A ward-based procedure for assessment of fluid status in peritoneal dialysis patients using bioimpedance spectroscopy. *Perit Dial Int,* Vol. 25. Suppl. 3 (2005), pp. S46–S48.

Lindley EJ, Stragier A, De Vos JY, Lahuis K, Shaldon S, Green D, McLaren P, Pegoraro M, Küntzle W, Tattersall JE & López-Gómez J. (2005) Summary of the EDTNA/ERCA Journal Club discussion of López-Gómez et al (Kidney Int 2005) 'Interdialytic fluid gain as a marker of blood pressure, nutrition, and survival in hemodialysis patients'. *EDTNA-ERCA Journal,* Vol. 31 (2005), pp. 164-168.

Lopot F, Nejedly B, Novotná H, Macková M & Sulková S. (2002) Age-related extracellular to total body water volume ratio (ECV/TBW) - can it be used for "dry weight" determination in dialysis patients? Application of multifrequency bioimpedance measurement. *Int J Artif Organs,* Vol. 25 (2002), pp. 762–769.

Marrón B, Remón C, Pérez-Fontán M, Quirós P & Ortíz A. (2008) Benefits of preserving residual renal function in peritoneal dialysis. *Kidney Int,* Vol. 73 Suppl. 108 (2008), pp. S42-S51.

Machek P, Jirka T, Moissl U, Chamney P & Wabel P. (2010) Guided optimization of fluid status in haemodialysis patients. *Nephrol Dial Transplant,* Vol. 25 (2010), pp. 538-544.

Mhurchu CN, Capelin C, Dunford EK, Webster JL, Neal BC & Jebb SA (2011) Sodium content of processed foods in the united kingdom: analysis of 44,000 foods purchased by 21,000 households. *Am J Clin Nutr,* Vol. 93 (2011), pp. 594-600.

Middleton RA & Allman-Farinelli MA. (1999) Taste sensitivity is altered in patients with chronic renal failure receiving continuous ambulatory peritoneal dialysis. *J Nutrition,* Vol 129 (1999), pp. 122-125.

Mitra S, Chamney P, Greenwood R & Farrington K. (2004) The relationship between systemic and whole-dody hematocrit is not constant during ultrafiltration on hemodialysis. *J Am Soc Nephrol,* Vol. 15 (2004), pp. 463–469.

Moissl UM, Wabel P, Chamney PW, Bosaeus I, Levin NW, Bosy-Westphal A, Korth O, Müller MJ, Ellegård L, Malmros V, Kaitwatcharachai C, Kuhlmann MK, Zhu F & Fuller NJ. (2006) Body fluid volume determination via body composition spectroscopy in health and disease. *Physiol Meas,* Vol. 27 (2006), pp. 21–33.

Ok E & Mees EJ. (2010) Unpleasant truths about salt restriction. Semin Dial. Vol 23 (2010), pp. 1-2.

Penne EL, Levin NW & Kotanko P. (2010) Improving volume status by comprehensive dietary and dialytic sodium management in chronic hemodialysis patients. *Blood Purif,* Vol. 30 (2010), pp. 71-78.

Piccoli A, Rossi B, Pillon L & Bucciante G. (1994) A new method for monitoring body fluid variation by bioimpedance analysis: the RXc graph. *Kidney Int,* Vol. 46 (1994), pp. 534-539.

Piccoli A, Nigrelli S, Caberlotto A, Bottazzo S, Rossi B, Pillon L & Maggiore Q. (1995) Bivariate normal values of the bioelectrical impedance vector in adult and elderly populations. *Am J Clin Nutr,* Vol. 61 (1995), pp. 269–270.

Reddan DN, Szczech LA, Hasselblad V, Lowrie EG, Lindsay RM, Himmelfarb J, Toto RD, Stivelman J, Winchester JF, Zillman LA, Califf RM & Owen WF Jr. (2005) Intradialytic blood volume monitoring in ambulatory hemodialysis patients: a randomized trial. *J Am Soc Nephrol,* Vol. 16 (2005); pp. 2162-2169.

Rupp JW, Stone RA & Gunning BE. (1978) Sodium versus sodium-fluid restriction in hemodialysis: control of weight gains and blood pressures. *Am J Clin Nutr* Vol. 31 (1978), pp. 1952-1955.

Santos SF & Peixoto AJ. (2008) Revisiting the dialysate sodium prescription as a tool for better blood pressure and interdialytic fluid gain management in hemodialysis patients. *Clin J Am Soc Nephrol,* Vol. 3 (2008), pp. 522-530.

Sezer S, Ozdemir FN, Arat Z, Perim O, Turan M & Haberal M. (2002) The association of interdialytic fluid gain with nutritional parameters and mortality risk in hemodialysis patients. *Ren Fail,* Vol. 24 (2002), pp. 37-48.

Titze J. (2008) Water-free Na+ retention: interaction with hypertension and tissue hydration. *Blood Purif,* Vol. 26 (2008), pp. 95-9.

Tomson CR. (2001) Advising dialysis patients to restrict fluid intake without restricting sodium intake is not based on evidence and is a waste of time. *Nephrol Dial Transplant,* Vol. 16 (2001), pp. 1538-1542.

US Department of Agriculture. Sodium content of selected foods per common measure. http://www.nal.usda.gov/fnic/foodcomp/Data/SR18/nutrlist/sr18a307.pdf (accessed May 2011).

US National Heart, Lung, and Blood Institute. (2006) Your guide to lowering your blood pressure with DASH. http://www.nhlbi.nih.gov/health/public/heart/hbp/dash/new_dash.pdf (accessed May 2011).

Van Biesen W, Williams JD, Covic AC, Fan S, Claes K, Lichodziejewska-Niemierko M, Verger C, Steiger J, Schoder V, Wabel P, Gauly A & Himmele R; for the EuroBCM Study Group. (2011) Fluid status in peritoneal dialysis patients: the European Body Composition Monitoring (EuroBCM) study cohort. *PLoS One,* Vol. 6 (2011), e17148.

van der Wal WM, Noordzij M, Dekker FW, Boeschoten EW, Krediet RT, Korevaar JC & Geskus RB; for the NECOSAD Group. (2011). Full loss of residual renal function causes higher mortality in dialysis patients; findings from a marginal structural model. *Nephrol Dial Transplant,* (2011). Epub ahead of print.

Vilar E, Wellsted D, Chandna SM, Roger N. Greenwood RN & Farrington K. (2009) Residual renal function improves outcome in incremental haemodialysis despite reduced dialysis dose. *Nephrol Dial Transplant,* Vol 24 (2009), pp. 2502–2510.

World Health Organisation. (2010) Creating an enabling environment for population-based salt reduction strategies. Report of a joint technical meeting held by WHO and the Food Standards Agency, United Kingdom, July 2010. http://whqlibdoc.who.int/publications/2010/9789241500777_eng.pdf (accessed May 2011).

12

Cell-Free Nucleic Acids as Biomarkers of Biocompatibility in Dialytic Process

Marie Korabečná[1] and Aleš Hořínek[2]
First School of Medicine, Charles University in Prague
Czech Republic

1. Introduction

In this review we describe what is recently known about the origin of free nucleic acids in human circulation, which processes can cause the elevations of their total concentrations and the alterations in the ratios among different types of circulating nucleic acids in human plasma and serum. We focus on the inflammatory response and apoptosis with regard to changes in the quantity and quality of circulating nucleic acids pool. We discuss the use of cell-free nucleic acids as biomarkers in patients with renal failure not only in hemodialysis but also in peritoneal dialysis with regard to future perspectives on the field of cell-free nucleic acids.

2. Origin and clearance of free nucleic acids in human circulation

The phenomenon of cell-free DNA circulating in human plasma was discovered in 1948 (Mandel &, Metais, 1948,). The authors detected DNA and RNA in blood plasma of healthy control and patients. With regard to the lack of biological understanding of such a finding their work remained unnoticed. During next thirty years only two studies focusing on cell-free DNA appeared. The patients with lupus erythematosus (Tan et al., 1966, in Swarup & Rajeswari, 2007) and the patients with rheumatoid arthritis (Ayala et al., 1951) were studied and elevated levels DNA in circulation were reported. The medical importance of cell-free nucleic acids was recognized when the decreasing levels of these nucleic acids were reported in cancer patients after successful chemotherapy (Leon et al., 1977).

In 1994, mutated oncogene K-ras was discovered in the pool of circulating DNA in pancreatic cancer patients (Sorenson at al., 1994). In 1997 the circulating DNA of fetal origin was found in plasmas of pregnant women (Lo et al., 1997). Till today numerous studies were performed not only to understand the nature and biological meaning of cell-free DNAs and RNAs but mainly to establish their diagnostic use under different clinical conditions such as cancer, autoimmune disorders, pregnancy related disorders and trauma (for review Tong & Lo, 2006).

Although recent molecular biology and genetics employ very broad spectrum of sophisticated methods, the complete understanding of biology of cell-free nucleic acids was so far not achieved. As there are speculations concerning the regulatory function of circulating nucleic acids in plasma, the clinical laboratory research and practice stream to develop approaches allowing the analytic use of these molecules. The main sources of nucleic acids in plasma are necrosis, apoptosis and active release by living, non-apoptotic cells. All mentioned processes will be discussed in details in following sections. Cell-free nucleic acids in human plasma present very heterogeneous material with heterogeneous function – there are for example fragments of genomic DNA, mitochondrial DNA, but also mRNAs and microRNA. The forms in which they circulate are studied also with regard to the development of effective extraction methods for clinical laboratories.

2.1 Necrosis and apoptosis as sources of cell-free DNA

From the methodological point of view, it is difficult to exactly distinguish between the apoptotic derived fraction of cell-free DNA and the necrotic-derived one in plasma. Veiko et al. (2008) developed a method for in vivo evaluation of cell death in patients with acute and/or chronic heart disease. The main parameters evaluated in the study by Veiko et al. were: total concentrations of cell-free DNA (cfDNA) in the blood (or serum), concentration of serum ribosomal repeat (rDNA), content of rDNA in total cfDNA, but also factors involved in clearance of cfDNA such as nuclease activity and anti-DNA antibodies.

The authors clearly demonstrated significant increase in the concentration of rDNA in the cfDNA pool in patients with acute myocardial infarction. Such an accumulation of rDNA within cfDNA may be caused by the resistance of rDNA to the fragmentation by serum endonucleases, because the nuclease activities in the serum of both acute and chronic coronary disease patients were elevated in comparison to healthy individuals. The titers of anti-DNA antibodies were also higher in the patients group. The anti-DNA antibodies were predominantly bound to cfDNA. It seems that the release of rDNA fragments into the blood may reflect cellular death in the body (Veiko et al., 2008).

Another clinical situation connected with massive cellular death is represented by the multiple-organ dysfunction syndrome (MODS). In MODS, the initial insult damages target organs and leads to tissue necrosis. The necrosis induces a systemic inflammatory response and an alteration of hemodynamics, microcirculation and oxygen metabolism. As a consequence, distant organs may be damaged by necrosis or apoptosis.

The prognostic role of elevated levels of plasma cfDNA in critically ill patients was demonstrated by Wijeratne et al. (2004). Pachl et al. (2005) developed an assay allowing to distinguish between DNA released from apoptotic and necrotic cells. The assay is based on electrophoretic separation of isolated plasma cfDNA fragments on agarose gel. The DNA from apoptotic cells (aDNA) is represented by fragments of typical size resembling the ladder on an electrophoretic gel, but DNA derived from necrotic cells (genomic - gDNA) does not provide this typical pattern when subjected to electrophoretic separation. The authors applied their assay on the samples of plasma cfDNA obtained from intensive care unit patients. They found that the contribution of aDNA to the amount of total plasma DNA in the critically ill patients was 16 fold greater than the contribution of gDNA from necrotic cells. The levels of aDNA were highest on the day of admission and declined thereafter, but the levels of gDNA altered in the opposite manner.

The concentration of apoptotic DNA in samples collected from patients on the day of admission significantly differentiated survivors and non-survivors (Pachl et al., 2005). The study by Pachl confirmed the results of previous research performed on rats (Guan et al., 2002). The most surprising fact in this context is represented by the finding of the highest concentration of cfDNA of apoptotic origin at the time of patient admission to the intensive care unit. The possible explanation for this fact can be found in the induction of apoptosis by the activation of the intrinsic pathway caused by the affection of mitochondria as a consequence of cellular damage caused by primary insult (Crouser et al., 2002).

According to the results obtained in an animal study (Guan et al., 2002) and the first human study (Pachl et al., 2005) it seems that primary insult induces apoptosis in the relationship to its severity and necrotic DNA originates from secondary organ damage therefore it can be detected with later onset during the course of the illness (Pachl et al., 2005).

Muscle injury caused by athletic overtraining leads also to elevation of plasma cfDNA concentrations as reported by Fatouros et al. (2006). The study demonstrated increase of cfDNA levels in proportion to training load. Overtraining causes an acute breakdown with subsequent repair of skeletal muscle and it is characterized by changes in the functionality of immune system resulting in increased susceptibility to infections. The correlation of plasma cfDNA with creatinine kinase but not with C-reactive protein was reported in this study.

The results achieved by Fatouros and coworkers are in good agreement with the results of an earlier study (Atamaniuk et al., 2004) in which long-distance runners were examined and 9- to 17.5 fold increase in concentrations of cfDNA was found immediately after the run. With regard to these reports, the extent of physical activities of examined subjects before the sampling procedure must be taken in account when evaluating the results of cfDNA based studies. The problems concerning the clearance of plasma cfDNA will be discussed in one of the following sections.

2.2 Active release of nucleic acids by cells

Necrosis and apoptosis were originally sought to be the only sources of cell-free nucleic acids in the circulation. The pioneer study by Stroun (2001a) clearly demonstrated the active release of fragmented DNA from cells in culture where apoptosis has been inhibited. Anker with coworkers (Anker et al., 1976) provided evidence about the release of newly synthesized DNA from human leucocytes. They reported that the release process is unrelated to cell death and is regulated by a homeostatic mechanism. Precursor incorporation into the DNA was inhibited by DNase, RNase, Pronase, and actinomycin D in their experiments.

The original hypothesis that the tumor specific cfDNA originates from lysis of tumor cells on the interface between the tumor and circulation is not more viable with regard to the high concentration of cancer specific cfDNA in circulation. Sorenson (1997, in Stroun et al., 2001a) calculated that 1000 cancer cell per milliliter would be necessary to provide the amount of DNA found in the plasma of pancreatic cancer patients. Later, the extraction methods for cfDNA were improved, and it has been demonstrated that the concentrations of cfDNA in plasma of cancer patients are even ten times higher than originally sought.

The tumors are not able to supply the circulation with 10 000 cells per each milliliter therefore the active release of nucleic acids by tumor cells is recently accepted as the main source of cell-free nucleic acids in cancer patients.

Cell-free DNA can occur in different forms in circulation. It may be transported by vesicle based particles, nucleosomes and virtosomes. The extracellular DNA bound in all mentioned structures forms the so called nucleome (Peters & Pretorius, 2011). The sequences contained in the nucleome were compared with genomic DNA sequences (Stroun et al., 2001; van der Vaart & Pretorius, 2008; Beck et al., 2009; Puszyk et al., 2009). Beck et al. studied the nucleome of 50 healthy individuals and concluded that practically no gene sequence is highly overrepresented here in comparison with genomic DNA.

The overrepresentation of non-coding sequences - *Alu* repeats - in the nucleome was repeatedly reported in studies of this type (Stroun et al., 2001; van der Vaart & Pretorius, 2008; Beck et al., 2009). Next generation sequencing (high-througput sequencing) has been used to analyze and compare the nucleome of healthy controls and patients with breast cancer. The higher representation of certain repetetive elements in the nucleomes of breast cancer patients was found and the finding was validated with regard to the diagnostic use for staging and outcome prediction (Beck et al., 2010).

During apoptosis DNA and RNA are packed in separate apoptotic bodies which are rapidly ingested by adjacent cells and professional phagocytes. The contribution of apoptotic DNA under physiological conditions to the pool of cfDNA is probably insignificant because DNA from apoptotic bodies is completely digested by DNAseII in lysosomes of phagocyting cells (Peters & Pretorius, 2011).

Cell-free DNAs are mostly in complex with histones in the form of nucleosomes. The association with histones can play the key role in the translocation of cfDNA across cell membrane. The binding of cfDNA with histone H3K27me2b was described, this histone could be crucial for externalization and stabilization of cfDNA in plasma (Beck et al., 2009).

It is known for longer time that regulated release of newly synthetized DNA/RNA – lipoprotein complexes requires energy. The newly synthetized particles contain DNA, RNA DNA-dependent DNA and RNA polymerases, lipoproteins and are referred as virtosomes. Synthesis of DNA for virtosomes probably takes place mainly in the G0 or G1 phase - it seems not to be limited to the mitosis (Peters & Pretorius, 2011).

Not only cell-free DNA can be detected in human plasma, but there is also broad spectrum of mRNA and microRNA. Surprisingly, these RNA molecules due their relative stability can be also isolated from patient plasma and analyzed in clinical laboratories. Their relative stability within the plasma samples is linked to the form in which they are released into circulation. These RNA molecules are enclosed in small vesicles referred as exosomes. Exosomes are 40 - 100 nm membrane bound vesicles of endocytic origin secreted by most cell types *in vivo*. More than 2,300 proteins and 270 microRNAs have been linked with exosomes derived from different biological fluid (Taylor et al., 2011). Exosomes were found *in vivo* in body fluid such as blood, urine, amniotic fluid, malignant ascites, bronchoalveolar lavage fluid, synovial fluid and breast milk (Simpson et al., 2008).

Recently it is not exactly known, if exosomes contains DNA or not. According to the research done by García-Olmo et al. (2000) it seems that exosomes can also carry DNA containing complexes.

The advent of genomic and proteomic technologies contributed to the understanding of the molecular composition of exosomes, but their biological functions remain still unclear. It is becoming apparent that they may be involved in the transfer of both mRNA and microRNA to the distant target cells to modulate their expression and behavior. The secretion of exosomes by tumor cells and their implication in the transport and propagation of infectious cargo such as prions and retroviruses provide the evidence that exosomes are important participants of different pathological processes (Simpson at al., 2008).

The group of García-Olmo demonstrated in an animal study that plasma from tumor-bearing rats was able to stably transfect cultured cells. The authors proposed a hypothesis that the metastasis might occur via transfection of susceptible cells located in distant target organ with dominant oncogenes circulating in plasma (García- Olmo et al., 1999) and called such a putative phenomenon "genometastasis."

One of the most common alterations of tumor related cfDNA is its hypermethylation. The methylated DNA fragment have been shown to be taken up by HeLa and human umbilical vein endothelial cells twice as efficiently as unmethylated fragments (Skvortsova, Vlassov & Laktionov, 2008).

Recent progress in immunology suggests that nucleic acids are active modulators of the immune system. Both RNA and DNA molecules can be detected by specific receptors - the so called Toll-like receptors, RIG-I-like receptors and NOD-like receptors (Koyama S. et al., 2010). All above mentioned facts contribute to the understanding of cell-free nucleic acids in human plasma as important tools in complex regulatory mechanisms involved in homeostasis and immune response under frequently changing endo- and exogenous conditions.

2.3 Clearance of circulating nucleic acids in human plasma

Cell-free nucleic acids circulate in plasma in different forms as described in previous sections. Their clearance and turnover represent very probably complex mechanism which is known only superficially. The equilibrium between nucleome and genome forms probably the base of genetic homeostasis (Peters & Pretorius, 2011). The individual cells from different organs can not only contribute to the pool of nucleic acids in plasma but also take part in their turnover using them for regulation of intracellular events in variable extent depending on the cell type and physiological state. The live span of the individual molecules and complexes determines the area of their effect in which the group of cells can benefit from horizontal gene transfer (Peters & Pretorius, 2011).

Our study (Horinek et al., 2008) brought an indirect evidence for the existence of homeostatic mechanisms between nucleic acids released into circulation and taken up by cells or digested by nucleases. We measured the concentrations of total cfDNA and fetal cfDNA in plasma of healthy pregnant women during pregnancy. Although the concentrations of total cfDNA were kept at the same level through the entire pregnancy, the fractions of cfDNA of fetal origin in the pool of total maternal cfDNA elevated from the first trimestr toward the labor. Lo et al. (1999) reported that fetal DNA is undetectable 2 hours postpartum, with a mean half-life of 16.3 min.

Under pathological conditions, the clearance of cfDNA can be affected as demonstrated in the study by Lau et al. (2002) where higher half-life of fetal DNA in preeclamptic (median 114 min) women was observed compared to healthy controls (median 28 min). Impaired clearance of cfDNA can be expected under other pathological conditions, for example in cancer patients. It has been actually documented that the activities of nucleases in cancer patient are lowered (Cherepanova et al., 2008).

It seems that cfDNA in human circulation is present predominantly in the form of nucleosomes (Holdenrieder et al., 2001). Liver, macrophages and immune system are mainly involved in the clearance of DNA bounded in nucleosomes as has been documented in animal model (Burlingame et al., 1996). Kupfer cells are able to degrade the naked DNA on their surfaces in a saturable process (Gauthier et al., 1996; Kobayashi et al., 2001). Botezatu et al. (2000) demonstrated that kidney is not the main route of elimination of cfDNA from the body, only 0,5 % – 2% of the cfDNA passes from bloodstream through kidney into urine. This group showed the presence of Y- chromosome sequences in the urine of pregnant women carrying male fetuses and detected KRAS mutations in the urine of patients with pancreatic and colorectal cancers.

The study by Chan et al (2010) confirmed that transrenal excretion of cfDNA is very low. Sequences of the Epstein- Barr virus they are present in plasma of patients suffering with nasopharyngeal carcinoma in high concentrations were used as model system to make the detection of cfDNA in urine more robust. Only minor fraction of DNA representing EBV sequences was found in the urine of examined patients, this fraction represented 0,0028% - 0,00018% of the clearance of creatinine.

The finding that the cfDNA is stable for at least 4 hours in urine (Su et al., 2005) is important for management of clinical samples and translation medicine based on examination of cfDNA quantity and quality. From the results of our pilot study (Korabecna et al., 2011) it would appear that plasma DNAse II (which is not inhibited in blood samples stabilized by EDTA) makes only minor contribution to the degradation of circulating DNA *in vitro.* If heparin is used for sample stabilization nucleases are not inhibited and cfDNA is degraded very quickly.

3. Concentrations of cell-free nucleic acids in human plasma in health and disease

3.1 Cancer patients

Numerous studies provided evidence for the value of cfDNA quantification in cancer diagnostics and the therapy monitoring. Healthy individuals have in most cases lower cfDNA concentrations than cancer patients.

Today, the study of cell-free DNAs and RNAs in cancer patients is the most fertile area of free-nucleic aids research (8180 articles for key words "cell free nucleic acids and cancer" on PubMed till April 2011)

The qualitative alterations reported in cfDNA in cancer patients include mutations of oncogenes and tumor suppressor genes, microsatellite alterations, promoter hypermethylation of different cancer related genes and mitochondrial variation. In plasma of cancer patients, the existence of tumor specific RNAs detectable with recent methods was reported.

Detection of circulating RNA in tumor biology has the advantage over DNA-based approaches as transcripts can be both tumor and tissue-specific and therefore the origin and location of the tumor can be followed. For comprehensive review concerning different aspects of the use of circulating nucleic acids as biomarkers in cancer see Vlassov, Laktionov & Rykova (2010).

3.2 Pregnancy related disorders

Qualitative analysis of fetal cfDNA in maternal circulation has been used for fetal gender determination using detection of Y- chromosomal specific sequences, for the detection of single gene mutations in fetuses with achondroplasia, myotonic dystrophy, congenital adrenal hyperplasia, thalassemia, cystic fibrosis and Huntington disease. Recently, the fetal cfDNA is routinely examined to detect the RhD positive fetuses in RhD negative mothers.

Quantitative aberrations in the concentrations of total levels of cfDNA were found to be associated with different pregnancy related disorders such as preeclampsia, various placental pathologies, preterm labor, intrauterine growth retardation, polyhydramnion, and ectopic pregnancy. Some studies described the elevated values of total cfDNA in maternal circulation in pregnancies with aneuploid fetuses, but such results were not satisfactory confirmed by others (for review Hořínek et al., 2008).

3.3 Other diseases

Elevated plasma levels of cfDNA have been reported to correlate with the severity of injury in patients with polytrauma (Lo et al., 2000; Rainer & Lam, 2006) and with the severity of stroke (Rainer & Lam, 2006). Another study proposed to use the concentrations of cfDNA in plasma for outcome prognosis in acute myocardial infarction (Antonatos et al., 2006). Strong correlations were also found between increase of cfDNA in plasma and the outcome of intensive care unit patients (Rhodes et al., 2006; Saukkonen et al., 2007).

The elevated plasma levels of cfDNA were described to be an excellent marker for graft rejection in patients after renal transplantation (García-Moreira et al., 2010).

3.4 Inflammatory response

Due to well documented increase in cfDNA levels during inflammatory process (Fatouros et al., 2006) it is necessary to take in account the actual health status of control subjects and patients with complex clinical diagnosis. The elevated levels of cfDNA interpreted without the clinical context can not indicate pathological situations. The actual physical activity of examined subjects may also contribute to the elevations of total cfDNA in plasma and serum (Atamaniuk et al., 2004; Fatouros et al., 2006).

The mechanism of immune response to increased amount of nucleosomes in circulation was examined in systemic lupus erythematosus (SLE). In this rheumatic autoimmune disease of unknown etiology numerous autoantibodies against circulating nucleosomes are produced. The production of anti-dsDNA autobodies serves as disease marker for SLE.

Polymorphonuclear cells, dendritic cells and monocytes strongly bind nucleosomes on their surfaces, the binding of nuckeosomes to lymphocytes is weaker. Circulating nucleosomes are endocyted in polymorphonuclears, dendritic cells and monocytes. It has been shown in polymorphonuclear cells that the nucleosomes are not translocated into nucleus. Polymorphonuclear cells represent the link between innate and adaptive immunity therefore the perturbations in the regulation of their function could lead to the development of autoimmunity (Lindau et al., 2011).

The role of the receptor TLR9 in the binding of circulating DNA and development of SLE is not fully understood. It is known that the TLR9 plays an important role in recognition of dsDNA in extracellular space and in its internalization (Lindau et al., 2011) but the internalized DNA molecules may stimulate the production of IFN I in dendritic cells also in the TLR9–independent pathway (Martin & Elkon, 2006).

After a hemodialytic procedure, the concentrations of cfDNA in patients are dramatically elevated as has been demonstrated in numerous studies (Atamaniuk et al., 2006; Garcia-Moreira et al., 2006; Korabecna et al., 2008; Horinek et al. 2011). Garcia-Moreira et al. reported quite rapid normalization to normal values during 30 min after the end of the procedure. The problems associated with the well documented increase of cfDNA during the dialytic procedure will be discussed in the following sections.

The interpretations of each cfDNA based study must be performed carefully with the respect to clinical data concerning the presence of autoimmune disease, malignancy, renal transplantation or acute infection in examined subjects. All mentioned conditions must be used as exclusion criteria.

For total plasma concentrations of different types of circulating ribonucleic acids, similar clinical data are urgently needed.

4. Cell-free nucleic acids as biomarkers in dialytic process

During hemodialysis, the interaction of dialyzer membrane with patient´s blood leads to the activation of alternate pathway of complement. The biologically active complement component C5A is generated and activates the aggregation of neutrophils and their adherence to the endothelial surfaces. Neutrophils harvested during hemodialysis exhibit altered oxidative response, chemotaxis, aggregation, and adherence (Lewis & Van Epps,

1987). Neutrophils have short half-live - under normal conditions they spend approximately 12h in the circulation and then migrate into normal tissues or are attracted by chemotactic stimuli to inflamed tissues. Once in tissues, they do not return back to circulation but undergo apoptosis and are cleared by phagocytosis (Savill 1997).
Direct contact of cell with membranes in dialyzer can also induce apoptosis (Carracedo et al., 1995). Interaction of cell-surface protein of monocytes with dialysis membrane can stimulate mononuclear cells to interact with neutrophils and induce their apoptosis (Nahar et al., 2001).
Interaction between dialysis membrane and blood leads not only to complement activation but also to cytokine synthesis and release. Certain cytokines, such as tumor necrosis factor (TNF) and interleukin (IL)-1β 1, component C5a and bacterial lipopolysacchride (LPS) can increase neutrophil survival (Colotta et al., 1992; Lee et al., 1993).
As some interleukins are generated during hemodialysis and activation of monocytes occurs it seems that hemodialysis effects are comparable to the pathophysiological mechanisms of inflammation and hypersensitivity response (García-Moreira et al., 2006).
The survival of leucocytes during hemodialysis is influenced by numerous factors therefore an analyte which would mirror the complex character of biological events during hemodialysis with regard to the impact of the procedure on immune system of each individual patient may be very helpful. The study of cell-free nucleic acids seems to be a promising approach. In the next sections, the first attempts in this newly arising field will be presented.

4.1 Cell-free nucleic acids in hemodialyzed patients

The first study focused on the examination of cfDNA was carried out in 1977 by means of semiquantitative counter-immunoelectrophoresis (Steinman & Ackad, 1977). It is till today the only one study examining the appearance of cfDNA in vitro experiment using circulation of fresh blood through dialysis coil. The authors conclude that the passage of blood through the coil itself can account, at least in part, for circulating DNA and speculate about the leucocytes as the main source of this DNA.
Fournie et al. (1989) used the detection method based on incorporation of radiolabeled nucleotide in nick translation reaction and confirmed the results obtained by Steinman & Ackad (1977). In the study by Fournie and coauthors, 45 patients during 99 sessions of hemodialysis or hemofiltration were followed. Independently on the method of treatment, during the first 3 h of the session the elevations of plasma DNA were observed. The authors concluded that the dialytic procedure induces the death of leucocytes on the artificial surfaces and the release of their DNA into blood thus is responsible for elevated values of extracellular DNA. In this study plasma DNA levels were increased in interdialytic interval in 41 out of 99 samples, among samples with elevated cfDNA levels were 18 out of 24 samples collected from hepatitis B infected person.
The study performed by Rumore et al. (1992) used the same cfDNA detection method as Steinman & Ackad (1977) and exploited the possibilities of the visualization of radiolabeled DNA on electrophoretic gels to demonstrate that in the blood of hemodialyzed patients the electrophoretic patterns known from patients with lupus erythematosus (SLE) are clearly recognizable. This study documented also by immunoprecipitation that at least the large fraction of cfDNA in the blood of hemodialyzed patients circulates in the form of nucleosomes like in the patients with lupus erythematosus. The autoradiograms provided the picture of DNA samples fragmented in the typical manner with predominance of bands corresponding to DNA of 150-200, 400 and in some cases 600 bp.

The authors calculated also very carefully the half-live of this fraction of cfDNA and its rate of clearance. Their study was limited by selection of patients with postdialytic concentrations of cfDNA high inough for performance of experiments. The half-life of cfDNA in blood of hemodialyzed patients immediately after hemodialysis was determined as 4 minutes in this study. The rate of cfDNA clearance from circulation calculated by authors is equivalent to the DNA content of approximately 15 g of a solid tissue such as liver or of the leucocyte content of 600 ml of whole blood at WBC of 5000/mm^3 per day (Rumore et al., 1992).

Although the nucleosomes were found in the blood of patients after hemodialysis in similar amount as in the patients with lupus erythematosus, the hemodialysis itself does not induce any autoimmune response. According to their results, Rumore et al. (1992) hypothesized that in patients with lupus erythematosus an impairment of mechanism of nucleosome clearance contribute to the development of autoimmune disease.

Atamaniuk et al. (2006) investigated the levels of cfDNA in hemodialyzed patients together with markers of early and late apoptosis in leucocytes. For detection of early and late apoptosis flow cytometric measurements of annexin V expression in combination with 7-amino-actinomycin D (7AAD) were used. Annnexin V has high affinity for phosphatidylserine which is translocated during early apoptosis from the inner to the outer surface of the plasma membrane. The nuclear 7AAD staining is possible only in the late apoptosis or in dead cells because the plasma membrane is desintegrated in such stages and allows the throughput of the stain into the nucleus. Employing this methodology, the leucocyte can be classified as normal (annexin V- and 7AAD-), early apoptotic (annexin V+ and 7AAD -), and apoptotic (annexinV + and 7AAD+). Ten patients hemodialyzed on synthetic polymer membranes [Fresenius Polysulfone Capillary dialyzers (F6) low-flux] and 30 healthy subjects were examined in the study. Blood samples from hemodialyzed patients were obtained before hemodialysis (HD), after 20 min of HD, at the end of HD. The concentrations of cfDNA in plasma samples were measured using Vistra Green and human placental DNA calibrators. The emitted fluorescent signals were measured in the LightCycler at 530 nm and reported in picograms per microliters.

In HD patients the cfDNA levels before hemodialysis were slightly higher than in controls. The significant increase was detected after 20 min of HD. The highest values of cfDNA concentrations were determined at the end of HD. The cfDNA samples isolated from plasma of patients were subjected to agarose gel electrophoresis. In pre-HD samples and in samples taken after 20 min of HD the weaker ladders than in samples after HD were observed.

The fraction of leucocytes in early apoptosis was significantly higher in predialytic interval in patients than in controls. The number of apoptotic leucocytes increased during HD. The authors conclude that the apoptosis induced by the contact of leucocytes with dialysis membrane may be the main source of elevated concentrations of cfDNA during HD sessions.

Different types of dialysis membrane were examined in the study by García-Moreira et al. (2006) performed with regard to their influence on the cfDNA levels in plasma. In this study, concentrations of cfDNA were measured first time using real-time quantitative PCR. The sequence of β-*globin* gene was amplified to quantify the total amount of cfDNA in plasma samples. To establish the range of normal values, the samples from 100 healthy voluntary blood donors were examined.

Thirty patients on regular HD were studied in 52 sessions. Chronic renal failure in patients was caused by diabetic nephropathy (7 patients), glomerulosclerosis (6 patients), nephroangioesclerosis (6 patients), chronic pyelonephritis (3 patients), polycystic kidney disease (2 patients), primary amyloidosis (1 patient), renal artery stenosis (1 patient), renal transplantation (1patient), and unknown causes (3 patients).The study was designed to compare high-flux (n=37) vs. low-flux (n=15) and polysulfone (n=42) vs. modified cellulose (n=10) membranes, seven different membranes were used: Arylane H, Tricea 210, HF-80, Arylane M6, FX-60, FX-80, and P160. The effect of the dialysis length on cfDNA concentration after HD was evaluated.

Although correct interpretation of the results is difficult with regard to many variable factors, cfDNA levels increased more than four-fold in 75% of the patients after HD. The study by García-Moreira et al. (2006) has two priorities: 1/ the real-time PCR method was used for the first time to quantify cfDNA; 2/ clear data about the clearance of elevated cfDNA concentrations after HD were provided to scientific community. The authors reported a rapid decline to normal values within 30 minutes of completing a hemodialysis session.

In our study (Korabecna et al., 2008), we determined not only pre- and post-dialytic cfDNA concentrations in patients on hemodialysis (n=17) but we also examined non-dialyzed patients with chronic kidney disease (n=20) and patients on peritoneal dialysis (n=18) in comparison with healthy volunteers (n=20). We measured the total cfDNA levels using real-time PCR on GADPH gene. All patients involved in our study were hemodialyzed on high-flux polysulfone membrane.

In HD patients, we found elevated postdialytic cfDNA values and reported high interindividual variability. We found also patients with lowered cfDNA values after hemodialysis. The levels of cfDNA in HD patients in pre-dialytic interval were significantly increased when compared with patients with chronic kidney disease and patients on peritoneal dialysis but there was no significant difference in comparison with healthy persons probably due to the very broad range of cfDNA concentrations obtained in our control group.

It seems that the study of quantitative and qualitative cfDNA parameters with regard to the process of hemodialysis can bring very interesting insights into the biological aspect of the treatment with important clinical consequences.

4.2 Cell-free nucleic acids in patients on peritoneal dialysis

In our study mentioned above (Korabecna et al., 208), we use real-time PCR based on the GAPDH gene sequence amplification for quantification of cfDNA in plasma and overnight dialysate in patients on peritoneal dialysis. We determined the ratio of dialysate cfDNA/plasma cfDNA (P/D ratio) and discovered that this ratio inversely correlates with the duration of period for which the person is treated by peritoneal dialysis. The values of P/D ratio lower than one were found in patients dialysed for longer time (median 17 months).

Ozkaya et al. (2009) studied the plasma cfDNA in children on peritoneal dialysis and found significantly elevated values in comparison to healthy children and positive correlation with C- reactive protein levels in treated children.

Samples of peritoneal effluent with regard to their content of cfDNA were examined in the study by Pajek et al. (2009) to analyze the impact of PD solution with different biocompatibility and cytotoxic properties on the peritoneal membrane cells. Two PD solutions were tested: a conventional lactate buffered, acidic solution and a novel, bicarbonate/lactate buffered, neutral solution low in glucose degradation products. A significant decrease in appearance of cfDNA in effluent was observed with the novel PD solution.

5. Future perspectives

The study of cell-free nucleic acids in connection with hemodialysis promises new clinically important findings. Application of new methods - mainly the technology of Next Generation Sequencing (NGS) in combination with bionformatics - will bring huge amount of qualitative and quantitative data and allow the study of tiny fractions of specific sequences on the total circulating nucleic acids background. Recently, no studies focused on analysis of microRNA and mRNA in the plasma of hemodialyzed patient are available. Probably, such studies will be managed in near future.

It has been reported that some interleukins are generated during hemodialysis. It is known that activated monocytes during HD liberate certain mediators of immune response (Kim et al., 2011) therefore the study of individual mechanisms of immune response in patients may be very helpful in the process of individualized treatment. Insights into the current character of immune response can be achieved through the analysis of the methylation status of selected genes using existing arrays technologies. Such high throughput technologies will lead to the comparison of hemodialysis effects on the character of immune response in different groups of patients with different comorbidities.

DNA methylation patterns determined at the level of cfDNA in hemodialyzed patiens may be predictive of response to specific drugs and drug combinations.

The clinical studies performed on hemodialyzed patients can also improve the theoretical knowledge about the clearance and turnover of circulating nucleic acids in connection to the regulatory functions of this extremely interesting class of molecules.

6. Conclusion

Today, there are various methodological approaches allowing the quantitative and qualitative characterization of cell-free nucleic acids in circulation of hemodialyzed patients. The study od cfDNA in plasma during the hemodialysis began 30 years ago and brought interesting results concerning the apoptotic origin of at least an important fraction of this DNA and increase of its plasma concentration during the hemodialysis session regardless of the used membranes and duration of session. In the past decade, the clearance of cfDNA from plasma was studied not only in hemodialyzed patients, and it was concluded, that it is very rapid (the half-life is given in minutes) and kidney does not play the major role in this process. In last years, the attention is paid to the examination of cell-free ribonucleic acids in the circulation with regard to their use as biomarkers under different pathological conditions. The application of such methodologies in the field of hemodialysis is still awaiting for the researchers, as well as the application of high throughput technologies likes Next Generation Sequencing and array technologies of different design. The connection of new technologies with clinical studies will result not only in clinical benefit but also in deeper insight into basic biological mechanisms of intracellular communication, epigenetic regulation and modulation of immune function at the individualized level leading to truly personalized medicine.

7. Acknowledgment

This work was supported by the grant of Ministry of Education of the Czech Republic no. MSM 0021620807.

8. References

Anker, P.; Stroun, M.; Maurice, P.A. (1976). Spontaneous Extracellular Synthesis of DNA Released by Human Blood Lymphocytes. *Cancer Research*, Vol. 36, No. 4, (August 1976), pp. 2832-2839, ISSN 0008-5472

Antonatos, D.; Patsilinakos, S.; Spanodimos, S.; Korkonikitas, P.; Tsigas, D. (2006). Cell-Free DNA Levels as a Prognostic Marker in Acute Myocardial Infarction. *Annals of New York Academy of Science*, Vol. 1075 (September 2006), pp. 278-281, ISSN 00778923

Atamaniuk, J.; Vidotto, C.; Tschan, H.; Bachl, N.; Stuhlmeier, K.M.; Müller, M.M. (2004) Increased Concentrations of Cell-Free Plasma DNA after Exhaustive Exercise. *Clinical Chemistry*, Vol. 50, No. 9, (September 2004), pp. 523–526, ISSN 0009-9147

Atamaniuk, J.; Ruzicka, K.; Stuhlmeier, K.M.; Karimi, A.; Eigner, M.; Mueller, M.M. (2006). Cell-Free Plasma DNA: a Marker for Apoptosis During Hemodialysis. *Clinical Chemistry*, Vol. 52, No. 3, (March 2006), pp. 523–526, ISSN 0009-9147

Ayala, W.; Moore, L.W. & Hess, E.L. (1951). The Purple Color Reaction Given by Diphenylamine Reagent. I. With Normal and Rheumatic Fever Sera. *Journal of Clinical Investigation*, Vol. 30, No. 7, (July 1951), pp. 781-785, ISSN 0021-9738

Beck, J.; Urnovitz, H.B.; Riggert, J.; Clerici, M.; Schutz, E. (2009). Profile of the Circulating DNA in Apparently Healthy Individuals. *Clinical Chemistry*, Vol. 55, No. 4, (April 2009), pp. 730–738, ISSN 0009-9147

Beck, J.; Urnovitz, H.B.; Mitchell, W.M.; Schütz, E. (2010). Next Generation Sequencing of Serum Circulating Nucleic Acids from Patients with Invasive Ductal Breast Cancer Reveals Differences to Healthy and Nonmalignant Controls. *Molecular Cancer Research*, Vol. 8, No. 3, (March 2010), pp. 335-342, ISSN 1541-7786

Botezatu, I.; Serdyuk, O.; Potapova, G.; Shelepov, V.; Alechina, R.; Molyaka, Y.; Ananév, V.; Bazin, I.; Garin, A.; Narimanov, M.; Knysh, V.; Melkonyan, H.; Umansky, S.; Lichtenstein, A.(2000). Genetic Analysis of DNA Excreted in Urine: a New Approach for Detecting Specific Genomic DNA Sequences from Cells Dying in an Organism. *Clinical Chemistry*, Vol. 46, No. 8, (August 2000), pp. 1078–1084, ISSN 0009-9147

Burlingame, R.W.; Volzer, M.A.; Harris, J.; Du Clos, T.W. (1996). The Effect of Acute Phase Proteins on Clearance of Chromatin from the Circulation of Normal Mice. *Journal of Immunology*, Vol. 156, No. 12, (June 1996), pp. 4783–4788, ISSN 0022-1767

Carracedo, J.; Ramirez, R.; Pintado, O.; Gomez-Villamandos, J.C.; Martin-Malo, A.; Rodriguez, M.; Aljama.P. (1995). Cell Aggregation and Apoptosis Induced by Hemodialysis Membranes. *Journal of the American Society of Nephrology*, Vol. 9, No.1, (January 1995), pp. 1586–1591, ISSN 1046-6673

Chan, K.C.; Leung, S.F.; Yeung, S.W.; Chan, A.T.; Lo, Y.M. (2008). Quantitative Analysis of the Transrenal Excretion of Circulating EBV DNA in Nasopharyngeal Carcinoma Patients. *Clinical Cancer Research*, Vol. 1, No. 14(15), (August 2008), pp. 4809-4813, ISSN 1078-0432

Cherepanova. A.V.; Tamkovich, S.N.; Bryzgunova, O.E.; Vlassov, V.V.; Laktionov, P.P. (2008) Deoxyribonuclease Activity and Circulating DNA Concentration in Blood Plasma of Patients with Prostate Tumors. *Annals of Nex York Academy of Sciences*, Vol. 1137, (August 2008) pp. 218-221, ISSN 00778923

Colotta, F.; Re, F.; Polentarutti, N.; Sozzani, S.; Mantovami, A. (1992). Modulation of Granulocyte Survival and Programmed Cell Death by Cytokines and Bacterial Products. *Blood,* Vol. 80, No. 8, (October 1992), pp. 2012–2020, ISSN 0006-4971

Crouser, E.D.; Julian, M.W. & Blaho, D.V. (2002). Endotoxin-Induced Mitochondrial Damage Correlates with Impaired Respiratory Activity. *Critical Care Medicine,* Vol. 30, No. 2, (February 2002), pp. 276-284, ISSN 0090-3493

Fatouros, I.G.; Destouni, A.; Margonis, K.; Jamurtas, A.Z.; Vrettou, C.; Kouretas, D., Mastorakos, G.; Mitrakou, A.; Taxildaris, K.; Kanavakis, E.; Papassotiriou, I. (2006). Cell-Free Plasma DNA as a Novel Marker of Aseptic Inflammation Severity Related to Exercise Overtraining. *Clinical Chemistry,* Vol. 52, No. 9, (September 2006), pp. 1820–1824, ISSN 0009-9147

Fournie, G.J.; Lule, J.; Dueymes, J.M.; Laval, F.; Delobbe, I.; Verner. I., Pourrat, J.P. (1989). Plasma DNA in Patients Undergoing Hemodialysis or Hemofiltration: Cytolysis in Artificial Kidney is Responsible for the Release of DNA in Circulation. *American Journal of Nephrology* , Vol. 9, No. 5, pp. 384–391, ISSN 0250-8095

García-Olmo, D.; García-Olmo, D.C.; Ontañón, J.; Martinez, E.; Vallejo, M. (1999). Tumor DNA Circulating in the Plasma Might Play a Role in Metastasis. The Hypothesis of the Genometastasis. *Histology and Histopathology,* Vol. 14, No. 4, (October 1999), pp. 1159-1164, ISSN 0213-3911

García-Olmo, D.; García-Olmo, D.C.; Ontañón, J.; Martinez, E. (2000). Horizontal Transfer of DNA and the "Genometastasis Hypothesis". *Blood,* Vo. 95, No. 2, (January 2000), pp. 724-725, ISSN 0006-4971

García-Moreira, V.; Prieto García, B.; Baltar Martín, J.M.; Ortega Suárez, F.; Alvarez, F.V. (2009). Cell-Free DNA as a Noninvasive Acute Rejection Marker in Renal Transplantation. *Clinical Chemistry,* Vol. 55, No. 11, (November 2009), pp. 1958-1966, ISSN 0009-9147

Gauthier, V.J.; Tyler, L.N.; Mannik, M. (1996). Blood Clearance Kinetics and Liver Uptake of Mononucleosomes in Mice. *Journal of Immunology,* Vol. 156, No. 3, (February 1996), pp. 1151–1156, ISSN 0022-1767

Guan, J.; Jin D.D.; Jin, L.J. (2002). Apoptosis in Organs of Rats in Early Stage after Polytrauma Combined with Shock. *Journal of Trauma,* Vol. 52, No 1, (January 2002), pp, 104-111, ISSN 1529-8809

Holdenrieder, S.; Stieber, P.; Bodenmuller, H.; Busch, M.; Von Pawel, J.; Schalhorn, A.; Nagel. D.; Seidel, D. (2001). Circulating Nucleosomes in Serum. *Annals of New York Academy of Sciences,* Vol. 945, (September 2001), pp. 93–102, ISSN 00778923

Horinek, A.; Korabecna, M.; Panczak, A.; Ulcova Gallova. Z.; Nouzova, K.; Calda, P.; Hancarova. M. (2008). Cell-Free Fetal DNA in Maternal Plasma During Physiological Single Male Pregnancies: Methodology Issues and Kinetics. *Fetal Diagnosis and Therapy,* Vol. 24, No. 1, (May 2008), pp. 15-21, ISSN 1015-3837

Horinek , A.; Panczak, A.; Mokrejsova, A.; Rocinova, K.; Korabecna, M; Cerny, D.; Tesar, V. (2011). Comparison of Plasma Cell-Free DNA Levels with Gene Expression Profiles of Peripheral Blood Cells During Hemodialysis. In: *Circulating Nucleic Acids in Plasma and Serum,* P.Gahan, (Ed.), 159-163, Springer, ISBN 978-90-481-9381-3

Kobayashi, N.; Kuramoto, T.; Yamaoka, K.; Hashida, M.; Takakura,Y. (2001). Hepatic Uptake and Gene Expression Mechanisms Following Intravenous Administration of Plastid DNA by Conventional and Hydrodynamics-Based Procedures. *Journal of*

Pharmacology and Experimental Therapeutics, Vol. 297, No. 3, (June 2001), pp. 853–860, ISSN 0022-3565

Kim, H.W.; Yang, H.N.; Kim, M.G.; Choi, H.M.; Jo, S.K.; Cho, W.Y.; Kim, H.K. (2011). Microinflammation in Hemodialysis Patients Is Associated with Increased CD14CD16(+) Pro-Inflammatory Monocytes: Possible Modification by On-Line Hemodiafiltration. *Blood Purification*, Vol 31, No. 4. (January 2011) pp. 281-288, ISSN 0253-5068

Korabecna, M.; Opatrna, S.; Wirth, J.; Rulcova, K.; Eiselt, J.; Sefrna, F.; Horinek, A. (2008). Cell-Free Plasma DNA During Peritoneal Dialysis and Hemodialysis and in Patients with Chronic Kidney Disease. *Annals of New York Academy of Sciences*, Vol. 1137, (August 2008), pp. 296-301, ISSN 00778923

Korabecna, M.; Horinek, A.; Bila, N.; Opatrna, S. (2011). Circadian Rhytmicity and Clearance of Cell-Free DNA in Human Plasma. In: *Circulating Nucleic Acids in Plasma and Serum*, P.Gahan, (Ed.), 159-163, Springer, ISBN 978-90-481-9381-3

Koyama, S.; Akira, S.; Ishii, K.J. (2010) Immune Recognition of Nucleic Acids and Their Metabolites. In: *Extracellular Nucleic Acids*, E.Y, Rykova, Y. Kikuchi (Eds.), Springer ISBN: 3642126162, Berlin, Germany

Lau, T.W.; Leung, T.N.; Chan, L.Y.; Lau, T.K.; Chan, K.C.; Tam, W.H.; Lo, Y.M. (2002). DNA Clearance from Maternal Plasma is Impaired in Preeclampsia. *Clinical Chemistry*, Vol. 48, No. 12, (December 2002), pp. 2141–2146, ISSN 0009-9147

Lee, A.; Chyte M.K.B. & Haslett, C. (1993). Inhibition of Apoptosis and Prolongation of Neutrophil Functional Longevity by Inflammatory Mediators. *Journal of Leukocyte Biology*, Vol. 54, No. 4, (October 1993), pp. 283–288, ISSN 0741-5400

Leon, S.A.; Shapiro, B.; Sklaroff, D.M.; Yaros, M.J. (1977). Free DNA in the Serum of Cancer Patients and the Effect of Therapy. *Cancer Research*, Vol. 37, No. 3, (March 1977), pp. 646-650, ISSN 0008-5472

Lewis, S.L. & Van Epps, D.E. (1987). Neutrophil and Monocyte Alterations in Chronic Dialysis Patients. *American Journal of Kidney Diseases*, Vol. 9, No. 5, (May 1987), pp. 381–395, ISSN 0272-6386

Lindau, D.; Rönnefarth, V.; Erbacher, A.; Rammensee, H.G.; Decker, P. (2011). Nucleosome-Induced Neutrophil Activation Occurs Independently of TLR9 and Endosomal Acidification: Implications for Systemic Lupus Erythematosus. *European Journal of Immunology*, Vol. 41, No. 3, (March 2011), pp. 669-681, ISSN 0014-2980

Lo, Y.M.; Corbetta, N.; Chamberlain, P.F.; Rai, V.; Sargent, I.L.; Redman, C.W.; Wainscoat, J.S. (1997). Presence of Fetal DNA in Maternal Plasma and Serum. *Lancet*, Vol 350. No. 9076, (August 1997), pp. 350-487, ISSN 0140-6736

Lo Y.M.D.; Zhang, J.; Leung, T.N.; Lau, T.K.; Chang, A.M.; Hjelm, N.M. (1999) Rapid Clearance of Fetal DNA from Maternal Plasma. *American Journal of Human Genetics*, Vol. 64, No. 1, (January 1999), pp. 218–224, ISSN 0002-9297

Lo, Y.M.; Rainer, T.H.; Chan, L.Y.; Hjelm, N.M.; Cocks, R.A. (2000). Plasma DNA as a Prognostic Marker in Trauma Patients. *Clinical Chemistry*, Vol. 46, No. 3, (March 2000), pp. 319–323, ISSN 0009-9147

Martin, D. A. & Elkon, K. B. (2006). Intracellular Mammalian DNA Stimulates Myeloid Dendritic Cells to Produce Type I Interferons Predominantly Through a Toll-Like Receptor 9-Independent Pathway. *Arthritis and Rheumatism*, Vol 54, No. 3, (March 2006), pp. 951–962, ISSN 0004-3591

García-Moreira, V.; de la Cera Martínez, T.; Gago González, E.; Prieto García, B.; Alvarez Menéndez, F.V. (2006). Increase in and Clearance of Cell-Free Plasma DNA in Hemodialysis Quantified by Real-Time PCR. *Clinical Chemistry and Laboratory Medicine*, Vol. 44, No. 12, pp.1410–1415, ISSN 1434-6621

Nahar, N.; Shah, H.; Siu, J.; Colvin, R.; Bhaskaran, M.; Ranjan, R.; Wagner, J.D.; Singhal, P.C. (2001). Dialysis Membrane-Induced Neutrophil Apoptosis is Mediated Through Free Radicals. *Clinical Nephrology*, Vol. 56, No. 1, (July 2001), pp. 52–59, ISSN 0301-0430

Pachl, J.; Duska, F.; Waldauf, P.; Fric, M.; Fanta, J.; Zdárský, E. (2005). Apoptosis as an Early Event in the Development of Multiple Organ Failure? *Physiological Research*, Vol. 54, No. 2, (2005), pp. 697-699, ISSN 0862-8408

Pajek, J.; Kveder, R.; Gucek, A.; Skoberne, A.; Bren, A.; Bucar, M.; Cerne, D.; Lukac-Bajalo, J. (2010). Cell-free DNA in the Peritoneal Effluent of Peritoneal Dialysis Solutions. *Therapeutic Apheresis and Dialysis*, Vol. 14, No. 1, (February 2010), pp. 20-26, ISSN 1744-9979

Peters, D.L. & Pretorius, P.J. (2011). Origin, Translocation and Destination of Extracellular Occurring DNA - A new Paradigm in Genetic Behaviour. *Clinica Chimica Acta*, Vol. 412, No. 11-12, (May 2011), pp. 806-811, ISSN 0009-8981

Puszyk, W.M.; Crea, F.; Old, R.W. (2009). Unequal Representation of Different Unique Genomic DNA Sequences in the Cell-Free Plasma DNA of Individual Donors. *Clinical Biochemistry*, Vol. 42, No. 7-8, (May 2009), pp. 736–738, ISSN 0009-9120

Rainer, T.H. & Lam, N.Y.L. (2006). Circulating Nucleic Acids and Critical Illness. *Annals of New York Academy of Sciences*. Vol. 1075, (September 2006), pp. 271–277 , ISSN 00778923

Rhodes, A.; Wort, S.J.; Thomas, H.; Collinson, P.; Bennett, E.D. (2006). Plasma DNA Concentration as a Predictor of Mortality and Sepsis in Critically Ill Patients. *Critical Care*. Vol 10, No. 2, (April 2006), pp. R60, ISSN 1466-609X

Rumore, P.; Muralidhar, B.; Lin, M.; Lai, C.; Steinman, C.R. (1992). Haemodialysis as a Model for Studying Endogenous Plasma DNA: Oligonucleosome-Like Structure and Clearance. *Clinical and Experimental Immunology*, Vol. 90., No. 1, (October 1992), pp. 56-62, ISSN 0009-9104

Saukkonnen, K.; Lakkisto, P.; Varpula, M.; Varpula, T.; Voipio-Pulkki, L.M.; Pettilä, V.; Pulkki, K. (2007). Association of Cell-Free Plasma DNA with Hospital Mortality and Organ Dysfunction in Intensive Care Unit Patients. *Intensive Care Medicine*, Vol. 33, No. 9, (September 2007), pp. 1624–1627, ISSN 0342-4642

Savill, J. (1997). Apoptosis in Resolution of Inflammation. *Journal of Leukocyte Biology*, Vol 61, No. 4, (April 1997), pp. 375–380, ISSN 0741-5400

Simpson, R.J.; Jensen, S.S; Lim. JW. (2008). Proteomic Profiling of Exosomes: Current Perspectives. *Proteomics*, Vol. 8, No.19, (October 2008), pp. 4083-4099, ISSN 1615-9853

Skvortsova, T.E.; Vlassov, V.V., Laktionov, P.P. (2008). Binding and Penetration of Methylated DNA into Primary and Transformed Human Cells. *Annals of New York Academy of Sciences*, Vol. 1137, (August 2008), pp. 36-40, ISSN 00778923

Sorenson, G.D.; Pribish, D.M.; Valone, F.H.; Nemolí, V.A.; Bzik, D.J.; Yao, S.L. (1994). Soluble Normal and Mutated DNA Sequences From Single-Copy Genes in Human Blood.

Cancer Epidemiology, Biomarkers & Prevention, Vol. 3, No. 1, (January-February 1994), pp. 67-71, ISSN 1055-9965

Steinman, C.R. &, Ackad A. (1977). Appearance of Circulating DNA During Hemodialysis. *American Journal of Medicine*, Vol. 62, No. 5, (May 1977), pp. 693–697, ISSN 0002-9343

Stroun, M.; Lyautey, J.; Lederrey, C.; Olson-Sand, A.; Anker, P. (2001a). About the Possible Origin and Mechanism of Circulating DNA Apoptosis and Active DNA Release. *Clinica Chimica Acta*. Vol. 313, No. 1-2, (November 2001), pp. 139-142, ISSN 0009-8981

Stroun, M.; Lyautey, J.; Lederrey, C.; Mulcahy, H.E.; Anker, P. (2001b). Alu Repeat Sequences are Present in Increased Proportions Compared to a Unique Gene in Plasma/Serum DNA: Evidence for a Preferential Release from Viable Cells? *Annals of New York Academy of Sciences*, Vol. 945, (September 2001), pp. 258-264, ISSN 00778923

Su,Y.H.; Wang, M.; Aiamkitsumrit, B.; Brenner, D.E.; Block, T.M. (2005). Detection of a K-ras Mutation in Urine of Patients with Colorectal Cancer. *Cancer Biomarkers*, Vol. 1, No. 2-3, (August 2005), pp.177-182, ISSN 1574-0153

Swarup, V. & Rajeswari, M.R. (2007). Circulating (Cell-Free) Nucleic Acids - a Promising, Non-Invasive Tool for Early Detection of Several Human Diseases. *FEBS Letters*, Vol. 581, No. 5, (March 2007), pp. 795-799, ISSN 0014-5793

Taylor, D.D.; Zacharias, W.; Gercel-Taylor, C. (2011) Exosome Isolation for Proteomic Analyses and RNA Profiling. *Methods in Molecular Biology*, Vol. 728, (2011), pp. 235-246. ISSN 1064-3745

Tong, Y.K. & Lo, Y.M. (2006). Diagnostic Developments Involving Cell-Free (Circulating) Nucleic Acids. *Clinica Chimica Acta*, Vol. 363, No. 1-2, (January 2006), pp. 187-196, ISSN 0009-8981

van der Vaart, M. & Pretorius, P.J. (2008). A Method for Characterization of Total Circulating DNA. *Annals of New York Academy of Sciences*, Vol. 1137, (August 2008), pp. 92-97, ISSN 00778923

Veiko, N.N.; Bulycheva, N.V.; Roginko, O.A.; Veĭko, R.V.; Ershova, E.S.; Ozdoba, O.A.; Kuz'min, V.A.; Vinogradov, A.M.; Iudin, A.A.; Speranskii, A.I. (2008). Ribosomal Repeat in the Cell Free DNA as a Marker for Cell Death. *Biomeditsinskaja Khimia*. Vol. 54, No. 1, (January-February2008), pp. 78-93, ISBN 0042-8809

Vlassov, V.V.; Laktionov, P.P.& Rykova, E.Y. (2010). Circulating Nucleic Acids as a Potential Source for Cancer Biomarkers. *Current Molecular Medicine*, Vol. 10, No. 2, (March 2010), pp. 142-165, ISSN 1566-5240

Wijeratne, S.; Butt, A.; Burns, S.; Sherwood, K.; Boyd, O.; Swaminathan, R. (2004). Cell-free plasma DNA as a Prognostic Marker in Intensive Treatment Unit Patients. *Annals of New York Academy of Sciences*, Vol. 1022, (June 2004), pp. 232-238, ISSN 00778923

13

Measuring System of Urea in Blood by Application in Recirculation for Hemodialysis Treatment

G.A. Martinez
Department of Nephrology
Hemodialysis Subsection
Military Hospital Center
México D.F.

1. Introduction

End stage renal disease (ESRD) is one of the most common life-threatening diseases. The number of patients accepted for renal replacement therapy including hemodialysis (HD), peritoneal dialysis, and kidney transplantation in developed and developing countries increases each year and imposes a major social and economic burden on these communities.(1)
With an increasing number of elderly patients as well as patients with co-morbid conditions such as vascular disease and diabetes mellitus in the hemodialysis (HD) population, a well functioning mature arteriovenous fistula (AVF) is essential for the delivering HD in these patients. [1],[2] Malfunction of permanent vascular accesses remains a cause of frequent and costly morbidity among these patients. [3]
Stenosis of the HD vascular access is common with an occlusion rate of 17–45% at one year. [4],[5] Therefore, periodic monitoring of the access is recommended; early detection and correction of stenotic lesions can reduce the frequency of thrombosis and the need for high-risk therapy, increase the life of the access and help to reduce the rate of access failure. [1],[5]
A variety of techniques such as physical examination, venous pump pressure, percent access recirculation, transonic flow and others are helpful in detecting vascular access dysfunction and improve assessment of the vascular access site. [4],[6] There is currently no consensus as to the optimum method of screening for stenosis; the most widely used method of screening for stenosis has been the percent access recirculation (%AR) measurement. [4]
Vascular access recirculation (AR) is defined as the return of dialyzed blood to the arterial segment of the access bypassing the systemic recirculation, thereby resulting in reducing the efficiency of dialysis. [7] High degrees of recirculation can lead to a significant discrepancy between the amount of HD prescribed and the amount of HD delivered.[8] Some investigators have suggested that AR of *15%* or higher reliably suggests significant stenosis. [4]
The usually method for recirculation measuring is the Doppler Effect and the different technical based in the circulation blood sense of through the needles. These procedures have the great advantage to be carried by the medical and infirmary personal.
At the moment some automatic systems estimate the recirculation rate with used hemodilutión technical that consist in the administration of saline serum in the return line,

as well the employment of differences sensors in the arterial line for example; they measure of transmission the ultrasounds speed, the changes in the hematocrit conductivity or the temperature in blood.
The investment of lines also produces changes in the increases of the hematocrit induced by abrupt increments of the ultra filtration rate, constituting the base of our procedure to measure the flow of the vascular access.
There are hemodialysis monitors that incorporate the automatic reading of the ionic dialisance by conductivity analysis in the dialysis liquid. This measuring is effectuated to input and output in the dialysis filter. The ionic dialisance is equivalent to urea clearing (clearing of the dialyzed corrected by the total recirculation) that variation in the ionic dialisance is depends on the flow in the vascular access and it allows the calculation of the same one without having to dilute the blood by the administration of saline serum.
At the moment some automatic systems estimate the recirculation rate with used hemodilutión technical that consist in saline serum administration, as well the employment of differences sensors (ultrasounds, conductivity or the temperature) in the arterial line.
Example of the previous things is that some hemodialysis monitors that incorporate the automatic reading based of the ionic dialisance and conductivity analysis in the dialysis liquid.
This measuring is effectuated to input and output in the dialysis filter. The ionic dialisance is equivalent to urea clearing (clearing of the dialyzed corrected by the total recirculation) that variation in the ionic dialisance is depends on the flow in the vascular access and it allows the calculation of the same one without having to dilute the blood by the administration of saline serum.
We are studying the possibility to recirculation measure in fixed and permanent vascular access by On-Line mensuration of the Urea in blood (BUN) by employ the optical sensor in visible range, this results which compare by laboratory technical based in the method recirculation of two needles.
The purpose of the present study was to evaluate AR in chronic renal failure patients for early detection of access stenosis and subsequent intervention or revision to prolong the life of the access.
It is well established that one of cause of inadequate dialysis in HD patients is arterio-venous (A-V) fistula access recirculation (AR). Hemodialysis AR is diagnosed when dialyzed blood returning through the venous side reenters the dialyzer through the arterial needle, rather than returning to the systemic circulation and as a result, the efficiency of HD is reduced.(8) Thus the aim of the study was to investigate the prevalence and causes of A-V fistula recirculation in HD patients in Military Hospital Center in Mexico City.

2. Material and methods

From February 2008 to August 2009, this cross sectional study was conducted on adult ESRD (End-stage Renal Disease) patients in HD of Military Hospital Center, Mexico City. A standardized questionnaire was used to collect demographic data, cause of ESRD, the date of HD onset, the type of access for HD, the date of creation and use of A-V fistula and history of a kidney transplant.
The ESRD was defined as permanent and irreversible loss of renal function requiring renal replacement therapy. They were included in the work all the patients in the Hemodialysis program in the Military Hospital Centre.

The study was practice in 37 patient's 15 males and 22 women, with ages 14 and 59 years and the time in hemodialysis treatment between 1 month and 4 years. Mean age of patients was 54.7±15 years, male 55.9±15.2 years and female 52.9±14.7 years. Causes of ESRD of our patients included high blood pressure, diabetes mellitus, glomeronephritis, obstructive uropathy, polycystic kidney and other causes.
HD was performed for 3-4 Hrs, three times a week, using synthetic (polysulfone) dialyzer membranes, and bicarbonate-based dialysate at a delivered bicarbonate concentration of 35 mEq/L. Blood flow rate was maintained at 250-350mL/min, and the dialysate flow rate at 500 mL/min. Then the degree of recirculation was measured with Urea based two needle method from the following formula (9):

2.1 Two needles technique

The analytic form in the recirculation access is based in the urea molecule mensuration or BUN (Nitrogenous Urea in Blood) this estimation is quantified by in employment of the following formulates.

$$R = \frac{(S-A)}{(S-V)} \text{ x } 100\% \tag{1}$$

Where;
S: Urea concentration in blood to take in Peripheral line a low fluid.
A: Urea Concentration in blood to take in arterial line a constant fluid.
V: Urea Concentration in blood to take in venous line a constant fluid.
Arterial (A) and Venus (V) samples to same time and Peripheral (P) obtained with the slow-stop-flow method; obtained A and V; the flow in peristaltic bomb to decrease at 50 ml/min, exactly 10 seconds. Then stop the bomb and immediately clampear the arterial line above the place samples extraction one the sample of blood S or systemic. Then the dialysis is restarted. It is the denominated method of the two needles. To make these determinations recommending 5 to 30 minutes of initiate the dialysis.
The following protocol was used for blood sampling.

1. The ultrafiltration was turned off approximately 30 minutes after the initiation of HD and then arterial and venous line samples (A and V in the above formula) were obtained.
2. Access blood flow was reduced to 50mL/min and 15 to 30 seconds later, the systemic blood sample (P in the above formula) from the arterial blood line was obtained (two-needle" techniques).
3. The samples are reported via the laboratory and they are compared with those registered by On-Line system, we compared the statistical results the recirculation percentage and the KT/V estimate.

2.2 Online measurement system in blood urea

We arranged optical custom measurement system based on photodiodes arrays connected to a PIC16F876 microcontroller, which implemented the acquisition and the physical interface between the optical sensors and the display and computer. The system is formed by an array of 128 photodiodes (Texas Instruments); the light source is a LED diode with a single wavelength of 620 nm.

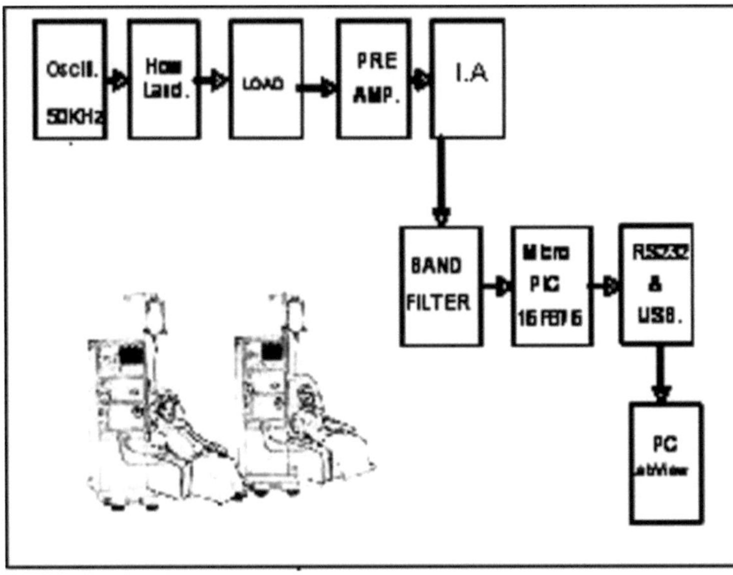

Fig. 1. Schematic diagrams the on line system for urea in blood and LabView programming to connection a PC via RS-232 Protocol used in recirculation measurement during Hemodialysis treatment.

The physical construction system consists on a small dark chamber where the source of light (LED) and the semiconductor device used as sensor (photodiode array) are placed. They are located lengthwise regarding the probe of transparent plastic through which the liquid samples are passed. The linear disposition of photodiodes gives a better rejection of stray light conduced through the tube walls. The voltage resulting of integrating the current of each photodiode during a controlled time is used as the input signal of the 10 bit microcontroller A/D converter. The captured data are then transmitted via RS-232 to a personal computer.
The user interface is developed with Visual Basic ver.6.0, and Lab view Programming performing the data graphical representation to determination the constant of the time.

A. On line Recirculación Systems

1. Oscillator: The oscillator used to generate a Sine wave, was the bridge Howland composed at four resistance and two capacitors. The configuration its low distortion and effective stabilization amplitude, used the TL081 circuit.
2. Tranconductance amplifier (OTA): Generate the current in LED (light-emitting diode), is implemented to LM3080 circuit, which has a gain control.
3. Instrumentation Amplifier (IA): AD624 instrumentation amplifier. The tension in the optical sensor (Array 128 photodiodes) adds to Voltage continuous in 1.25 V.
4. Filtered / Conditioning: The filter function is used TL081 Operational amplifiers, for passes band filter in 45-55 KHz.
5. Microcontroller: PIC16F876 microcontroller, with the internal A/D converter for Sine signal Voltage, and transmission RS-232 communication protocol.

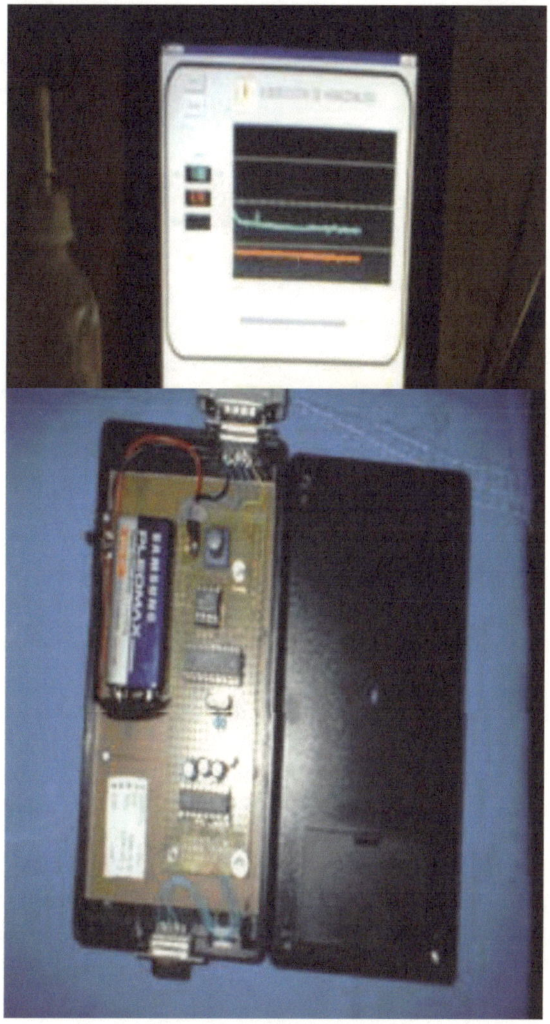

Fig. 2. Experimental Prototype by using PIC16F8767 Microcontroller and connection in the Hemodialysis machine

B. Operation Mode

The optical system consists on a small dark chamber where the source of light (LED) and the semiconductor device used as sensor (photodiode array) are placed. They are located lengthwise regarding the probe of transparent plastic through which the liquid samples are passed. The linear disposition of photodiodes gives a better rejection of stray light conduced through the tube walls. The voltage resulting of integrating the current of each photodiode during a controlled time is used as the input signal of the 10 bit microcontroller A/D converter. The captured data are then transmitted via RS-232 to a personal computer; this date is used to calculations urea concentration. Finally the parameters they show in the graphics interface.

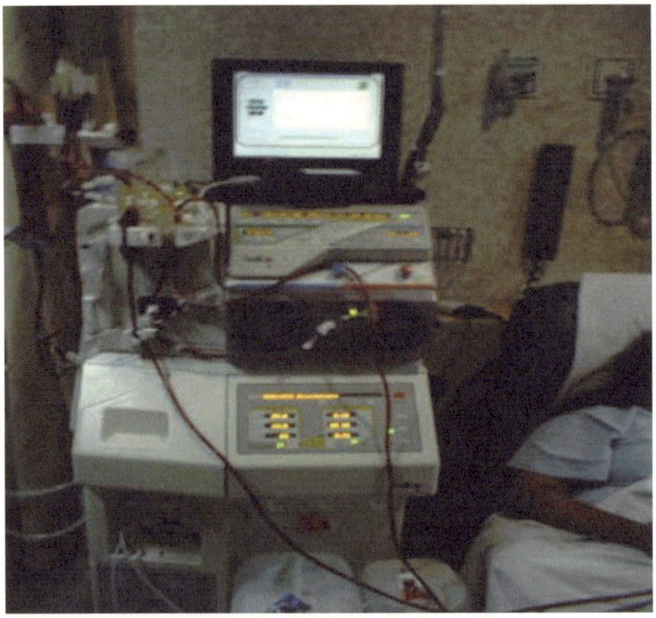

Fig. 3. Experimental systems with both the optical absorbance probe in patients in hemodialysis treatment.

2.3 Measure process of urea concentration in blood in laboratory technical

We used the two needles technique for the recirculation measure in the vascular access. In hemodialysis session, the flow in the vascular access is measured by employs the optical sensor for practice the on-line measure of Urea in blood and blood samples for evaluation in laboratory.

To treatment started the flow is the 400 ml/min after 30 min. We proceed to taking of samples in blood in the arterial (A) and venues (V) line in a simultaneous way, next time diminishes the flow to 50 ml/min during 30 seconds, which this proceeds to a second blood sample in the arterial line (S), concluded this activity with continues the hemodialysis session to the arterial flow prescribed.

The all measurements samples were evaluated in laboratory and on line measurement prototype for urea in hemodialysis treatment. The patients were divided into two groups, group 1 patients without recirculation and group 2 patients with recirculation.

For each patient distances between arterial and venous needles and distances of needles from A-V fistula and its directions was recorded. The findings were analyzed by SPSS statistical program. Chi square test or Fisher Exact test were used for qualitative data. For two group's quantitative data, the means were compared by using student's t test.

Association between risk factors and recirculation rate was evaluated by COX regression model. Statistical significance was assessed at the 0.05 probability level in all analyses.

3. Results

Overall, thirty seven patients 15 male (40.54%) and 22 female (59.45%) were on HD therapy in our centers. From them, thirty seven patients have an A-V fistula and they were on HD more than three months that they enrolled for the study.

3.1 Experimental system

The direct results obtained with the prototype display the optical transmittance in the range of 600-620 nm, corresponding to a Red LED show the evolution in the urea concentration estimated during the experimental Hemodialysis procedure in a patient. In the Figure 4 show the recirculation evolution of the urea concentration during Hemodialysis treatment in a patient shows values in the A-V fistula.

3.2 Clinical measurements

To verify the functioning system, we comparing the urea concentration values obtained with the online prototype values versus Laboratory. Successive measurements under same conditions (connectors, power, temperature, etc.) observing a small dispersion.

The results obtained with optical system and Laboratory (Dade Behring equipment) was coherent. In the Figure 5 we can observe that statistic factor between laboratory and prototype for recirculation percentage in Permanent Vascular Access (PVA). The average estimation for recirculation percentage impermanent accesses via laboratory is 3.57 ± 2.28 %, with optical system is 4.55±2.35%The Figure 6 we can observe that statistic estimation for recirculation percentage in Permanent Hemodialisys Catheter (PHC)

The average accesses via laboratory is 6.25 ± 4.16 %, with optical system is 8.77±5.13%. The show results indicate good correlation in average and standard deviation, the equal forms both measurement systems show wide dispersion The correlation coefficient between optical system and laboratory in the recirculation measurement in permanent accesses is $R^2 = 0.69$ was temporary accesses $R^2 = 0.66$

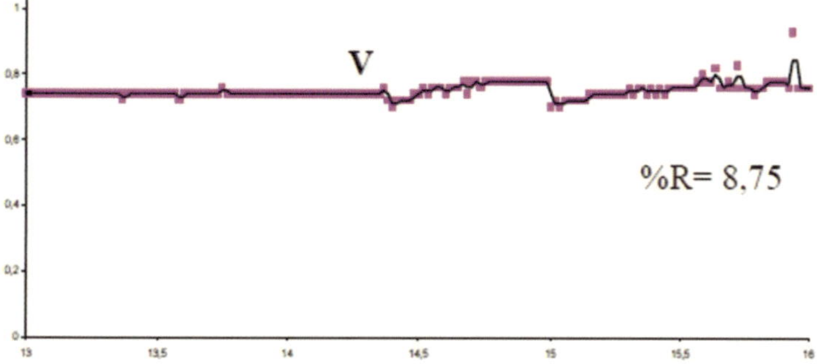

Fig. 4. Recirculation measurement by optical system, the calculation is based in the voltages estimation during Hemodialysis Treatment, Peripheral (S), Arterial (A) and Venous (v) blood samples when two needles technique.

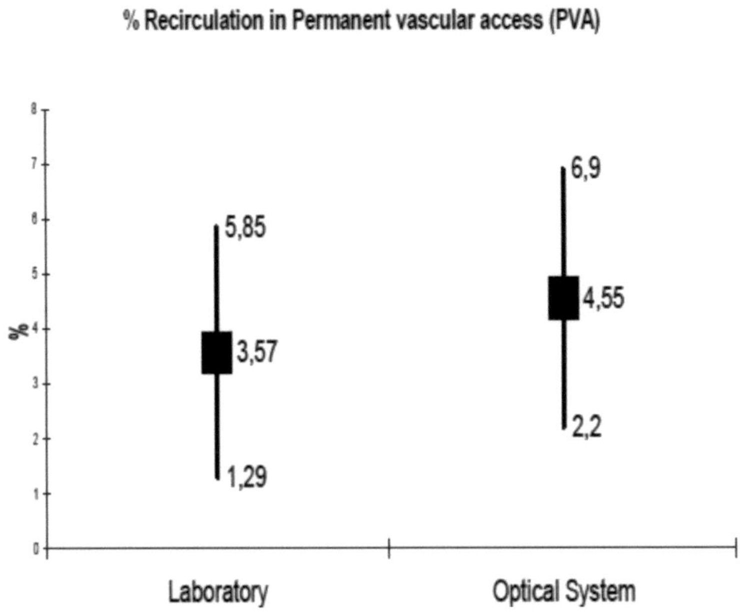

Fig. 5. Results obtained by Laboratory vs. Optical system for recirculation percentage in Permanent Vascular Access (PVA).

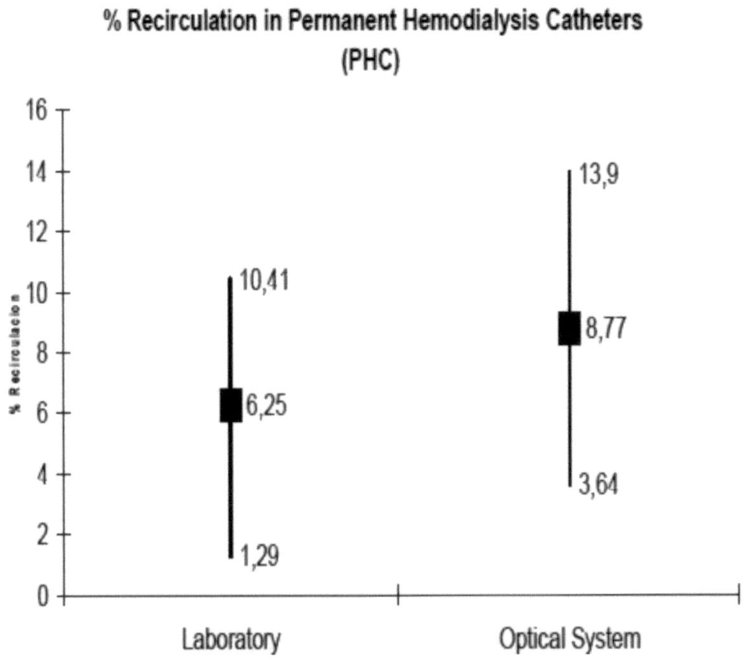

Fig. 6. Results obtained by Laboratory vs. Optical system for recirculation percentage Permanent Hemodialisys Catheter (PHC).

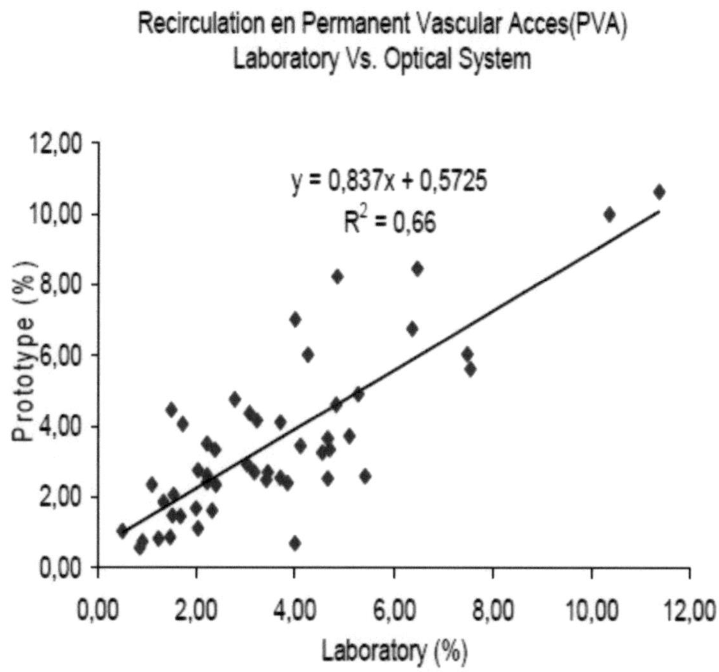

Fig. 7. Correlation between the laboratory analysis and optical system results for recirculation measurement in Permanent Vascular Access (PVA) is $R^2 = 0.66$.

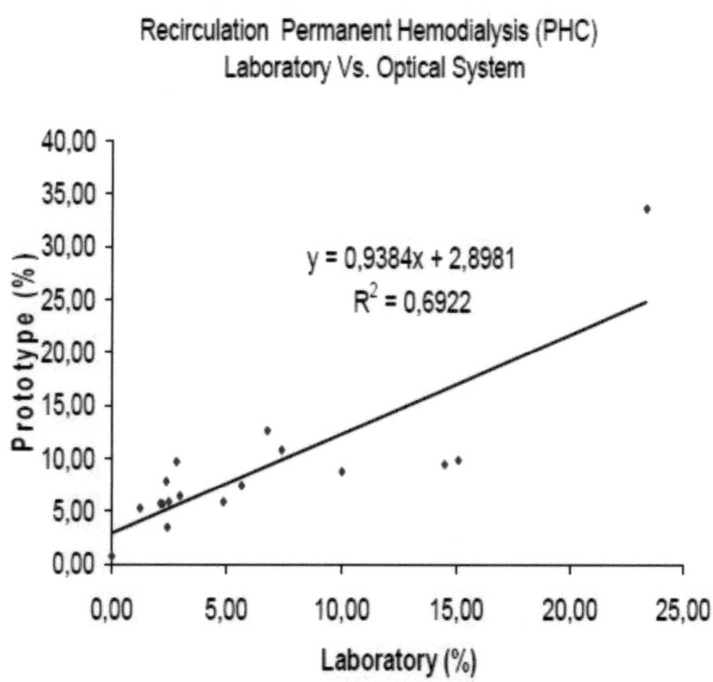

Fig. 8. Correlation between the laboratory analysis and optical system results for recirculation measurement in Permanent Hemodialisys Catheter (PHC) is $R^2 = 0.69$

There was no statistically difference in the recirculation between diabetic versus non diabetic (P =0.28) and hypertensive versus normotensive (P =0.21%) hemodialysis patients.
The distances between arterial and venous needles were 5.53±2.69 cm and 13.17 ± 3.38 cm respectively. It represents that there is a significant association between distances of needles (P=0.002) and improper needle placement (P=0.000) with degree of recirculation.
The average time between creation and use of A-V fistula were 71±31 days and 46 ± 13 days. There were also a significant difference between them (P=0.043).
The length of time of A-V fistula use was 26.59± 9.37 months and 33.20± 7.35 months.
The mean A-V fistula flow rate in both groups was more than 400 ml/min. The mean A-V fistula flow rate was significantly (p = 0.001).

4. Discussions

The measurement of A-V Fistula Recirculation in HD patients is an important issue, since it appears to be an important cause of inadequate HD. In addition, some clinical guidelines are suggested regular monitoring of HD vascular access by methods such as vascular access recirculation for early detection and correction of access dysfunction.[10]
An accurate assessment of access fistula recirculation can be made by urea-based method as the same as the present study and nonurea-based techniques by ultrasound dilution technique, conductivity, or potassium-based dilutional method.[11, 12, 13]
In urea-based method, it's usually measured by comparing the systemic and dialyzer inlet blood urea concentration. Urea concentration in blood entering the dialyzer (A in the above formula) is assumed to be equal to the systemic urea concentration (P in the above formula) if there is no recirculation.
There are different protocols for systemic blood urea sampling in the urea-based method measurement of access recirculation. In the three-needle or traditional method, the systemic urea concentration has been obtained from a peripheral vein in the contralateral arm. However, it is now recognized that this approach is inaccurate and tends to overestimate access recirculation because the BUN obtained from a peripheral vein is often higher than the BUN in the blood entering the dialyzer inlet, even in the absence of recirculation.[14]
Two factors contribute to this problem: Cardiopulmonary recirculation and veno/venous disequilibrium.[15, 16, 17] Thusthree-needle method dose not routinely use due to its requirement for additional venipuncture, unpredictable manner, and overestimation of access recirculation.
Sampling peripheral arterial blood eliminates the effects of both cardiopulmonary recirculation and venovenous disequilibrium. However arterial puncture during HD is not also practical and does not recommended.
Preferred alternatives to the peripheral vein or three-needle method and arterial puncture is two needle technique as same as use in the present study. In the study, systemic urea concentration is obtained from the dialyzer blood inlet line after slowing the blood pump to 50mL/min for about 30 seconds (P in the above formula).[18] This "two-needle" technique as opposed to the use of three needles are presumably more accurate for the determination of access recirculation.[19]
In our study, the average degree of A-V fistula recirculation was 9.56±2.32 percent and it was almost similar to findings of salimi et al in 2008, Bay et al in 1998, Besarab et al in1997. These groups used two needle technique urea-based method as same as present study for measurement of recirculation. The average degree of recirculation in these groups were 8.7%, 11.8 ± 9.9% and 5.5 ± 0.8% respectively.[20, 21, 22]

Depner et al have measured recirculation by ultrasound dilution technique and they reported recirculation rate of 8.82% during 34 HD session in 28 patients.(23).

The most common causes of A-V fistula recirculation in HD` patients are the presence of high-grade venous stenoses, improper needle placement, inadequate arterial inflow and congestive heart failure.(24, 25)

Moderate to sever venous stenoses can obstruct or restrict venous outflow from A-V fistula and as a result some dialyzed blood reenters to the dialytic circuit through the arterial needle for some times, thereby blood entering the dia-lyzer can become diluted with blood that has just left the dialyzer.Thus it can re-duce the effective clearance obtained in the course of a dialysis session.

Backflow or recirculation may increase with improper needle placement.(25) Close proximity and or misdirection of needles will increase the reentry of dia-lyzed blood into the arterial needle. Unfortunately, the role of misplacement of needles in recirculation, usually ignore but according to the present study it was the most common source of recirculation.

Some other centers have also reported that improper needle placement is a common source. Schneditz, for example, reported that improper needle place-ment is a common cause of A-V fistula recirculation, even after such placement had been previously recognized.(25)

Therefore we should have more emphasis on specific training and education of HD nursing staffs. HD staffs should also know anatomy and physiology of A-V fistula and A-V fistula recirculation.

On the other hand, access recirculation can also be facilitated by inadequate arterial inflow.(24) In this setting, backflow from the venous side of the access is necessary to support the dialytic blood flow rate set by the blood pump. It appears that inadequate arterial inflow was not a cause in our study because although A-V fistula flow rate was between 400- 500ml/min in four patients, dialytic blood flow rate was lower and it was maintained at 300 mill/min.

5. Conclusions

The measurement of A-V Fistula Recirculation has important diagnostic implications in Hemodialysis patients because it is an important cause of inadequate dialysis. According to the study it was a common occurrence. Although, the role of improper arterial and venous needles placement in recirculation usually ignore, it was the most common cause in our HD patients. Therefore we should have more emphasis on education and training of Hemodialysis staffs.

6. References

[1] USRDS: The United States Renal Data System: Overall hospitalization and mortality. Am J Kidney Dis 2003; 42 (6 suppl 5): S136-40.

[2] Beladi Musavi, SS, Hayati, F, Alemzadeh Ansari, MJ, et al. Survival at 1, 3, and 5Years in Diabetic and Nondiabetic Hemodialysis Patients. IJKD 2010; 4; 74-7.

[3] USRDS: The United States Renal Data System. Excerpts from the USRDS 2008 annual data report: Atlas of end-stage renal disease in the United States. Am J Kidney Dis 2009; 1 (Suppl 1): S1.

[4] Mailloux, LU, Bellucci, AG, Napolitano, B. Survival estimates for 683 patients starting dialysis from 1970 through 1989: Identification of risk factors for survival. Clin Nephrol1994; 42: 127.

[5] Murphy, SW, Foley, RN, Barrett, BJ. Comparative mortality of hemodialysis and peritoneal dialysis in Canada. Kidney Int 2000; 57: 1720-6.
[6] Goodkin, DA, Bragg-Gresham, JL, Koenig, KG, Wolfe, RA. Association of comorbid conditions and mortality in hemodialysis patients in Europe, Japan, and the United States: the Dialysis Outcomes and Practice Patterns Study (DOPPS). J Am Soc Nephrol 2003; 14: 3270.
[7] Miskulin, DC, Meyer, KB, Martin, AA. Comorbidity and its change predict survival in incident dialysis patients. Am J Kidney Dis 2003; 41: 149.
[8] Sherman, RA. The measurement of dialysis access recirculation. Am J Kidney Dis 1993; 22: 616.
[9] Michael, B, Thomas, AG, therodore, WP, Peter , JB. Arterovenous fistula recirculaton in hemodialysis, UP to date ver 17.2
[10] K/DOQI Clinical Practice Guidelines and Clinical Practice Recommendations 2006 Updates Hemodialysis adequacy Peritoneal Dialysis Adequacy Vascular Access. Am J Kidney Dis 2006; 48 (Suppl 1): S1.
[11] Brancaccio, D, Tessitore, N, Carpani, P. Potassium-based dilutional method to measure hemodialysis access recirculation. Int J Artif Organs 2001; 24: 606.
[12] Bosc, JY, LeBlanc, M, Garred, LJ. Direct determination of blood recirculation rate in hemodialysis by a conductivity method. ASAIO J 1998; 44: 68.
[13] Alloatti, S, Molino, A, Bonfant, G. Measurement of vascular access recirculation unaffected by cardiopulmonary recirculation: evaluation of an ultrasound method. Nephron 1999; 81: 25.
[14] Sharman RA: Recirculation revisited. Semin Dail 4: 221-223, 1991.
[15] Schenditz D. Polaschegg HD. Levin NW. Cardiopulmonary recirculation in dialysis- An underrecognized phenomenon. ASAIO J 38: M 196. 1992.
[16] Schenditz D. Kaufman AM, Polaschegg HD. Cardiopulmonary recirculation during hemodialysis. Kidney Int 42: 1450- 456,1992.
[17] Depner TA, Rizwan S, Sheer A, Wagner J: Peripheral urea disequilibrium during hemodialysis is temperature - dependent ASAIO Trans 37: 141-143, 1991.
[18] Sherman, RA. The measurement of dialysis access recirculation. Am J Kidney Dis 1993; 22: 616.
[19] Sherman, RA, Matera, JJ, Novik, L, CodyRP. Recirculation reassessed: The impact ofblood flow rate and the low-flow method reevaluated. Am J Kidney Dis 1994; 23: 846.
[20] Salimi J, Razeghi E, Karjalian H, et alPredicting Hemodialysis Access Failure with the Measurement of Dialysis Access Recirculation. Saudi J Kidney Dis Transpl 2008; 19:781-4.
[21] Bay WH, Henry ML, Lazarus JM, et al. Predicting hemodialysis access failure with color flow Doppler ultra-sound. Am J Nephrol 1998; 18 (4): 296-304.
[22] Besarab A, Sherman R. The relationship of recirculation to access blood flow. Am J Kidney Dis 1997; 29 (): 223-9.
[23] Depner, Thomas A.; Krivitski, Nikolai M.; MacGibbon, David. Hemodialysis Access Recirculation Measured by Ultrasound Dilution. ASAIO Journal 1995; 41 (suppl 3).
[24] Sherman R, Levy SS: Rate- related recirculation: the effect of altering blood flow on dialysis- an underrecognized phenomenon. ASAIO J 38: M194- M196; 1992.
[25] Schneditz, D. Recirculation, a seemingly simple concept. Nephrol Dial Transplant 1998; 13: 2191.
[26] NKF-DOQI clinical practice guidelines for vascular access XII Recirculation methodology, limit, evaluation and follow up. Am J Kidney Dis 2001; 37 (supply 1): s155.

14

Acetate Free Biofiltration with Potassium Profiled Dialysate (AFB-K)

R.I. Muñoz, I. Gallardo and J. Montenegro
Hospital de Galdakao-Usansolo, Bilbao
Spain

1. Introduction

Hyperkalaemia is a common, significant electrolyte disorder in uremia. Patients with chronic renal failure (CRF) undergoing haemodialysis (HD) accumulate potassium during the interdialysis period, and clearance of this potassium is one of the functions of haemodialysis. A sudden decrease in blood potassium levels during haemodialysis can induce or worsen arrhythmias, (Cupisti et al., 1999) particularly in patients already suffering arrhythmia or with risk factors for developing arrhythmia, such as heart disease of any origin, old age and diabetes mellitus, disorders which are highly prevalent in our dialysis units. Acetate Free Biofiltration with Potassium Profiled Dialysate (AFB-K) is a new haemodialysis technique that uses a potassium profiled dialysate (high at the start and low at the end of dialysis), so that by maintaining a constant potassium gradient between dialysate and blood, the decrease in blood potassium is slower - thereby contributing to prevent the appearance of arrhythmia (Santoro et al., 2002).

2. Description of the AFB technique

Acetate Free Biofiltration (AFB) is a haemodiafiltration technique (combining diffusion and convection) that uses a dialysate without acetate or bicarbonate, and in which post-dilution sodium bicarbonate is infused (145 or 167 mmol/L) throughout dialysis (Santoro et al., 2007) (Figure 1).

The primary characteristic of this haemodialysis technique is the absence of acetate. It must be taken into account that in conventional bicarbonate haemodialysis we continue to use 4 mmol/L of acetate to stabilise the acid part of the dialysate. This leads serum acetate levels to increase in conventional bicarbonate haemodialysis. Acetate is not used in AFB.

The advantages of this technique comprise improved haemodynamic stability and a reduction in the number of hypotensive episodes (Cavalcanti et al., 2004), the correction of metabolic acidosis, and improved clearance versus conventional haemodialysis (Santoro et al., 2007). Haemodynamic stability is improved by avoiding acetate (related to cytokine production, vasodilation and negative inotropic action); a solution is supplied with a high sodium content in reinfusion throughout dialysis (thereby improving vascular filling) (Tsutomu et al., 2011); the temperature is lowered (through sodium bicarbonate reinfusion at room temperature); and convection is employed (this involving the use of highly-permeable biocompatible membranes). These advantages prove more evident in patients susceptible to suffering hypotension during dialysis, such as diabetics or elderly subjects with autonomous nervous system disorders, heart disease or liver disease, and subjects with significant comorbidity (Tsutomu et al., 2011, Sato et al., 2011). In a literature review, Santoro et al. (Santoro., 2007) described a reduction in hypotension events in AFB vs bicarbonate haemodialysis: the probability of intradialysis hypotension with AFB was reported to be close to 40% of the probability of intradialysis hypotension in the case of conventional bicarbonate haemodialysis.

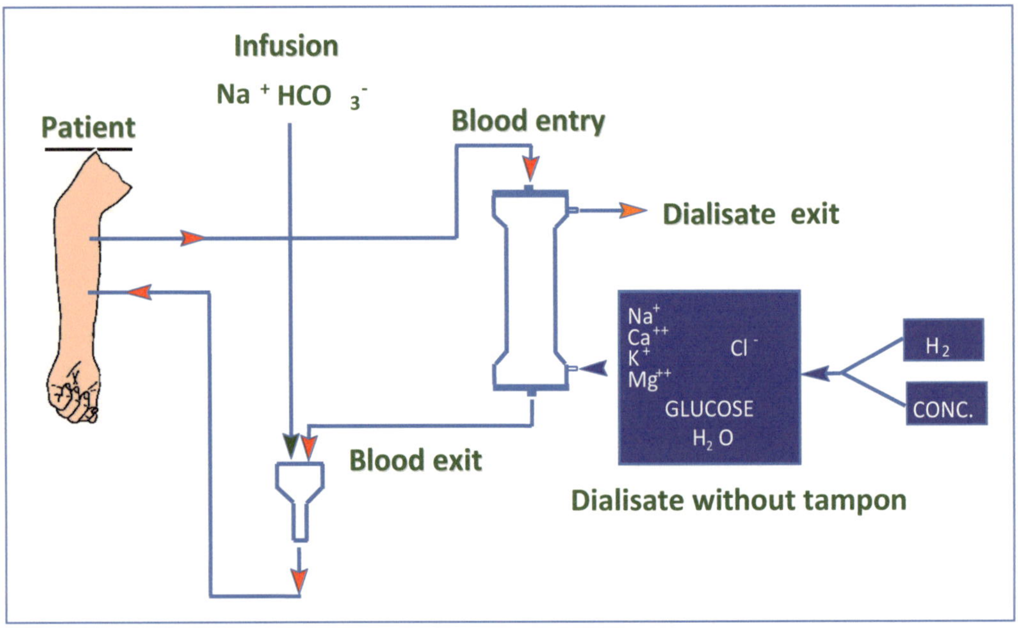

Fig. 1. AFB dialysis circuit.

3. Description of the AFB-K technique

Acetate Free Biofiltration with Potassium Profiled Dialysate (AFB-K) is the same haemodiafiltration technique free from acetate as that described above, with the addition of a potassium profiled dialysate. This is achieved with a double bag of concentrate (Santoro et al., 2002) - one bag with potassium and the other without it (Figure 2).

The dialysis machine takes concentrate from one bag or the other to form a potassium profiled dialysate: high at the start of dialysis and low at the end. The initial and final K^+ values of the dialysate are established individually for each patient (e.g., 4 mmol/L at the start of dialysis and 1 mmol/L at the end), according to a series of guidelines supplied by the manufacturer, and based on the needs of each patient. The aim is to maintain a constant K^+ gradient between the blood and dialysate bath, in order to prevent sudden K^+ reductions (Santoro et al., 2002).

The slow decrease in K^+ during dialysis is added to the advantages inherent to AFB. Dialysis with high K content in the dialysate cannot adequately reduce patient hyperkalaemia, though symptomatically it is very well tolerated. Dialysis with low K content in the dialysate adequately reduces patient hyperkalaemia, but proves highly arrhythmogenic and is poorly tolerated by the patients. With AFB-K we are able to adequately reduce hyperkalaemia without causing arrhythmia, since blood K is gradually reduced. The patients who stand to benefit most from this dialysis technique are those with significant comorbidity and therefore with an increased risk of suffering arrhythmia.

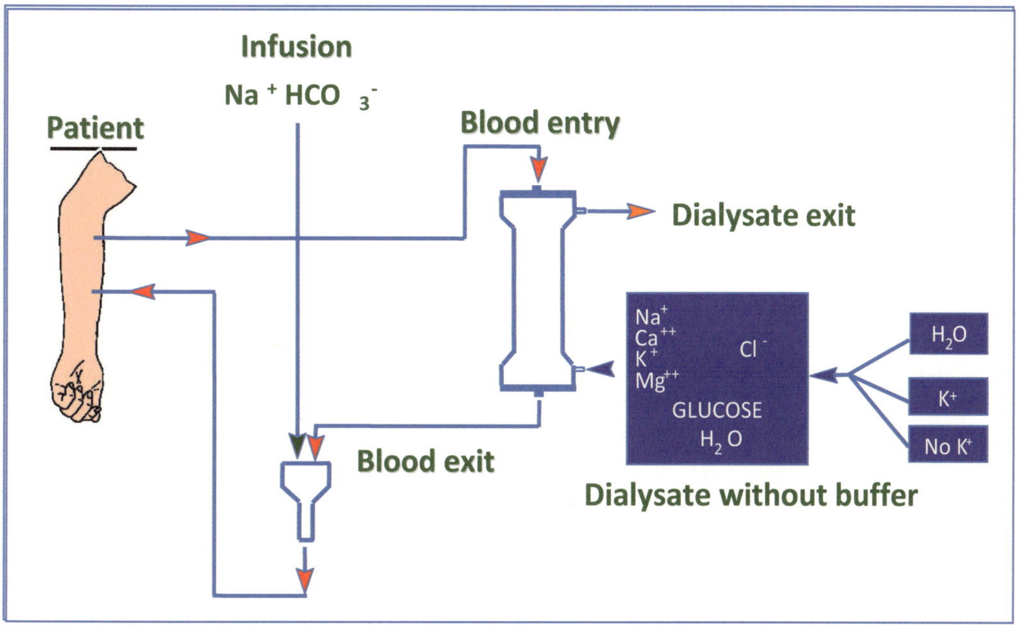

Fig. 2. AFB-K dialysis circuit.

4. Arrhythmia in patients on dialysis

Arrhythmias are very common in patients with CRF undergoing dialysis, and they are the cause of a significant percentage of sudden deaths of cardiac origin (Meier et al., 2001). Arrhythmias are more common in certain groups of patients: subjects with heart disease, left ventricular hypertrophy, coronary disease, heart valve disorders, high blood pressure or diabetes, and elderly patients.

Haemodialysis causes an arrhythmogenic effect (Meier et al., 2001). Dialysis is known to be related to QT prolongation in the ECG tracing (this being a risk marker for serious ventricular arrhythmia) (Genovesi et al., 2003).

Arrhythmia in dialysis may be related to sudden ion or blood pressure fluctuations. K^+ is a particularly arrhythmogenic ion (Kovesdy et al., 2007), related to the membrane potential, which is involved in cardiac cell depolarisation. K+ experiences sudden changes during haemodialysis, and a sharp drop can induce arrhythmia (Cupisti et al., 1999). In some cases, and despite diet advice or medical therapy, patients arrive for their dialysis session with high serum K+ levels, and experience a sudden decrease during the early part of the session. This has been related to the appearance of arrhythmias or to the worsening of pre-existing arrhythmias: induction or worsening of ventricular extrasystoles, QT prolongation (Cupisti et al., 1999, Floccari et al., 2004) and onset of paroxysmal atrial fibrillation have been described.

Acetate Free Biofiltration with Potassium Profiled Dialysate (AFB-K) is a haemodialysis technique that attempts to obviate this problem, avoiding sudden potassium reductions during the haemodialysis session, but with due correction of the hyperkalaemia of the patients (Santoro et al., 2005).

5. Development of AFB-K

One of the first studies on potassium profiled haemodialysis was published by Readelli (Readelli et al., 1996). This multicenter, randomised, cross-over, prospective study evaluated 42 patients with a known increase in Premature Ventricular Complexes (PVC) during dialysis (Holter-ECG recording). The author compared a haemodialysis model with constant K^+ in the dialysate versus a model with decreasing K^+ that maintained a constant K^+ gradient between the blood and dialysate. A significant reduction of over 30% in PVC was recorded (both in terms of the number of PVC/h and as regards the PVC couplets/h) when performing potassium profiled dialysis. This PVC decrease is observed particularly in the first hour of dialysis, which corresponds to the greatest reduction in blood K^+ values in the case of dialysis with constant K^+. The result is obtained without affecting the K^+ levels compared with conventional constant K^+ haemodialysis.

Subsequently, Santoro (Santoro et al., 2002) published a study including 125 patients from a single centre in which dialysis with two techniques - one comprising AFB with constant K^+ and another with potassium profiled dialysate (AFB-K) - resulted in slower K^+ reduction with the latter technique (serum K^+ being greater in the first hour of dialysis with the potassium profiling procedure). Both techniques reached the same final serum K^+ levels. This study recorded a reduction in the number of intra-dialysis arrhythmias, particularly in those patients with a significant presence of ventricular ectopic beats. In conclusion, the safety and easy application of the AFT-K technique was confirmed, as well as the possibility of adapting the profile to each individual patient. In addition, this treatment was shown to reduce the impact upon repolarisation homogeneity and thus prevent cardiac arrhythmia.

Buemi et al. (Buemi et al., 2005) studied a series of 28 patients undergoing haemodiafiltration with constant K^+ (HDF), compared with HDF involving variable K (HDFK). The authors examined the ECG tracings at different times during dialysis to measure the QT-interval, and analysed serum K, intra-erythrocyte K and the electrical membrane potential at rest. Intra-erythrocyte K remained constant. The electrical membrane potential at rest decreased over time, though the reduction proved significantly greater in HDF versus HDFK. In turn, the ECG tracing showed a reduction in QT dispersion and in the QT-interval with HDFK. The authors concluded that the risk of arrhythmia may be lower when using haemodialysis with variable K.

Subsequently, Santoro (Santoro et al., 2008) published a multicenter, randomised, cross-over, prospective study in which 30 patients susceptible to arrhythmia were dialysed in a cross-over design with AFB involving constant K^+ (2.5 mEq/L) or AFB with decreasing K in the dialysate bath (AFB-K). A tendency towards fewer arrhythmias is observed with AFB-K that becomes significant in the case of patients sensitive to dialysis. A reduction in the number of PVC per hour is observed both during dialysis and hours after the end of dialysis (with a maximum reduction in the number of PVC 14 hours after dialysis). In the first hour of treatment the serum K^+ levels of the patients were lower in AFB than with AFB-K. The study concluded that the slow clearance of K^+ may exert a protective effect.

6. Our study

Our group conducted a pilot study (Muñoz et al., 2008) at the start of the introduction of the AFB-K technique. The purpose of this study was to evaluate its efficacy and safety, analyse the decrease in blood K^+, and establish whether a decrease in arrhythmias occurs compared with AFB involving constant K^+ (AFB). We subsequently used the technique as an additional dialysis procedure in our Unit.

Twelve patients were included in the study (mean age 79 years; 5 males and 7 females). The subjects had arrhythmia or were at high risk of developing it, because of their old age, with high blood pressure (n=12), left ventricular hypertrophy (n=12), valve disease (n=8), coronary heart disease (n=3), diabetes mellitus (n=3) or paroxysmal atrial fibrillation (n=2).

A cross-over design was used, each subject serving as his or her own control. The subjects were dialysed for three weeks with AFB involving constant K^+, and for three weeks with potassium profiled AFB. At first dialysis in week 3 with each technique we conducted laboratory tests and performed ECG and Holter recordings (starting before the session and continuing until the next session).

The following dialysis regimen was prescribed: Integra® monitor (Novacor, Rueil-Malmaison, France), AN69 dialyser (Nephral® 500, Hospal), blood flow 300-350 mL/min, dialysate flow 500 ml/min and sodium bicarbonate reinfusion rate 167 mmol/L from 2100 to 2300 mL/h. The dialysate with constant K^+ was 2 mmol/L, while potassium profiling was 3.2-4 mmol/L ingoing and 1-1.3 mmol/L outgoing.

Both techniques were found to be easy to use, safe and without complications. There were no special technical requirements, and the procedures were well accepted by the nursing personnel. Patient haemodynamic tolerance was good with both techniques, with no differences in blood pressure or heart rate.

The pre- and post-dialysis results were similar with both techniques. We only observed a difference in blood K^+ determined half-way through the dialysis session, with higher values in the AFB-K group (4.0 mmol/L) than with AFB (3.6 mmol/L) ($P<0.0001$).

The ECG parameters in turn showed a significant difference in QTc (QT corrected for heart rate) after dialysis between the two techniques, with better results for AFB-K (448.8 24.2 ms vs 456.8 24 ms, $p=0.039$).

The mean PVC in the Holter recording was lower with AFB-K (163.5 range 21-900) versus AFB (444.5, range 23-13,565), though statistical significance was not reached ($p=0.06$) (Figure 3).

PVCs proved less severe (Lown grades I-II) with the AFB-K technique than with AFB involving constant K^+ (grades I-V).

All these findings were more obvious in patients with higher blood K^+ values at the start of dialysis.

In summary, K^+ decreased more slowly with AFB-K than with AFB, and a tendency towards decreased PVCs and their severity was noted (statistical significance probably not being reached because of the limited sample size), as well as a susceptibility to QTc reduction. All this is indicative of fewer arrhythmias. Our findings are similar to those previously reported by other authors (Santoro et al., 2002, Severi et al., 2003, Santoro et al., 2008).

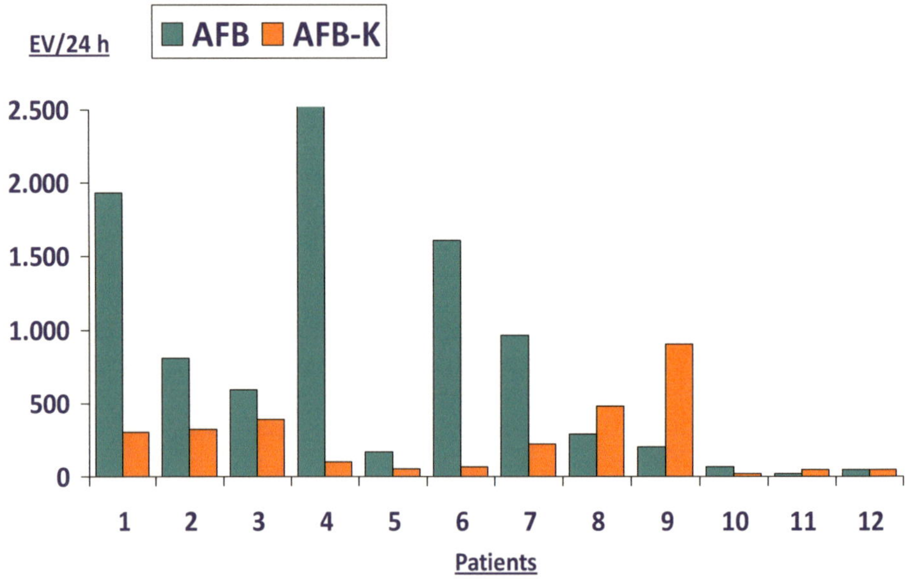

Fig. 3. PVC/24 h with both techniques (AFB and AFB-K).

In view of the results obtained, we decided to incorporate the technique to our Unit. We have indicated AFB-K in 27 patients who have been on dialysis for up to 5 years with the same technique.

We concluded that patients with arrhythmia or at risk of suffering arrhythmia benefited from potassium profiled dialysis, particularly those subjects with hyperkalaemia. Larger studies are required to confirm this reduction in arrhythmias, which could imply improved survival for patients with such a high cardiovascular risk.

7. Indications of AFB-K

Based on the literature reviewed, AFB-K is seen to be a dialysis technique offering the possibility of modulating potassium reduction according to the needs of each individual patient, with a view to ensuring slower reductions and thus preventing the appearance of arrhythmias. The indications therefore would be the following:

1. Patients with known arrhythmia, related or not to dialysis (e.g., ventricular extrasystoles detected around dialysis).
2. Patients with arrhythmia risk factors, such as subjects with heart disease of any origin, diabetes mellitus, old age, etc.
3. Patients susceptible to experiencing predialysis hyperkalaemia and markedly symptomatic dialysis sessions at the start, leading us to doubt the presence of arrhythmia.
4. Patients with indications for AFB and susceptibility to predialysis hyperkalaemia.

8. Requirements of AFB-K

The AFB-K technique has no added requirements with respect to AFB – only a different dialysate concentrate bag (double bag). AFB-K does not imply overburdening of the Dialysis

Unit or of the attending nephrologists, since it is very simple to prescribe, and likewise does not pose an added workload for the nursing personnel, since the technique is simple and easy to schedule.

9. Conclusions

One of the advantages afforded by this technology is the possibility of individualising the prescription of dialysis with a view to improving patient tolerability and prognosis (Phipps et al., 2010). Potassium profiling of the dialysate with AFB-K allows us to advance in this direction. The reduction of arrhythmias and the improved haemodynamic stability can contribute to improve the cardiovascular prognosis and survival of the patients. Larger studies (which are also more difficult to carry out) are needed to confirm improved patient survival with the new, attractive dialysis techniques.

10. References

Cupisti A, Galetta F, Caprioli R et al. Potassium removal increases the QTc interval dispersion during hemodialysis. Nephron 1999; 82: 122-6.

Santoro A, Mancini E, Fontanazzi F, Paolini F, Potassium profiling in acetate-free biofiltration. Contrib Nephrol 2002; (137):260-267.

Santoro A, Guarnieri F, Ferramosca E, Grandi F. Acetate Free Biofiltration Contrib Nephrol 2007, vol 158: 138-152.

Cavalcanti S, Ciandrini A, Severi S, et al. Model-based study of the effects of the hemodialysis technique on the compensatory response to hypovolemia. Kidney Int 2004; 65: 1499-1510.

Tsutomu Kuno. Who needs Acetate-Fre Biofiltration? Contrib Nephrol 2011, 168:188-194

Sato T, Taoka M, Miyahara T. Improvement of Autonomic Nervous Regulation by blood purification therapy using acetate-free dialysis fluid- Clinical evaluation by Laser Doppler Flowmetry. Contrib Nephrol 2011, 168:195-203.

Meier P, Vogt P, Blanc E Ventricular arrhytmias and sudden cardiac death in end.Stage Renal Disease patients on chronic hemodialysis Nephron 2001; 87:199-214.

Genovesi S, Rivera R, Fabbrini P, et al. Dynamic QT interval analysis in uraemic patients receiving chronic haemodialysis: Journal of Hypertension 2003; 21(10):1921-1928

Kovesdy C, Regidor D, Mehrota R et al. Serum and dialysate potassium concentrations and survival in hemodialysis patients. Clin J Am Soc Nephrol 2007; 2: 999-1007.

Floccari F, Alisi E, Nostro L, et al. Qtcinterval and QTc dispersion during haemodiafiltration. Nephrology 2004;9: 335-340.

Santoro A, Mancini E, Gaggi R, et al. Electrophysiological response to dialysis: the role of dialysate potassium content and profiling. Contrib Nephrol 2005; 149: 295-305

Redaelli B., Locatelli F., Limido D., et al. Effect of a new model of haemodialysis potassium removal on the control of ventricular arrhythmias. Kidney Int. 1996 (5): 609-617.

Buemi M, Aloisi E, Coppolino G, et al. The effect of two different protocols of potassium haemodiafiltration on QT dispersion. Nephrol Dial Transplant 2005; 20: 1148-1154

Santoro A, Mancini E, London G, et al. Patients with complex arrhythmias during and after haemodialysis suffer from different regimens of potassium removal. Nephrol Dial Transplant 2008; 23:1415-1421.

Muñoz R.I , Montenegro J, Salcedo A, et al. Effect of acetate-free biofiltration with a potassium-profiled dialysate on the control of cardiac arrhytmias in patients at risk: a pilot study. Hemodialysis International 2008; 12:108-113.

Severi S, Vecchietti S, Cavalcanti S, et al. Electrocardiographic changes during hemodiafiltration with different potassium removal rates. Blood Purif 2003; 21: 381-388.

Phipps L, Harris D. Review: modelling the dialysate. Nephrology 2010; 15: 393-398.

15

Blood Volume Regulation

Roland E. Winkler[1], Fabio Grandi[2] and Antonio Santoro[3]
[1]*Department Nephrology and Dialysis-PDA Rostock*
[2]*Gambro S.p.A.*
[3]*Department of Nephrology, Dialysis and Hypertension*
Policlinico S. Orsola-Malpighi
[1]*Germany*
[2,3]*Italy*

1. Introduction

Cardiovascular death remains the most frequent cause of mortality of dialysis population. Among the risk factor of cardiovascular mortality low blood pressure has been investigated by several authors even though not all the author conclude that low blood pressure per se, not adjusted for concomitant factors like age, and the presence of diabetes can be seen as independent predictor of mortality (Tisler et al., 2003; Iseki et al., 1997; Port et al., 1999).
In particular, the presence of low blood pressure and the intradialytic fall in the systolic and diastolic blood pressure seems to predict mortality in the dialysis population (Sohji et al., 2004). Some other authors found that not only low predialysis systolic blood pressure but also high values (J shape theory) expose patients at higher risk of mortality (Port et al, 1999).
Nevertheless, the fall in systolic blood pressure seems to be to date the most common intradialytic complication accounting for up to 30 % of dialysis related symptoms, despite the several improvement of dialysis techniques in terms of biocompatibility of the material used, more convection and quality of dialysis fluid. But hypertension is indeed the most frequent chronic co morbidity affecting dialysis patients.
Predialysis hypertension does not prevent hypotension episodes and not having targets for blood pressure control will not necessarily reduce its onset. When improved control of blood pressure is desired, modifications to the dialysis treatment itself should be considered as part of the management strategy (Davenport et al., 2008).
Hypo- as well hypertension are then the most challenging complications which dialysis has to face with. Several strategies are available to prevent hypo and hypertension like longer or more frequent dialysis regimen, diffusive-convective therapies, and assessment of dry body weight. Not all of them can be used in routine practice due to infrastructural or financial constraints while some others give in a certain extent opposite's effects like assessment of dry body weight beneficial for the hypertensive status, but which can lead to an increase of intradialytic symptoms (Davenport et al., 2008). Among the tools today available, the biofeedback systems, those devices able to adapt the operative condition of dialysis to the dynamic changes of the patients status along the dialysis, seems to be promising for contributing a step forward in the patients well-being (Locatelli et al., 2005) Among these devices the Hemocontrol Biofeedback System (HBS) has been extensively studied by several

authors as a tool to contribute in lowering the hypotension incidence but also as a further utility to control or normalize the blood pressure.
This review will summarize all the contributions given by the several studies about the cardiovascular stability in HBS dialysis.

2. HemocontrolTM biofeedback system

It is well known that blood volume behavior during dialysis is affected by several factors among which the ultrafiltration and changes in dialysate sodium level are the most relevant. Ultrafiltration should be adapted to the rhythm of plasma water removal respect to the patient's refilling capabilities, but the main limitation relies in the inability to maintain the total planned weight loss within the preset dialysis time except for long lasting dialysis treatments. The dialysate sodium can also promote the mobilization of water from the extravascular space reconstituting the plasma lost during ultrafiltration. Moreover, the modification of the intravascular sodium level can increase the activity of the autonomic nervous system, with a better hemodynamic response from the peripheral vascular resistance. However, the intradialytic sodium balance must be taken under tight control to avoid any sodium overload leading in turn a fluid overload especially in the interdialytic period. The blood volume control system (Hemocontrol) has been developed bearing in mind these three aspects (hemodynamic stability, fluid and sodium balance). The system is designed as feedback controller with three controlled variables (blood volume, total weight loss and average dialysate sodium level) and two actuators, the ultrafiltration and actual dialysate sodium level (Paolini & Bosetto, 1999) (Figure 1).

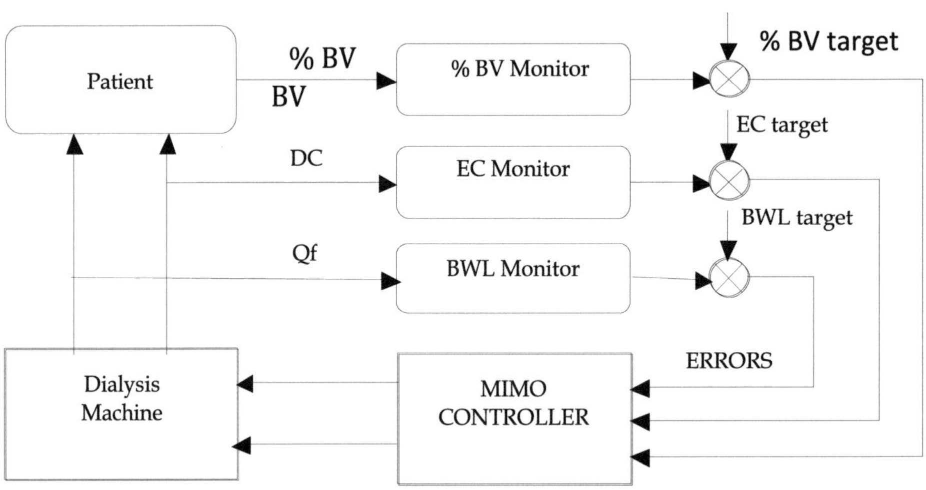

Fig. 1. Schematic representation of the Hemocontrol Biofeedback System. The MIMO controller processes three different controlled variables (blood volume reduction, average dialysate conductivity, body weight loss) through the errors between the actual and the desired values. The two actuators, reacting to the errors, are the actual dialysate conductivity and the weight loss rate (Santoro et al., 1998).

In Particular, the multi-input multi-output controller processes the errors between the actual continuously measured values of BV, weight loss and average dialysate sodium and their desired values, and reacts by adjusting the ultrafiltration and actual dialysate sodium to keep all the controlled variables as close to the target values as possible, however within pre-specified degree of tolerance. The desired blood volume reduction is set according to the total amount of fluid to be removed during dialysis (BV/UF volume). In fact, the blood volume reduction is a function of the overall water removal (Mancini et al, 1995), then its reduction per liters of water removal should be an invariant for any patient and then can take into account for the long or short interdialytic period. Since the actual dialysate sodium level is adjusted from the controller to regulate the blood volume time pattern, another parameter is set at the beginning of dialysis, that is the average dialysate sodium level. This value must prevent any sodium overload or abrupt depletion during the treatment (Moret et al., 2002).

All the actuators, that is the ultrafiltration and actual dialysate sodium, are always limited within safety operating regions. In particular the ultrafiltration rate is upper limited from the max UF rate at the beginning of dialysis to the average weight loss rate at the end and it is lower limited by the minimum UF rate (100 mL/h). The maximal initial UF rate is prescribed by the nurse according to patients characteristics and it is usually set at a value 20% to 50% higher than the average UF rate. The dialysate sodium is again upper limited from a maxi initial sodium content to the lowest value at the end of the treatment and the user can set the most appropriate range for the patients (Figure 2).

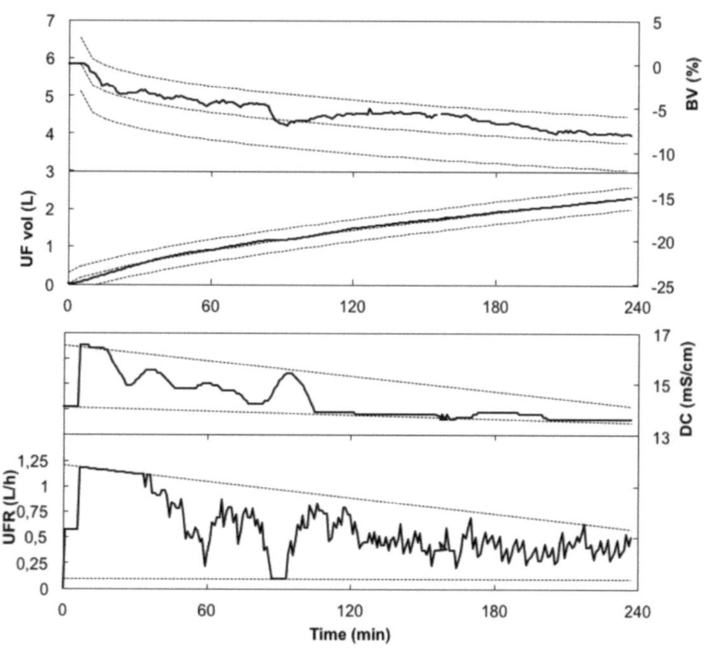

Fig. 2. Example of a HBS dialysis. The time course of the controlled variables (BV, %, UF volume, L), are shown on the top panel, while the actuators (DC, mS/cm and Ultrafiltration rate rate, L/h) are shown at the bottom. According to the desired BV and UF vol time pattern (the dashed mid line in 1 and 2) the UFR and DC are adjusted time by time by the controller to minimize the error between the desired and actual values. At any time their maximum and minimum values are maintained within safety limits (dashed lines in the bottom panel) As long as the BV, UF Vol and average DC are within the pre-set tolerances (dashed lines in the top panel) there is no need to change any set-point (Santoro et al., 2002).

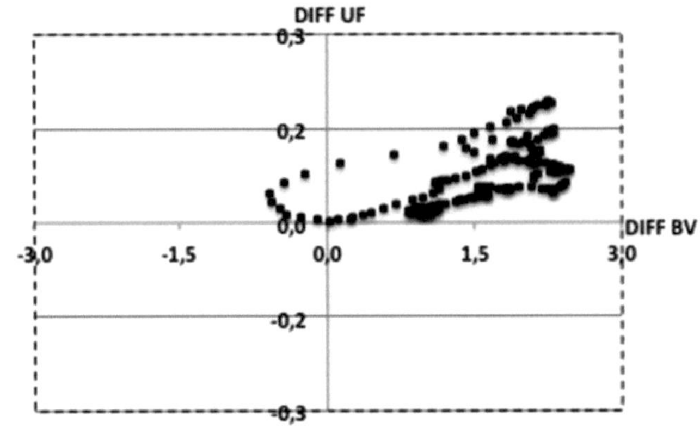

Fig. 3. State diagram of two out of the three controlled variables (BV and UF vol) during the sample dialysis shown in figure 2.

Thanks to the continuous adjustment of these parameters according to the dynamically changing clinical condition of the patient, the system is also useful to understand the refilling capacity of the patients. In fact, it can display the deviation from the set and forecasted end dialysis values respectively of the blood volume and UF volume to their set points (Figure 3). In particular, the diagram shows, on the horizontal axis, the difference between the forecasted end-dialysis BV and its set-point at any minute, while, on the vertical axis the difference between the forecasted end-dialysis UF volume and its set-point at any minute. It is worth to note that the deviation between the forecasted and set-point lies almost always in the upper right quadrant of the diagram. In this case, despite a forecasted higher UF volume, the blood volume does not fall down correspondingly, meaning that the patient's refilling capacity is higher than expected. On the contrary, when the state vector is in the lower left quadrant, the patient's refilling capacity seems to be less than expected
How much this can be attributable to the hydration status (over-hydration or under-hydration) is still matter of discussion even though there should be a physiological dependency behind.

3. Clinical studies on the hemocontrol™ biofeedback system

Since the first appearance of an abstract talking about the blood volume monitoring and control in the far 1991 Santoro et al., 1991, several studies and papers have been undertaken and written. The overall body of this literature is reported in Table 1.
Many of them are studies showing the clinical benefit of HBS in particular in the reduction of hypotension events, some others have been published to explain the underlying mechanisms for such a kind of results (Cavalcanti et al, 2004, Severi et al, 2006). We will review the results of original clinical trials, which are summarized in Table 2.
Fifteen studies were prospective, randomised, controlled trials lasting from four weeks to 48 weeks. In general, study objectives addressed haemodynamic stability during dialysis, cardiovascular effects, dialysis efficiency, interdialytic events and quality-of-life aspects. In total, the HBS has been used in more than 280 patients who were hypertensive, hypotension-prone or non-hypotension-prone. The studies were run in Canada and several European countries. Actually, 287 patients were treated in the demonstrated clinical studies, ratio between male and female was 2.2, the mean age 66.3 years +/- 6.3 years. Diabetes mellitus was

observed in 32.16% of all patients, Glomerulonephritis in 29.03%, interstitial nephropathy 14.3%, IgA nephropathy 7.1%, chronic pyelonephritis 3.6%, other 13.81%.

Author	Year	Journal	Type of publication
Santoro A et al	1994	ASAIO Trans	Clinical Trial
Santoro A	1995	Nephrol Dial Transplant	Editorial
Mancini E et al	1995	Int J Artif Organs	Clinical Trial
Santoro A et al	1996	Nephrol Dial Transplant	Review
Santoro A et al	1997	Int J Artif Organs	Editorial
Santoro A et al	1998	Am J Kidney Dis	Clinical Trial
Santoro A et al	1998	Nephrol Dial Transplant	Review
Paolini F et al	1999	Adv Ren Replace Ther	Review
Ronco C et al	2000	Kidney Int	Clinical Trial
Basile C et al	2001	Nephrol Dial Transplant	Clinical Trial
Zucchelli P et al	2001	Semin Nephrol	Review
Begin V et al	2002	ASAIO J	Clinical Trial
Pastore C et al	2002	EDTNA ERCA J	Clinical Trial
Santoro A et al	2002	Contrib Nephrol	Review
Santoro A et al	2002	Kidney Int	Clinical Trial
Wolkotte C et al	2002	Nephron	Clinical Trial
McIntyre CW et al	2003	Clin Nephrol	Clinical Trial
Santoro A et al	2003	J Nephrol	Review
Cavalcanti S et al	2004	Kidney Int	Clinical Trial
Franssen CF et al	2005	Hemodial Int	Clinical Trial
Selby NM et al	2006	Am J Kidney Dis	Clinical Trial
Moret K et al	2006	Nephrol Dial Transplant	Clinical Trial
Severi S et al	2006	Hemodial Int	Clinical Trial
Dasselaar JJ et al	2007	ASAIO J	Clinical Trial
Dasselaar JJ et al	2007	J Ren Care	Clinical Trial
Deziel C et al	2007	Clin J Am Soc Nephrol	Clinical Trial
Azar AT	2008	Saudi J Kidney Dis Transpl	Review
McIntyre CW et al	2008	Clin J Am Soc Nephrol	Clinical Trial
Nesrallah GE et al	2008	ASAIO J	Clinical Trial
Santoro A et al	2008	Contrib Nephrol	Review
Winkler RE et al	2008	Contrib Nephrol	Clinical Trial

Table 1. Full list of peer reviewed papers on HBS.

Author	**Patients**	**Study Design**	**Major Results with HBS Compared to HD**	***P***
Santoro et al, 1994	hypotension prone n=5	Prospective, cross-over HD(2wks) – HBS(2wks) – HD(2wks)	Intradialytic hypotension ↓ Intradialytic symptoms ↓	<0.05 n.s.
Santoro et al., 1998[1]	hypotension-prone n=8	Prospective, cross-over HD(4wks)–HBS(4wks)–HD(4 wks)	intradialytic stability (SAP)↑ hypotensive episodes ↓ intradialytic events ↓ isotonic saline ↓	<0.05 <0.05 - <0.05
Ronco et al., 2000[2]	hypotension-prone n=12	Prospective RCT, cross-over HD(2wks)–HBS(2wks) vs. HBS(2wks)–HD(2wks)	hypotensive episodes ↓ saline infusions ↓ rebound ↓ (eKt/V↑)	<0.001 <0.001 <0.001
Basile et al., 2001[3]	hypotension-prone n=19	Prospective, cross-over HD(6mo)–HBS(14-30mo) – HD(4*+3wks)–HBS(4*+3wks)	symptomatic hypotension ↓ muscle cramps ↓ post-HD-asthenia ↓(other symptoms n.s.) vascular refilling ↓	<0.002 <0.02 <0.0001 <0.05
Bégin et al., 2002[4]	hypotension-prone n=7	Prospective, cross-over 3x[HD(2wks)–HBS(2wks)]	event-free sessions ↑ mean postdialysis BP ↑	<0.01 -
Wolkotte et al., 2002	Unselected sample N=16	Prospective, cross-over HD(3wks) - HBS(3wks)	Intradialytic hypotension ↓ Intradialytic symptoms ↓	0.033 0.039
Santoro et al., 2002[5]	hypotension-prone n=36	Prospective RCT, cross-over 2x[HD(4wks)–HBS(4wks)] vs. 2x[HBS(4wks)–HD(4wks)]	intradialytic hypotension ↓ interdialysis symptoms ↓	0.004 <0.001
McIntyre et al., 2003[6]	non-hypotension-prone n=15	Prospective, cross-over HD(3wks)–HBS(2*+3wks)	symptomatic episodes ↓ reductions in systolic BP ↓ RBV falling >10% ↓ interdialytic weight gain ↓ eKt/V ↑, urea clearance ↑	<0.001 - <0.001 0.009 <0.01
Franssen et al., 2005[7]	hypotension-prone n=7	Prospective, cross-over HD(3wks)–HBS(3wks)–HBS(6wks)[1]	intradialytic hypotension ↓ systolic BP ↑ no effect on post-HD dry weight	<0.01 <0.05
Moret et al., 2006[8]	hypotension-prone n=12	Prospective RCT, cross-over 4 phases: HD, HBS, SP[§], PC[#2]	hypotensive episodes least frequent with HBS	n.s.
Selby et al., 2006[9]	hypotension-prone n=8	Prospective RCT, cross-over HD(1*+2wks)–HBS(1*+2wks) vs. HBS(1*+2wks)–HD(1*+2wks)	LV regional wall motion abnormalities ↓ EF ↑ haemodynamic data ↑	- 0.043 <0.05
Dasselaar et al., 2007[10]	hypertensive n=28	Prospective RCT HD(4*+12wks) vs. HBS(4*+12wks)	hypotensive episodes ↓ brain natriuretic peptide levels ↓ predialysis systolic BP ↓	<0.05 n.s. <0.05

Author	Patients	Study Design	Major Results with HBS Compared to HD	*P*
Déziel et al., 2007[11]	~50% hypotension-prone ~ 50% hypertensive n=36	Prospective RCT HD(4wks*+6mo) vs. HBS(4wks*+6mo)	systolic and diastolic BP ↓ intradialytic interventions ↓ QoL/KDQOL-SF (burden of kidney disease) ↑	n.s. 0.04 0.004
Nesrallah et al., 2008[12]	hypotension-prone n=60	Prospective RCT HD(4wks*+6mo) vs. HBS(4wks*+6mo)	no change in extracellular fluid volume intradialytic hypotension ↓ no change in QoL/dialysis-related symptoms quest.	- 0.04 -
Winkler et al., 2008[13]	hypotension-prone n=18	Retrospective HD–HBS(48wks)	hypotensive episodes ↓ muscle cramps ↓ eKt/V ↑ LVMI ↓ EF ↑ Antihypertensive drugs ↓	<0.01 <0.01 <0.05 <0.01 n.s n.s

*wash-out/run-in phase; § SP, sodium profiling; # PC, plasma conductivity controlled feedback; ↓, reduced; ↑, improved
1) during first HBS phase post-HD weight remained stable, during second phase reduced target weight
2) 11 consecutive treatments for each modality followed by 1 week of treatment with standard dialysis
Abbreviations: RCT, randomised controlled trial; HD: haemodialysis; HBS: Hemocontrol™ biofeedback system; SAP, systolic arterial blood pressure; n.s., not significant; BP, blood pressure, LV(MI), left ventricular (mass index); EF, cardiac ejection fraction.

Table 2. Summary of the main results of the clinical trias on HBS.

4. Intradialytic haemodynamic stability

Based on the European Best Practice Guidelines (EBPG) for hemodynamic instability (Kooman et al., 2007) the average incidence of hypotensive episodes during dialysis therapy is 20%. In some cohort studies, hypotensive events were observed in up to 33% of cases during dialysis therapy. Hypotensive episodes during the course of dialysis therapy are closely correlated with morbidity and mortality and play a fundamental role in the development of myocardial and cerebral ischemia. Frequent occurrences of hypotension lead to chronic over-hydration and have a negative impact on the clearance of dissolved substances due to water retention.

The first study on HBS was run by Santoro in 1994 which was addressed to check the feasibility of the system. They included a small sample of five patients in a HD-HBS-HD experimental set-up. The occurrence of dialysis complicated by severe hypotension was 8 in HD, 1 in HBS and 5 in the second HD period.

Subsequently, they did another clinical investigation on 8 hypotension-prone patients in a prospective crossover study including 8 hypotension-prone haemodialysis patients (Santoro et al, 1994). They compared conventional haemodialysis (HD) to the HBS, following a protocol with an HD1-HBS-HD2 sequence, with each treatment period lasting one month. Changes in predialysis to postdialysis systolic arterial pressure were lower in the HBS period (-12.4%) compared to both HD periods (-20% in HD1 and -17.5% in HD2; $P<0.05$), despite comparable total ultrafiltration rates and mean treatment times. A significant reduction in the number of severe hypotensive episodes (HBS: 3, HD1: 26, HD2: 16; $P<0.05$) and fewer intradialytic events, such as cramps and nausea, were observed. This resulted in a reduced need for therapeutic isotonic saline in each session (HBS: 60 mL, HD1: 160 mL, HD2: 95 mL; $P<0.05$).

The first randomised, controlled trial on HBS was published by Ronco (Ronco et al, 2000), who treated 12 hypotension-prone patients with either 2 weeks of HD followed by 2 weeks of HBS or *vice versa* (6 session per patient and 72 in total). They also observed fewer hypotensive episodes with HBS (24/72 vs 59/72 in HD; $P<0.001$). Saline infusion was required in 15 cases during HBS in comparison to 57 cases during HD ($P<0.001$).

Medium-term treatment with HBS was evaluated in a prospective study published by Basile (Basile et al., 2001). They investigated the efficacy and safety of HBS vs conventional HD in 19 hypotension-prone uraemic patients. After a period of 6 months on HD, patients switched to HBS for 14 to 30 months. A wash-out phase of 4 weeks was followed by a short-term treatment period of 3 weeks, first with HD and then after wash-out with HBS. The overall occurrence of symptomatic hypotension and muscle cramps was significantly reduced, with a decrease of 34% and 40% respectively (*P*-values: <0.002 and <0.02 respectively). In the short-term part of the study, the vascular refilling (residual BV%/ECV% ratio) was significantly higher during the HBS treatment.

Several other groups have been shown improvement in haemodialysis-induced hypotension in hypotension-prone patients [Santoro et al., 2002; Franssen et al., 2005; Selby et al., 2006; Moret et al., 2006; Dasselaar et al., 2007; Neshrallah et al; Winkler et al., 2008).

Ambulatory blood-pressure measurement in one prospective trial revealed that during the first 16 hours post-HD, systolic blood pressure was significantly higher with HBS in comparison to conventional HD (Franssen et al., 2005). Other trials showed a significant overall decrease in systolic blood pressure in both groups during the study period ($P=0.005$ vs the baseline) (Deziel et al., 2007). However, the difference between the HD and HBS arms was not significant.

Attempts to correct extracellular fluid volume (ECFV) with aggressive ultrafiltration often leads to intradialytic hypotension. Therefore, it was of interest to see whether HBS treatment could safely reduce ECFV in extracellular fluid-expanded patients (Neshrallah et al., 2008). However, the results of this randomised trial revealed no change with HBS, even after multivariate adjustment.

Bégin et al. investigated whether improvement in hypotension-related events can be explained by changes in dry weight (Begìn et al., 2002). In their prospective trial in 7 hypotension-prone patients, they observed the greatest improvement in event-free sessions (i.e. sessions not requiring therapeutic intervention for hypotension-related signs and symptoms) in patients who had the smallest changes in dry weight. This is supported by other studies, which revealed that HBS was not effective in reducing post-HD dry weight (Fransesen et al, 2005, Dasselaar et al., 2007). A randomised, controlled trial demonstrated that the best responders to HBS treatment were those with higher predialysis systolic blood-pressure values compared to poor responders ($P=0.04$) (Santoro et al., 2002).

While most data on HBS were obtained from the study of hypotension-prone patients, one trial was especially designed to look at the effects in non-hypotension-prone uraemic patients (McIntyre et al., 2003). During this prospective study, 15 patients received conventional HD over 3 weeks followed by a 2-week wash-out phase and an HBS-treatment phase over 3 weeks. There was a reduction in symptomatic episodes (per patient over 3 weeks) from 3 during HD to 0.13 with HBS (P<0.001). The number of treatments affected by a reduction of > 40% in systolic blood pressure decreased from 1.4 to 0.46 and episodes during which relative blood volume fell by > 10% were reduced from 6.3 to 1.13 per patient and treatment period (P<0.001). The treatment of 28 hypertensive patients with either standard HD or HBS in a randomised manner showed significantly fewer hypotensive episodes, lower brain natriuretic peptide levels (not significant) and a significant reduction in predialysis blood pressure in the HBS group (Neshrallah et al., 2008).

5. Pooled analysis about intradialytic cardiovascular stability

Since, most of the studies, addressed the intradialytic hypotension, we summarized the data about the cardiovascular instability (intradialytic hypotension and weight loss) in the following pooled analysis. We included all the studies of any type (random cross-over, random not cross over and not random), which reported available data in form of percentage of dialysis complicated by hypotensions or average frequency of hypotension events, disregarding this was or was not the primary response variable.

Intradialytic hypotension

Study or Subgroup	Weight	Mean Difference IV, Random, 95% CI
1994 Santoro (1)	5.7%	-19.00 [-31.21, -6.79]
1998 Santoro (2)	6.4%	-9.00 [-20.12, 2.12]
2000 Ronco	4.8%	-49.00 [-62.96, -35.04]
2001 Basile (3)	15.2%	-10.80 [-11.79, -9.81]
2002 Santoro	12.5%	-10.00 [-14.46, -5.54]
2002 Wolkotte	9.8%	-12.00 [-19.02, -4.98]
2003 McIntyre	11.4%	-8.00 [-13.49, -2.51]
2005 Franssen	2.4%	-27.00 [-48.66, -5.34]
2006 Moret (4)	8.4%	-8.00 [-16.56, 0.56]
2007 Dasselaar	0.6%	-44.70 [-93.15, 3.75]
2007 Deziel (5)	8.4%	-1.00 [-9.50, 7.50]
2008 Neshrallah	2.9%	-8.00 [-27.53, 11.53]
2008 Winkler	11.6%	-7.80 [-13.09, -2.51]
Total (95% CI)	**100.0%**	**-11.76 [-15.43, -8.09]**

Test for overall effect: Z = 6.28 (P < 0.00001)

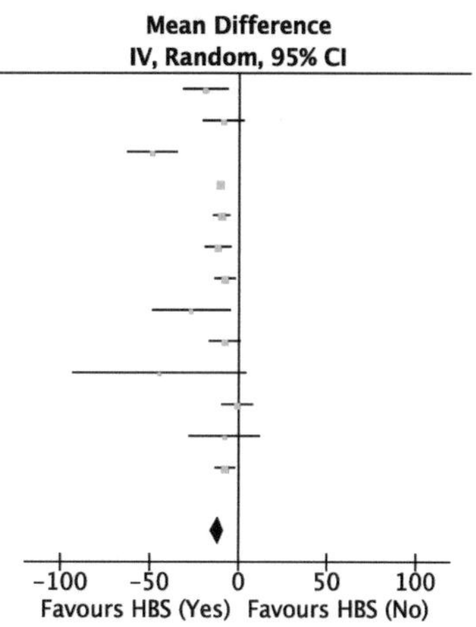

(1) Data pooled over A1, A2 study phases
(2) Data pooled over A1, A2 study phases
(3) Medium term study
(4) Data referred to the conventional vs HBS phases
(5) Data referred to 4 weeks recording (2 weeks at the beginning and 2 weeks at the end)

Fig. 4. Pooled analysis of intradialytic hypotensions. The figure shows the hypotension events expressed as mean ± SD over the total number of dialysis.

We did not include in the analysis those studies for which confounding factors like hemodiafiltration and/or acetate free biofiltration, cold dialysate temperature if not present both in the intervention and control treatments could interfere with data interpretation.

For each study we extracted the total number of treatments performed both with standard and HBS hemodialysis and the total events (dialysis complicated by hypotensions or major hypotension events) for each one, or the mean±SD hypotension events as reported in the paper.

Figure 4 shows the results of the pooled analysis about the intradialytic hypotension of the thirteen included studies in the analysis. The reported data refer to 2520 dialysis in HBS against 2130 dialysis in conventional dialysis.
The overall mean difference was nearly -12% favoring the HBS treatment with an estimated range between -15% and -8%. The range is almost narrow despite some studies showed wider ranges (Dasselaar et al., 2007).
Discrepancies between the single studies can be partially explained by: a) the difference in within study variance underlying the difference in the sample size (from 8 to 44 recruited patients), b) the difference in the study design (cross-over, parallel group, etc) c) the target population (hypotension prone, non-hypotension prone and hypertensive patients), d) the difference in the between study reflecting the difference in the primary response variable (blood pressure drop, fluid overload) leading sometimes to a bias in the dialysis complicated by hypotension variable, e) the length of follow up ranging from few weeks to two years.
These good results are emphasized by looking at the weight loss during dialysis in the two treatments as reported in Figure 5. The overall result shows a higher weight loss in HBS than in standard treatment equal to 160 g. All the authors reported this behavior even though some were not statistically significant. McIntyre indeed report the interdialytic weight gain, which could not properly reflect the weight loss during the follow-up.

Ultrafiltration volume (L)

Study or Subgroup	Weight	Mean Difference IV, Random, 95% CI
1994 Santoro (1)	11.7%	0.45 [0.29, 0.61]
1998 Santoro (2)	11.8%	0.35 [0.20, 0.50]
2000 Ronco	10.3%	0.05 [-0.18, 0.28]
2001 Basile (3)	6.3%	0.30 [-0.14, 0.74]
2002 Santoro	11.7%	0.10 [-0.06, 0.26]
2002 Wolkotte	11.6%	0.00 [-0.17, 0.17]
2003 McIntyre	10.8%	-0.30 [-0.50, -0.10]
2005 Franssen	5.2%	0.10 [-0.42, 0.62]
2006 Moret (4)	10.3%	0.20 [-0.03, 0.43]
2008 Neshrallah	10.5%	0.35 [0.13, 0.57]
Total (95% CI)	**100.0%**	**0.16 [0.01, 0.31]**

Test for overall effect: Z = 2.06 (P = 0.04)

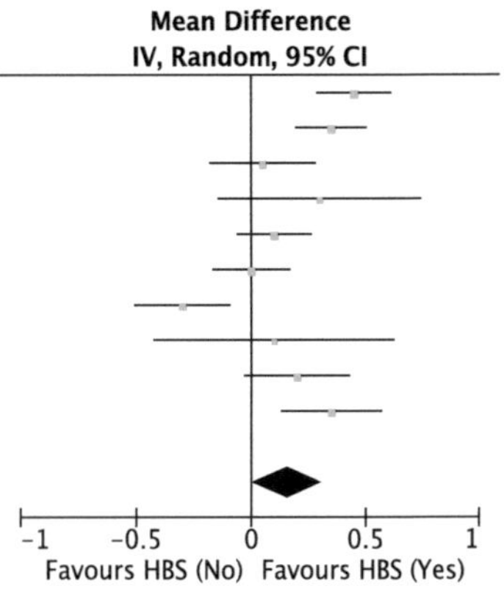

(1) Data pooled over A1, A2 study phases
(2) Data pooled over A1, A2 study phases
(3) Data reported are those averaged over the patients
(4) Data referred to the conventional vs HBS phases

Fig. 5. Body weight loss during dialysis. Data report the pre to post dialysis body weight change during dialysis (in Kg or L) expressed as mean ±SD over the total assessed dialysis.

Different alternatives are available to reduce or prevent the noticeable drop in blood pressure during the extracorporeal therapy. In this context, the time and frequency of dialysis play a significant role, but the time of dialysis cannot be infinitely expanded because of socioeconomic framework conditions. Regulating the blood temperature via dialysate temperature can also have a noticeable positive effect on the blood pressure management. To what extent the efficacy of the therapy is limited because of the higher peripheral overall resistance is the subject of further studies. On-line hemodiafiltration is another established possibility to prevent a drop in blood pressure during blood purification therapy. The high convective rate of this procedure is capable of achieving the stabilisation of the blood

pressure. However, during the first half of the therapy time with in-line hemodiafiltration, HBS is also characterised by a high convective dialysis rate. The recommended increase of the dialysate calcium concentration to 1.5 mmol/L should be considered with caution because it may result in a significant elevation of the calcium x phosphate product. HBS works with ultrafiltration control and sodium management to realise better refilling of the intravascular compartment.
The short reaction time of the MiMo (Multi input - Multi output) controller (Figure 2) guarantees the prevention of a hypotensive event or reduces its intensity. The underlying mechanisms should be found both in the fast reaction of the system to rapid blood volume drops and in the pre-set pathway which avoid the achievement of risky patient dependent blood volume thresholds.

6. Electrolyte implications

The electrolyte implication of HBS have been included in some of the studies and deeply investigated in one paper by Moret (Moret et al., 2006).
In this study they compared the effect of sodium manual profiling and automatic profiling versus standard treatment on the sodium mass balance measure through its surrogate variable, the ionic mass balance. It is interesting the comparison between standard dialysis prescribed at 140 mMol/L and biofeedback technologies (HBS and biofeedback on plasma conductivity) prescribed at equivalent values of 14.0 mS/cm. The manual profiling was indeed, prescribed with a linear time course starting at 15.0 mS/cm and ending at 14.0 mS/cm. The ionic mass balance in each study session was 423±166 mMol, 488±179 mMol and 409±109 mMol respectively in standard, HBS and plasma conductivity biofeedback.
Other studies on HBS reported data about the post dialysis natremia. Despite they did not investigated the actual sodium mass removal, they found no differences between standard versus HBS sessions. Santoro in 1998 reported end dialysis natremia equal to 146±1.5 mMol/L in standard hemodialysis and 146.2±1.1 in HBS. They did not showed the predialysis natremia then one cannot conclude that the ionic mass balance could have been similar in the two treatments. Moreover, this was a short term study and a potential sodium overload could not have been seen. Subsequently the same group published a multicenter study (Santoro et al, 2002) in which data about the pre and postdialysis natremia were shown. Pre and post-dialysis plasma sodium values were: 138.7±0.5 and 141.8±0.6 in standard HD and 138.8± .6 and 141.3±0.7 in HBS. Moreover, if we consider that actual weight loss, blood flow rate and treatment time were equal in both the treatment, we could argue that the sodium mass balance should have been similar in the two treatment. Similar results in short-term study were reported by Wolkotte (Wolkotte et al, 2002). Pre and Post dialysis sodium levels were 139.8±2.5, 141.2±1.8 in standard HD and 139.6±2.4, 141.3±1.8 in HBS respectively and corresponding to weight loss of 2.4±0.7 in HD and 2.5±0.8 in HBS. Mid-term results were reported only in the study by Dasselaar (Dasselaar et al., 2007). The follow-up lasted 12 week per group (HD and HBS) and the values were at the end of the follow-up were: 139.2±2.5, 139.8±2.1 in HD and 139.8±2.2, 139.9±2.1 in HBS. Then, they observed an increase of 1 mMol/L in the postdialysis natremia but, the actual wight loss was 2.7±6.7L in HD while 3.1±6.5L in HBS even though not statistically significant.
In conclusion, the several authors who investigated this aspect did not find any potential sodium overload in HBS. This is due to the underlying mathematical sodium kinetics model used to regulate the sodium mass balance in the form of equivalent conductance.

7. Cardiac effects of haemodynamic stability

Cardiac failure and the rate of cardiovascular mortality are extremely high in dialysis patients. One of the major causes of heart failure in these patients is probably recurrent subclinical myocardial ischemia. Selby et al. examined whether this occurs in response to stress of haemodialysis and whether it can be reduced by improved hemodynamic stability with HBS treatment (Selby et al., 2006). Eight hypotension-prone patients were included in a randomised cross-over trial to compare the development of left-ventricular regional-wall motion abnormalities during HBS treatment and standard HD. There were 42 regional-wall motion abnormalities during HD vs 23 during HBS (odds ratio 1.8; 95% CI: 1.1 to 3.0). The majority of these abnormalities improved in function within 30 minutes after dialysis (Figure 7). At peak stress, ejection fraction was significantly lower during HD (P=0.043). Haemodynamic parameters, such as pulse rate, stroke-volume decrease, cardiac output decrease, peripheral resistance and mean baroflex sensitivity, were all significantly improved during HBS vs HD. We noted comparable results in a retrospective analysis of 18 patients after 48 weeks of HBS treatment (Winkler et al., 2008): ejection-fraction increase, though not significant, and a decrease in left ventricular-mass index (P<0.05). In addition, the use of antihypertensive drugs decreased (Figure 7). Two other groups looked at the effect of HBS treatment on antihypertensive drug use (Dasselaar et al. 2007, Neshrallah et al., 2008). Dasselaar et al. showed that the defined daily dose (DDD) of antihypertensive drugs decreased (not significantly) in the HBS group, whereas it was stable in the control HD arm (Dasselaar et al., 2007). Nesrallah et al. observed no change in antihypertensive drug use in their randomised controlled trial (Neshrallah et al., 2008).

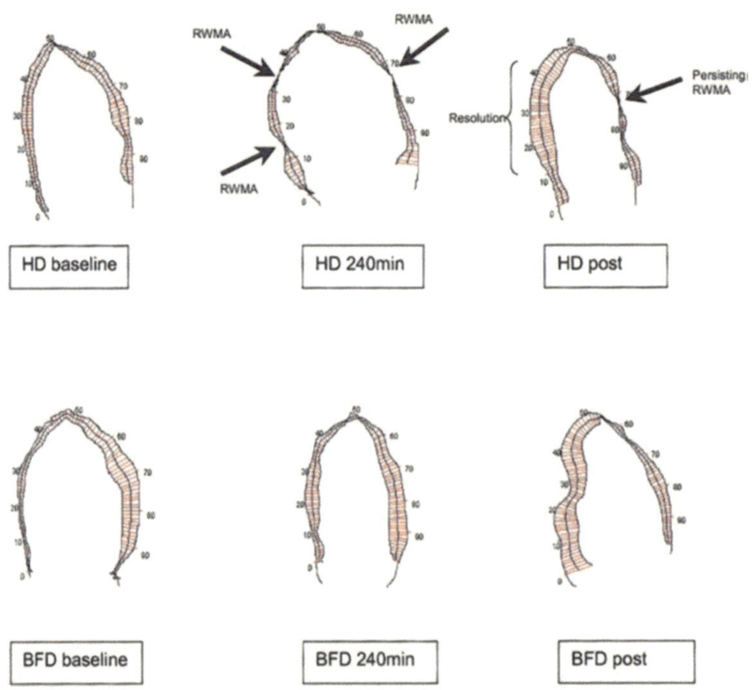

Fig. 6. Analysis of left ventricular wall motion in one patients during conventional (HD) and biofeedback dialysis (BFD). Arrows indicates the regional wall motion abnormalities which persist even after the end of the treatment (Selby et al., 2006).

8. Efficiency of treatment

Effects of the achieved cardiovascular stability were accompanied by an improved efficiency of treatment. A lower urea rebound was observed during the HBS sessions, resulting in a higher equilibrated Kt/V (eKt/V) as shown by several groups (Ronco et al., 2000, McIntyre et al., 2003, Dasselaar et al., 2007, Neshrallah et al., 2008, Winkler et al. 2008).
In hypotension-prone patients, total urea removed was significantly higher during HBS compared to HD sessions (Ronco et al., 2000). This was also demonstrated for non-hypotension-prone patients. The eKt/V ratio increased from 1.01 ± 0.03 to 1.13 ± 0.03 with HBS ($P<0.01$) (McIntyre et al., 2003) In this group of patients, the mass of urea removed increased from 24.9 to 32.7 ($P<0.01$).

9. Interdialytic events

The effect of HBS on interdialytic symptoms, such as muscle cramps, headache, dizziness, thirst, dyspnoe, angina, vomiting, itching, the need to lie down, anorexia and asthenia, was analysed by Santoro (Santoro et al., 2002) They looked at the number of symptoms between 2 consecutive sessions within the first 6 hours from the end of dialysis (early symptoms) and later until the beginning of the next dialysis session (late symptoms) and observed a 10% overall reduction ($P<0.001$) in symptoms after treatment with HBS.

10. Quality of life

Déziel et al. investigated the impact of HBS treatment on health-related quality of life (Deziel et al., 2007). They included 44 patients who were partially hypertensive and/or hypotension-prone in a 6-month randomised controlled trial comparing standard HD and HBS. Quality of life was assessed using the Kidney Disease and Quality of Life Short Form (KDQOL-SF) questionnaire. There was a significant improvement in the burden of

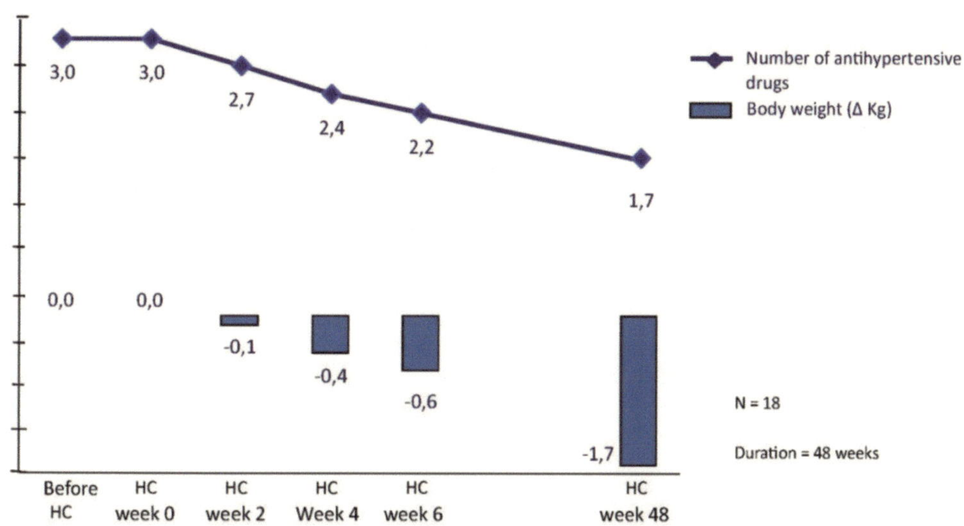

Fig. 7. Decrease of antihypertensive drug and end dialysis body weight over 48 months of follow-up.

kidney disease score in the HBS group, while there was a decrease in the control group (P=0.004). There was no other significant variation in quality-of-life items during the study. In another randomised trial comparing 6-month HD vs HBS treatment, a validated dialysis-related symptoms questionnaire was used to assess dialysis-related quality of life (Neshrallah et al., 2008). This questionnaire asked patients to rate the frequency and severity of dizziness, fatigue, muscle cramps, and other symptoms. None of these differed significantly between groups over time.

11. Conclusions

The growing number of patients with CKD/KDOQI stage 5D is characterised by higher age and increasing comorbidities such as arterial hypertension, diabetes mellitus, arteriosclerosis and atherosclerosis, coronary heart disease as well as peripheral arterial perfusion impairments. In the large majority of patients, age and morbidity-related vascular alterations result in a reduced refilling capacity from the extracellular and intracellular compartment into the intravasal compartment.

The divergence between ultrafiltration and absent refilling can lead to severe hypotensive events during the course of the dialysis. Incidence and intensity of hypotensive complications are correlated with morbidity, frequency of hospitalisation, myocardial and cerebral ischemia and consecutively with mortality.

The complications are preventable by increasing the dialysis time and frequency, decreasing the dialysate temperature, increasing the dialysate calcium concentration and/or with on-line hemodiafiltration. Nonetheless, dialysis time and frequency are finite, and affects the staff and unit workload, while elevated dialysate calcium concentrations could lead to positive mass balance with cumulative calcium overload exposing the patients to higher risk of valvolar and vascular calcification. Nevertheless, hemodiafiltration, due to the high efficiency and high solute extraction, can yield to transient electrolyte and osmolar disequilibrium (Ursino et al, 1997) opposing to plasma refilling and exposing to higher risk of electrical disequilibrium and cardiac dysrhythmias especially in fragile patients, Then, HBS lends itself as a gentle and effective procedure to improve the refilling capacity, to prevent hypotensive events and to optimize the post-dialysis weight. Under HBS, arterial hypertension was improved, dialysis therapy more effective, the body weight optimised, the myocardial function improved, the risk of intradialytic hypotension lower and the patients' quality of life during intradialytic and interdialytic intervals improved.

HBS is a treatment option for elderly, morbid dialysis patients.

12. References

Azar T A, Biofeedback systems and adaptive control hemodialysis treatment, Saudi J Kidney Dis Trasplant, 2008, 19, 6, 895-903.

Basile C, Giordano R, Vernaglione L et al. Efficacy and safety of haemodialysis treatment with the Hemocontrol™ biofeedback system: a prospective medium-term study. Nephrol Dial Transplant 2001; 16: 328-334.

Bégin V, Déziel C, Madore F. Biofeedback regulation of ultrafiltration and dialysate conductivity for the prevention of hypotension during hemodialysis. ASAIO Journal 2002; 48: 312-315.

Cavalcanti S, Ciandrini A, Severi S, Badiali F, Bini S, Gattiani A, Cagnoli L, Santoro A, Model-based study of the effects of the hemodialysis technique on the compensatory response to hypovolemia, Kidney Int, 2004, 65, 1499-1510.

Dasselaar JJ, Huisman RM, De Jong PE, Burgerhof JGM, Franssen CFM. Effects of relative blood volume-controlled hemodialysis on blood pressure and volume status in hypertensive patients. ASAIO Journal 2007; 53: 357-364.

Dasselaar JJ, Relative blood volume based biofeedback during dialysis, J of renal Care, 2007, XXXIII, 2, 59-65.

Davenport A, Cox C, Thuraisingham R. Achieving blood pressure targets during dialysis improves control but increases intradialytic hypotension. Kidney Int 2008; 73: 759–764.

Déziel C, Bouchard J, Zellweger M, Madore F. Impact of Hemocontrol on hypertension, nursing interventions, and quality of life: a randomized controlled trial. Clin J Am Soc Nephrol 2007; 2: 661-668.

Franssen CFM, Dasselaar JJ, Sytsma P, Burgerhof JGM, De Jong PE, Huisman RM. Automatic feedback control of relative blood volume changes during hemodialysis improves blood pressure stability during and after dialysis. Hemodialysis Int 2005; 9: 383-392.

Iseki K, Miyasato F, Tokuyama K, ey al, Low diastolic blood pressure, hypoalbuminemia, and risk of death in a cohort of chronic hemodialysis patients, Kidney Int. 1997, 51, 1212-17.

Kooman J, Basci A, Pizzarelli F, et al EBPG guideline on hemodynamic instability, Nephrol Dial & Transplan, 2007, 22, S2, i22-i44.

Locatelli F, Buoncristiani U, Canaud B, et al, Haemodialysis with on-line monitoring equipment: tool or toys? Nephrol Dial Tranpslant, 2005, 20, 22-33.

Mancini E, Santoro A, Spongano M, Paolini F, Zucchelli P, Effects of automatic blood volume control over intradialytic hemodynamic stability, Int J Artif Organs, 1995, 18, 6, 495-498.

McIntyre CW, Lambie SH, Fluck RJ. Biofeedback controlled hemodialysis (BF-HD) reduces symptoms and increases both hemodynamic tolerability and dialysis adequacy in non-hypotension prone stable patients. Clin Nephrol, 2003; 60: 105-112.

McIntyre CW, Burton JO, Selby NM, Leccisotti L, Korsheed S, Baker C, Camici P, Hemodialysis-induced cardiac dysfunction is associated with an acute reduction in global and segmental myocardial blood flow, Clin J Am Soc, 2008, 3, 19-26.

Moret K, Aalten J, Van den Wall Bake W et al. The effect of sodium profiling and feedback technologies on plasma conductivity and ionic mass balance: a study in hypotension-prone dialysis patients. Nephrol Dial Transplant 2006; 21: 138-144.

Nesrallah GE, Suri RS, Thiessen-Philbrook H, Heidenheim P, Lindsay RM. Can extracellular fluid volume expansion in hemodialysis patients be safely reduced using the Hemocontrol biofeedback algorithm? A randomized trial. ASAIO Journal 2008; 54: 270-274.

Paolini F, Bosetto A, Biofeedback system architecture, Adv in Renal Repl Therapy, 1999, 6, 3, 255-264.

Pastore C, Ruggeri G, Pastore A, Siliberto P, Cristofaro V, Daily use of the physio dialysis system: long-term experience, EDTNA/ERCA J, 2002, XXVIII, 2, 16-20.

Port, FK, Hulbert-Shearon TE, Wolfe RA, et al., Predialysis blood pressure and mortality risk in a national sample of maintenance hemodialysis patients, Am J Kidney Dis, 1999, 33 (3), 507-517.

Ronco C, Brendolan A, Milan M, Rodeghiero MP, Zanella M, La Greca G. Impact of biofeedback-induced cardiovascular stability on hemodialysis tolerance and efficiency. Kidney Int 2000; 58: 800-808.
Santoro A, Spongano M, Mancini E, Rossi M, Paolini F, Zucchelli P, Parameter estimator and adaptive controller to regulate intradialytic blood volume trends, Proceed of 32nd Congress of Italian Society of Nephrology,1992
Santoro A, Mancini E, Paolini F, Spongano M, Zucchelli P, Automatic Control of Blood Volume trends during Hemodialysis, ASAIO J, 1994, 40, M419-M422.
Santoro A, On-Line monitoring, Nephrol Dial & Transplant, 1995, 10, 615-618.
Santoro A., Mancini E., Paolini F., Zucchelli P., Blood volume monitoring and control, Nephrol Dial & Transplant, 1996 11, S2, 42-47.
Santoro A, Clinical significance of intradialytic blood volume monitoring, Int J Artif Organs, 1997, 20, 1, 1-6.
Santoro A, Mancini E, Paolini F, Cavicchioli G, Bosetto A, Zucchelli P. Blood volume regulation during hemodialysis. Am J Kidney Dis 1998; 32: 739-748.
Santoro A, Mancini E, Zucchelli, Ultrafiltration behaviour with different dialysis schedules, Nephrol Dial & Transplant, 1998, 13, S6, 55-61.
Santoro A, Mancini E, Blood volume monitoring systems and biofeedback, in Ronco C, La Greca, eds Hemodialysis Technology, Contrib to Nephrol, 2002, 137, 233-244.
Santoro A, Mancini E, Basile C et al. Blood volume controlled hemodialysis in hypotension-prone patients: a randomized, multicenter controlled trial. Kidney Int 2002; 62: 1034-1045.
Santoro A, Mambelli E, Canova C, Lopez A, Sestigiani E, Mancini E, Biofeedback dialysis, J Nephrol, 2003, 16, S7, S48-S56.
Santoro A, Ferramosca E, Mancini E, Biofeedback Driven Dialysis: where are we? In: Ronco C, Cruz DN (eds): Hemodialysis - from basic research to clinical trials. Contrib Nephrol. Basel, Karger 2008; 161: 199-209.
Selby NM, Lambie SH, Camici PG, Baker CS, McIntyre CW, Occurrence of regional left ventricular dysfunction in patients undergoing standard and biofeedback dialysis, Am J Kidney Dis, 2006, 47, 5, 830-841.
Severi S, Ciandrini A, Grandi E, Cavalcanti S, Bini S, Badiali F, Gattiani A, Cagnoli L, Cardiac response to hemodialysis with different cardiovascular tolerance: heart rate variability and QT interval analysis, Hemod Int, 2006, 10, 287-293.
Sohji T, Tsubakihara Y, Masamitsu F, et al, Hemodialysis-associated hypotension as an independent risk factor for two-years mortality in hemodialysis patients. Kidney Int. 2004, 66, 1212-20.
Tisler A, Akocsi K, Borbas B, et al, The effect of frequent or occasional dialysis-associated hypotension on survival of patients on maintenance hemodialysis, Nephrol Dial & Transplant, 2003, 18, 2601-05.
Winkler RE, Pätow W, Ahrenholz P. Blood volume monitoring. In: Ronco C, Cruz DN (eds): Hemodialysis - from basic research to clinical trials. Contrib Nephrol. Basel, Karger 2008; 161: 119-124.
Wolkotte C, Hassell DR, Moret K, Gerlag PG, van den Wall Bake AW, van der Sande FM, Blood volume control biofeedback and dialysis-induced symptomatology, Nephron, 2002, 92, 605-609.
Zucchelli P, Santoro A, Dry weight in hemodialysis: volemic control, Semin Nephrol, 2001, 21, 3, 286-290.
Ursino M, Innocenti M. Mathematical investigation of some physiological factors involved in hemodialysis hypotension. Artif Organs. 1997, 21(8), 891-902.

16

Acute Complications of Hemodialysis

Gülsüm Özkan and Şükrü Ulusoy
*Karadeniz Technical University, School of Medicine, Department of Nephrology
Turkey*

1. Introduction

Chronic kidney disease (CKD) is a common public health problem, which occurs in many countries with an increasing prevalence. Over 50 million people throughout the world are known to have CKD, and of these, more than 1 million require renal replacement therapies such as dialysis and renal transplantation. In recent years , the rising incidence of diabetes and hypertension, the most common two causes of CKD, cause an increase in the prevalence of CKD.

Hemodialysis, which is one of the renal replacement therapies, is a life-saving treatment. In the absence of this therapy, more than a million patients worldwide would have died within weeks. Hemodialysis was successfully performed for the first time in 1944 by Willem Kollf in patients with renal failure. However, hemodialysis is accompanied by several complications. During the first years following the introduction of hemodialysis, complications were common due to the technical drawbacks associated with the dialysis machines and water systems. Currently, the advances in technology, particularly those in the last 20 years, have reduced the complications. However, complications caused by the reasons other than the dialysis machine and water system remain as a significant cause of morbidity and mortality in hemodialysis patients.

Cardiovascular complications are currently the most common complication of hemodialysis. Among these complications, the rate of symptomatic intradialytic hypotension ranges between 20% and 50%, and it remains an important problem (Cruz DN et al., 1997). Another concern is the hemodialysis-associated arrhythmias, the rate of which was reported to be 5% to 75%. The common and lethal types of arrhythmias include ventricular arrhythmias and ectopies. The rate of hemodialysis-associated complex ventricular arrhythmia is around 35% (Burton JO et al., 2008). The second most common type of arrhythmia is the atrial fibrillation, the rate of which is 27% (Genovesi S et al., 2008). Sudden cardiac death accounts for 62% of cardiac-related deaths and it is usually attributed to arrhythmias (Herzog CA et al., 2008). The first year of hemodialysis is of vital importance with respect to sudden cardiac deaths, which was determined in 93 of 1000 patients in the first year of hemodialysis (Shastri S et al., 2010).

While cramps were observed in 24%-86% of the cases during the first years following the introduction of dialysis therapy, recently it has been shown that only 2% of the patients having ≥2 hemodialysis sessions in a week suffer from cramps (Kobrin SM et al., 2007). Other common complications include nausea, vomiting with a rate of 5%-15%, headache with a rate of 5%-10% and itching with a rate of 5%-10%(Jesus AC et al., 2009; Mettang T et al., 2002). Although cramps, nausea-vomiting, headache and itching do not result in mortality, they substantially deteriorate the quality of life of the patients. Although more

common during the first years following the introduction of dialysis, Disequilibrium syndrome and complications associated with dialyser, water systems and dialysis machines are currently uncommon but may have fatal consequences.
Hemodialysis cause many complications despite the advances in technology. It is of great importance to prevent the complications before they occur. Particularly, early recognition and correction of life-threatening complications save lives. Some complications may not threaten the patients' life but deteriorate the quality of life of the patients. The treatment of these complications provides a longer life and a better quality of life for the patients. Acute complications of hemodialysis can be classified as follows:

Complications associated with hemodialysis equipment

- Hemodialysis device-related complications
- Membrane-related complications
- Water system-related complications
- Vascular acces-related complications

Cardiovascular complications

- Hypotension
- Hypertension
- Arrhythmias
- Pericardial effusion
- Sudden death
- Chest pain

Neurological complications

- Disequilibrium syndrome
- Cerebrovascular accident
- Consciousness changes
- Headache
- Seizure
- Tremor

Complications associated with use of anticoagulant therapy

- Heparin associated thrombocytopenia
- Bleeding diathesis

Electrolyte abnormalities

Hematologic complications

Others

- Nausea
- Vomiting
- Itching

2. Complications associated with hemodialysis equipment

2.1 Hemodialysis device-related complications

The basic principles of hemodialysis were established many years ago. Technology that developed over many years enabled hemodialysis machines to better meet the needs of patients and reduce the amount of complications. However, the number of hemodialysis patients is increasing today and especially those with comorbid disorders need hemodialysis treatment. As a result of this situation, more research is being made to further develop the hemodialysis machine technology.

The functions of a hemodialysis machine include taking the patient's blood from the access by using a blood pump and extracorporeal tubing, passing it through the dialyzer and returning it to the patient, preparing the dialysate using purified water and concentration, circulating the dialysate along the dialyzer system and ultrafiltrating it, and enabling the blood and diaysate to circulate safely by means of control and alarm systems (Ward& Ronco,2006). Such control and alarm systems include an air detector, pressure monitor (for artery and vein pressure), heat detector, blood leakage detector, conductivity monitor, and ultrafiltration control systems.

With the developments in technology, some dialysis machines now display blood flow rates corrected port the pressure at the pump inlet using software algorithm (Depner et al.,1990). Moreover, low pressure-sensitive blood tubing sets have been produced recently (Ahmed et al.,2004). Despite all these developments, it is of vital importance to know and prevent the complications associated with the HD machines and equipment.

2.1.1 Air embolism

One of the much-feared fatal complications of the hemodialysis therapy is the air embolism. There are ultrasonographic air detectors in hemodialysis machine trapping air bubbles to prevent air embolism. Such detectors sense the air bubbles in certain volumes and diameters and activate the control systems. The most common cause of air embolism is air entering in the system mostly from the pre-pump section where there is a negative pressure system and the access points of artery needles (Barak et al.,2008). The symptoms of an air embolism depend on the position of the patient at that moment. If he/she is in a sitting position, neurologic complications occur because the embolus will go into the cerebral system whereas symptoms such as shortness of breath and chest pain occur when the embolus goes into the lungs in the supine position. The first step in treatment is to clamp the vein tubing and stop the pump. The patient then should be laid on his/her left with his/her head and chest facing downwards and 100% oxygen should be given. If the embolus is in the heart, it can be removed with a needle percutaneously and a hyperbaric oxygen therapy may also be used. The clinical signs and therapies we mentioned above are for large air emboli. Besides this, creation of micro-bubbles is also possible during a hemodialysis therapy. The contemporary hemodialysis machines cannot detect any doses of air infusions less than 0,1 ml/k/minutes in bolus infusions and 0,03 ml/kg/minutes in continuous infusions and thus fail to activate the alarm system (Polaschegg, 2007). Therefore, the hemodialysis machines today remain ineffective in preventing micro-bubbles to enter the venous system. Micro-bubbles usually do not result in acute symptoms in patients, but are thought to cause pulmonary hypertension in the lungs and chronic changes in the brain in the long run. Various filters have been developed to prevent micro-bubbles to penetrate the venous system during hemodialysis. However, routine use of such filters has not approved as they cause an extra resistance before the blood flow and the patient's blood becomes exposed to various chemicals contained in the filters (Barak et al.,2008). There are efforts in recent years to develop new technologies to detect and eliminate micro-bubbles through ultrasonographic methods. Works on the issue is still in progress (Palanchon et al., 2001; Versluis et al., 2010).

2.1.2 Complications resulting from manual setup of the machines or not following the instruction manual

Despite the technological developments in hemodialysis machine, some complications arise due to failure to follow their instruction manuals or setting the alarm limits manually by individuals (Davenport, 2006). For example, one of the errors is to set up artery tubing which does not fit the diameters of the blood pump. This may result in hemolysis by increasing the pre-pumping pressure. Another error occurs when lowering the temperature of the dialysate especially in patients with intradialytic hypotension. In such a case when the hemodialysis machine is reset to stop the alarm, the temperature changes may go unnoticed even at very high or low levels due to a problem in the machine. Very low temperatures make the patient feel cold and very high temperatures may cause serious hemolysis. Most of the hemodialysis machine can automatically perform disinfection through heat or chemicals, but if the user manually restricts the disinfection process, this may cause hemolysis and the resulting symptoms as some of the compounds used in disinfection cannot be removed adequately. In some instances, the venous needle comes loose, but the hemodialysis machine cannot sense this and give the necessary alarm in time, or when the venous alarm limits are changed or the alarm is disabled by the user, an abundant loss of blood from the patient may not be sensed. Considering the above mentioned complications, it would be advisable not to disable the alarm systems of the hemodialysis machine or in cases of necessity to employ close monitoring.

In a recent study, the effect of the age and maintenance status of a hemodialysis machine on the satisfactoriness of dialysis was examined. The study showed that technical maintenance of the machines in regular intervals had a significant effect on the efficacy of the hemodialysis therapy (Azar, 2009). Therefore, it should remembered that in order to reduce the number of complications and to give the patient the targeted dose of dialysis, calibrations and service maintenance of hemodialysis machine should be regularly made, the machines should be used according to their instruction manuals, and as manual adjustments may harm the patient, the patients in such situations should be monitored closely.

2.2 Membrane-related complications

During hemodialysis, the patient's blood passes through many extracorporeal compartments. These include the dialyzer, the blood tubing set, the chemicals used during sterilization of the dialyzer and the dialysate. The dialyzer contains a dialysis membrane and sterilization products used during its manufacturing. Dialyzers come in two geometries as hollow-fiber and parallel plate dialyzers according to their membrane structure. In hollow-fiber dialyzers with thousands of tiny hollow fibers, blood flows into the compartment at one end of the cylinder-shaped case and passes through thousands of tiny capillaries. Dialysis solution flows in the opposite direction of the blood flow around the capillaries. Blood passing through the capillaries is collected in the compartment at the other end of the dialyzer and returned to the patient.

Membranes also come in various types with respect to the material used in them; they can be cellulosic, cellulose/synthetic (semi-synthetic), synthetic and bioactive (in dialyzers covered by vitamin E). They can be referred to as being reusable or not and biocompatible or not in the terminology. The most commonly used ones are the synthetic membranes today.(Twardowski, 2008).

2.2.1 Dialyzer reactions

Hemodialysis-related anaphylactoid reaction was first reported in 1975. A well-documented prospective study on its incidence is not available. However, according to the data from the Food and Drug Administration, a severe hypersensitivity reaction was reported in 3.5 of 100.000 dialysis sessions in 1982 (Ebo et al., 2006). Such reactions consisted of a series of incidences involving both anaphylactic reactions and reactions with unknown causes. The classification made by Daugirdas JT and associates is the one most commonly used for these reactions. The classification involves Type-A (hypersensitivity) reactions and Type-B (non-specific) reactions (Daugirdas & Ing, 1988).

Type-A reactions

The symptoms may start with dyspnea, fear of death, and a sensation of heat in the fistula site or the whole body and end with a complete anaphylactic episode. In less severe cases, there may be symptoms such as itching, coughing, sneezing, nasal discharge, nausea and vomiting. These generally occur at the very beginning of dialysis, but may also appear between the 15th and 20th minutes. Such reactions are seen more in patients with atopy and/or eosinophilia (Walter &Taraba, 1991).

The criteria developed by Daugirdas and Ing. are mostly used in diagnosis. The major criteria include the reaction occurring in the first 20 minutes after the beginning of dialysis, dyspnea, sensation of burning or heating-up in the access site or diffused to the whole body and angioedema whereas the minor criteria include recurrence of the reaction during the next dialysis session when the same class or type dialyzer is used, urticaria, rhinorrhea or lacrimation, abdominal cramps and itching. Diagnosis is made when three major or two major and 1 minor criteria are met (Daugirdas & Ing, 1988).

It is mostly caused by sterilization using ethylene oxide, other reasons being the use of an AN69 membrane, reuse, complementary fragment release and eosinophilia (Shaldon & Koch, 1995).

Treatment

The dialysis must immediately be discontinued and the blood in the blood tubing set must not be given back to the patient. Antihistaminic, adrenalin or steroid may be administered depending on the severity of the reaction.

Prevention

It can be considered to sufficiently wash the dialyzers before using them for each patient, to use a dialyzer sterilized by γ-rays or steam if the reaction was due to the use of a dialyzer sterilized by ethylene oxide, to use a membrane that activates the complement more mildly or to make a transition from those using Angiotensin Converting Enzyme (ACE) inhibitor to those using Angiotensin Receptor Blockers (ARB) (Dumler et al., 1987; Daugirdas & Ing, 1988).

Type-B reactions

Their primary symptoms are chest pain and lower back pain. They appear after 20 to 40 minutes after the beginning of dialysis. The symptoms alleviate or disappear in the progressing hours of the dialysis. Complement activation may be blamed of them although the etiology is not fully known (Jaber&Pereira, 1997). The treatment is similar to that in type-A reactions and is adapted depending on the intensity of the symptoms.

2.2.2 Hemodialysis-related hypoxemia

During hemodialysis, Pa O_2 drops to approximately 10-20 mmHg. While such decrease does not lead to significant clinical problems in patients with normal oxygenation, may produce catastrophic results in those with poor oxygenation (De Backer et al.,1983; Hakim & Lowrie,1982). One of the factors that is blamed in the etiology of hypoxemia that emerge during hemodialysis is dialysate containing acetate (De Backer et al.,1983). However, it was demonstrated that it could also be observed in dialysate with bicarbonate. Dialysate with acetate may induce hypoxia in two ways, first by increased oxygen consumption during acetate bicarbonate conversion and second by intradialytic loss of CO_2 (Dolan et al.,1981; Oh et al.,1985). The biocompatibility of the membrane used is one of the most frequently blamed factors in hypoxemia (Graf et al.,1980). Especially the use of an acetate-containing dialysate together with a Cuprophan membrane increases hypoxemia (Vanholder et al.,1987). Hypocapnia associated with intradialytic loss of CO_2 and adaptation to chronic metabolic acidosis lead to periodic shortness of breath and a tendency to sleep apnea syndrome (De Broe & De Backer, 1989).

Treatment and prevention

Increasing the level of CO_2 in the dialysate by directly adding CO_2 to it or by using a dialysate containing bicarbonate,

Using biocompatible membranes (De Backer et al.,1983; Hakim & Lowrie,1982),

Making appropriate ventilator settings for the patients who are known to have hypoxemia prior to the dialysis and are administered mechanical ventilation, nocturnal hemodialysis may be appropriate for those with sleep apnea syndrome (Hanly&Pierratos, 2001),

2.2.3 Disadvantages of first-use dialyzers

New dialyzer syndrome, neutropenia and complement activation as well as reactions associated with the use of ethylene oxide are seen more often.

2.2.4 Disadvantages of reuse dialyzers

Reactions associated with the compounds used in chemical disinfection, side-effects of the volatile gases used during sterilization, allergic reactions, residual chemical infusion, sterilization in insufficient concentrations, pyogenic reactions, variations in the permeability of the membrane and failure to perform an efficient dialysis are seen more often (Twardowski, 2006).

2.3 Water system-related complications

Patients receiving hemodialysis therapy become exposed to 18000 to 36000 liters of water a year during hemodialysis. The formation of dialysate involves water purification, distribution of the purified water to individual hemodialysis machines, concentrate preparation (acidic and basic concentrate) and finally mixing the concentrates with the purified water. While the acidic concentrate is not suitable for bacterial growth, the basic concentrate creates an environment suitable for bacterial growth. For this reason, dry powder cartridges are being used as basic concentrates recently; this allows online preparation of fluid bicarbonate in individual dialysis machines (Ward, 2004). A large portion of the water used in preparing the dialysate is the purified water produced in the water system. In case the hemodialysis water system fails to produce the proper water, patients can be exposed to various chemicals, bacteria and toxic contaminations (Montanari

et al.,2009). The water system technology used in the hempdialysis process is being improved from day to day to reduce such unwanted effects. Two types of water purification systems are being used, the Pure Water and the Ultrapure Water systems. The Pure Water system is used in the conventional hemodialysis process. The Ultrapure Water purification system is used in many dialysis modalities including online hemodiafiltration, online hemofiltration and high flux dialysis ([No authors listed] 2002).
The conventional hemodialysis water system conveys the water taken from the water supply into the hemodialysis unit after passing it through the mechanical filter, water softener, carbon filter, reverse osmosis and UV. An endotoxin filter is also available in some systems. In units with no online processing, the purified water is kept in big tanks before carried to the patients and then distributed to the hemodialysis machine of the patients via water tubes. Every part of this system may constitute a reservoir for bacteria. Moreover, chemical contamination can also occur. For this reason, the European Pharmacopeia has developed the hemodialysis water standards. According to these standards, the levels of microbial contamination and bacterial endotoxin are recommended to be < 100 CFU/ml and < 0.25 IU/ml respectively in the conventional regular hemodialysis water system (Lindley & Canaud,2002) and < 0.1 CFU/ml and < 0.003 IU/ml in the ultrapure water system ([No authors listed] 2002). The chemical contents of the recommended hemodialysis water are given in the table 1.

Contaminant	Methods of analysis	Maximun concentration (mg/l)
Aluminum	Atomic absorption spectrometry	0.0100
Antimony	Atomic absorption spectrometry	0.0060
Arsenic	Atomic absorption spectrometry	0.0050
Barium	Atomic absorption spectrometry	0.1000
Beryllium	Atomic absorption spectrometry	0.0004
Cadmium	Atomic absorption spectrometry	0.0010
Calcium	Atomic absorption spectrometry	2 (0.05 mmol/l)
Chloramines	Colorimetry	0.1000
Chromium	Atomic absorption spectrometry	0.0140
Copper	Atomic absorption spectrometry	0.1000
Cyanide	Spectrophotometric	0.0200
Fluoride	Molecular photoluminescence	0.2000
Free chlorine	Colorimetry	0.5000
Lead	Atomic absorption spectrometry	0.0050
Magnesium	Atomic absorption spectrometry	2 (0.08 mmol/l)
Mercury	Atomic absorption spectrometry	0.0010
Nitrate	Colorimetry	2.0000
Potassium	Flame photometry	2 (0.08 mmol/l)
Selenium	Atomic absorption spectrometry	0.0900
Silver	Atomic absorption spectrometry	0.0050
Sodium	Flame photometry	50 (2.2 mmol/l)
Sulfate	Turbidimetric method	100
Thallium	Atomic absorption spectrometry	0.0020
Zinc	Atomic absorption spectrometry	0.1000

Table 1. Maximum water contaminant levels and methods of analysis recommended by the European Pharmacopoeia (No authors listed] 2002)

In spite of these standards, the complications related to production of water is still being significant with the increased use of high-flux dialyzers, which increase the back-filtration of the dialysate, and the increased use of online hemodiafiltration process, which is based on allowing the blood compartment to contact large amounts of purified water (Brunet & Berland, 2000). The problems associated with the water purification process lead to short and long term complications. In short term complications, a serious septic episode may develop accompanied by tremble, fever, nausea, myalgia, headache, debility and even hypotension and shock when the patient is exposed to excessive amounts of bacteria or endotoxins (Dinarello et al.,1987). Therefore, it is of vital importance to detect in time any contaminant in the dialysis fluid or any formation of biofilm in the parts of the system (Glorieux et al.,2009).

Some problems arise if the chemical contents of the water system are not in desired limits. For example, a low level of sodium may cause hypotension, cramps and hemolysis while a high level of sodium may result in thirstiness and a disequilibrium-like episode. While low and high levels of potassium lead to cardiac arrhythmia, low levels of calcium cause hypotension, hyperparathyroidism, fasciculation, tetany and petechiae. Low levels of magnesium may cause hyperparathyroidism and high levels of it may lead to osteoporosis and osteomalacia, nausea, visual disorders, muscle weakness, ataxia and hypotension (Floege & Lonnemann, 2000)).

It is advisable to check the levels of certain chemicals or contaminants when some symptoms and signs exist. For example, in the case of anemia, the levels of aluminum, chloramines, nitrate, lead, copper, zinc and silicon; in the case of hypertension, the levels of calcium, magnesium and sodium; in the case of hypotension, the levels of bacteria, endotoxins and nitrate; in the case of muscle weakness, the levels of calcium and magnesium; in the case of nausea and vomiting, the levels of bacteria, endotoxins, chloramines, pH, nitrate, sulfate, calcium, magnesium, copper and zinc; and in the case of a neurological disorder, the levels of aluminum, lead, calcium and magnesium may be checked (Hoenich& Levin, 2003).

Taking samples from the water system for microbiological and chemical analysis may be done once a week when the water system is newly set up, but the sampling should not be done immediately after the sterilization process. The frequency of analysis may be decreased after making sure that water quality, but it is recommended not to exceed once a month. The quality of the water tank should be checked at least twice a year. The water system should be sterilized in certain intervals. The frequency of such sterilization should comply with the instructions of the manufacturer. It is also advisable to replace the active carbon filters and the membranes in the reverse osmosis (RO) unit as frequently as advised by the manufacturer (Hoenich& Levin, 2003). The samples for microbiological inspection should be taken into sterile cups of 50 ml from the RO unit, softening unit and water tank, and then from the water system components right before the connection to the dialysis machine. If endotoxins will be checked, samples should be taken into cups with no endotoxines and placed in the culture medium within 30 minutes (Alter et al., 2004).

In conclusion, the necessary care should be taken for the quality of water used in hemodialysis, the allowed levels of chemical contaminants should be maintained, the limits of the European Pharmacopeia should not be exceeded in the levels of microbiological contaminants, and proper samples should be taken and analyzed from various sections of the dialysis water system unit in regular intervals.

2.4 Vascular acces-related complications

Hemodialysis therapy requires a safe vascular access from which an adequate blood flow can be obtained. This is made possible by using arteriovenous fistulae (AVF) or synthetic grafts (AVG) made of poytetrafluoroethylene in chronic dialysis patients whereas central venous catheters (CVC) are used in patients with acute or chronic kidney failure who must urgently undergo dialysis.

2.4.1 Use of central venous catheters, their complications and treatment

Although the The National Kidney Foundation Kidney Disease Outcomes Quality Initiative (NKF KDOQI) recommends that the use of catheters in hemodialysis should remain below 10%, they are being used today in increasing amounts reaching a level of 21% (Chan, 2008; Pisoni et al.,2002). The reason for their being used so much is because they are placed easily, can be used immediately and enable a pain-free dialysis (Chan,2008). There are mainly two classes of CVCs. One is temporary, dual lumen, mostly non-tunneled catheters and the other is long-term tunneled catheters. The temporary catheters are usually preferred in patients whose hemodialysis must be started immediately, whose fistula has not matured yet or whose fistula cannot be used due to a problem. The long-term tunneled catheters, on the other hand, are used in patients for whom an AVF cannot be opened or whose fistula is thought to take long to mature (Wadelek, 2010). Hemodialysis catheters are placed in internal jugular, external jugular or femoral veins respectively. In recent years, subclavian vein catheters are not recommended because of the high possibility of stenosis. However, if catheters cannot be placed in the above mentioned veins, a temporary catheter may be placed in the subclavian vein opposite the AVF *(*Trerotola et al.,1997*)*.

2.4.1.1 Early complications that develop during and after catheter placing

The catheter-related complications in hemodialysis usually develop during catheter placing. Such complications include cardiac arrhythmia, pneumothorax, pleural or mediastinal hematoma, air emboli, thoracic tract injury, nerve injury in the neck or thorax, puncture of the cardiac cavities or cardiac arrest (Chan,2008).

In a study made by Stuart RK et al atrial arrhythmia was seen in 41% of the cases and ventricular ectopia in 25% of the cases during placing of CVCs. Ventricular ectopia was more common in shorter patients in that study. Ventricular ectopia was seen in 43% of the cases when catheters were being placed in the right subclavian vein while it was seen in 10% of the cases when catheters were being placed in other areas. The patient's age and cardiac disease history, the procedure type or the levels of potassium did not affect the development of arrhythmia, but it was demonstrated that over-insertion of the guide wire triggered arrhythmia depending on the body structure of the patient (Stuart et al.,1990). The most important factor in preventing development of arrhythmia is to avoid over-insertion during catheter placing (Fiaccadori et al.,1996). First of all, the guide wire should be pulled back in a case of symptomatic dysrhythmia. A vagal maneuver should be attempted in supraventricular arrhythmia and if the arrhythmia persists, iv administration of adenosine or calcium channel blockers may be considered. A synchronized cardioversion may be attempted in patients with hypotension, lung edema or ischemic chest pain (Yavascan et al.,2009).

While pneumothorax was being observed in 1-6% of the cases when placing CVCs previously (Moini et al.,2009), the prevalence of it has been reduced considerably today as catheters are now placed with the help of ultrasonography. Farrell J et al, for example, did

not observe any pneumothorax when placing 460 internal jugular dialysis catheters (Farrell et al.,1997).
Carotid artery puncture and hematoma during placing of CVCs occur less frequently when they are placed with the help of USG as is the case in other complications. For example, in the study carried out by Farrell J et al, carotid artery puncture was seen 7.6% of the whole patient group and hematoma in 12% of it whereas carotid artery puncture was not observed in patients whose catheters were placed under USG (Farrell et al.,1997). In the study where Oguzkurt et al made 220 internal jugular vein catheterizations under USG, 78% of the patients were under risk in terms of catheter complications such as hematologic complications and incompatibility. Yet, a 100% technical success was achieved in that study and only 4% minor complications developed. Carotid artery puncture was observed in 1.8% of the cases, leakage-like bleeding around the catheter in 1.4% of the cases and minor hematoma in 0.4% of the cases (Oguzkurt et al.,2005).
Air embolus is a rare complication that is seen during placing of catheters. It is only mentioned as case reports in the literature (Heckmann et al.,2000; Yu & Levy,1997). Intense cardiovascular and pulmonary changes typically occur after air emboli. Symptoms usually vary according to the amount of air, its diffusion in the body and its location (Orebaugh, 1992). Cerebral air emboli may also develop in patients with left-to-right shunts (Yu & Levy,1997). When treating it, air intake should be stopped immediately, air should be aspirated from the right ventricle if the catheter is still in place, the patient should be brought to an upside-down, on-the-left-side position and resuscitation process including cardiopulmonary resuscitation and oxygen support should be initiated (Heckmann et al.,2000).
Therefore, while the occurrence of complications is around 6% even in competent hands (Bour & *Weaver,* 1990), it comes down to 0.8% with the use of USG (Trerotola et al., 1997). The said complication percentage is less in jugular vein catheterization than in subclavian vein catheterization (Feldman, 1996).
In addition to the complications developing during placing of catheters, the early catheter dysfunctions are usually associated with the patient's position, mechanical kink, bending of the catheter outside the right atrium and formation of fibrin sheaths. Fibrin sheaths are formed as a result of a pathologic process that follows the placing of a catheter, which is a foreign object for the body, in the vein and a damage occurring in vein endothelium. In general, a fibrin sheath develops within the first 24 hours after the placing of a catheter and in addition to inadequate functioning of the catheter, it may also result in a thrombus, catheter infection and pulmonary emboli after the catheter is removed (Alomari & Falk A, 2007). After any catheter malposition or kink formation is ruled out by radiological exam, 10 mg of saline is given through the catheter. Then the saline is aspirated. Fluid may be injected when a fibrin sheath is diagnosed, but it cannot be aspirated. Although formation of a fibrin sheath is observed as much as 100%, only a portion of them becomes symptomatic (Faintuch&Salazar, 2008). Prevention and treatment of fibrin sheath is similar to those of thrombosis (see below). In treating malpositioned catheters, repositioning or if appropriate replacement of the catheter through the sheath may be considered (National Kidney Foundation: K/DOQI Clinical Practice Guidlines for Vascular Access (NKF KDOQI), 2006).

2.4.1.2 Complications of central venous catheter at later stages

The CVC complications in later periods include thrombosis, infection and stenosis (Chan,2008).

2.4.1.2.1 Thrombosis in central venous catheter

Development of a thrombosis as a later-period complication of CVC is one of the significant causes of catheter malfunction. Catheter thromboses are divided into extrinsic and intrinsic thromboses. Extrinsic thromboses include mural thrombosis, central vein thrombosis and atrial thrombosis and intrinsic thromboses include intraluminal, catheter-type thrombosis and fibrin sheaths (Floege &Lonnemann, 2000). The percentage of catheter thromboses that may require removal of catheters is reported to be between 17 and 33% (Chan,2008). The risk factors involved in a catheter thrombosis are formation of a fibrin sheath, venous stasis, catheter malposition, a patient-related predisposing factor that creates tendency towards thrombosis, and failure to make sufficient heparinisation during the hemodialysis (Mandolfo et al., 2002; Dinwiddie, 2004). Central vein thrombosis is important in that it may prevent efficient dialysis in the clinic, produce tendency towards catheter infection and cause mortality and morbidity. Antiplatelet and anticoagulant drugs have been used in various trials to prevent catheter thrombosis. Buturovic et al compared heparin, citrate and polygeline for their efficacy in preventing catheter thrombosis and found that duration of using catheters was longer in the group taking citrate than in other groups (Buturovic et al., 1998). In a study conducted by Filiopoulos V et al, the efficacy of two groups of catheter lock solutions (gentamicin/heparin and taurolidine/citrate) in preventing catheter infection and thrombosis was assessed. Catheter-related bacteremia and thrombosis were seen in similar rates in both groups and catheters could be used for 3 months on the average without any thrombosis (Filiopoulos et al., 2011). Another trial investigated the efficacy of tPA in reducing catheter thrombosis and infection. The trial evaluated the difference between the use of heparin as a catheter lock solution 3 times a week and the use of rt-PA once a week plus heparin in the other days. It was observed after a 6-month monitoring that the rate of catheter-related thrombosis and bacteremia decreased with the use of rt-PA (Hemmelgarn et al.,2011). Another study assessed the efficacy of a solution containing 0.24 M (7.0%) of sodium citrate, 0.15% methylene blue, 0.15% methylparaben, and 0.015% propylparaben (C-MB-P) against heparin and revealed that the group taking C-MB-P experienced less catheter-related infection and thrombosis (Maki et al.,2010). It can be concluded that the use of catheter lock solutions may be appropriate in preventing catheter-related infection and thrombosis. In treating catheter thrombosis, thrombolytics are administered using either an intraluminal lytic, intradialytic lock protocol, or an intracatheter thrombolytic infusion or interdialytic lock (NKF KDOQI,2006). It is recommended that the use of anticoagulants after a thrombolytic treatment is decided on the basis of a potential benefit and harm assessment because they have plenty of side-effects (Mondolfo & Gallieni, 2010).

2.4.1.2.2 Central venous catheter infections

Bacteremia is seen in patients using CVCs 7.6 times as much when compared to patients using AVFs (Hoen et al., 1998). The average prevalence of catheter-related bacteremia is 3-4 episodes / 1000 catheter days; this rate is slightly higher in non-tunneled catheters (NKF KDOQI,2006; Battistella et al.,2011). Catheter-related bacteremia may often result in serious infections such as endocarditis, osteomyelitis, epidural abscess and septic arthritis (Hoen et al., 1998). In conclusion, the rate of mortality in patients using CVC was found to be 2.3 times as much in diabetic ones and 1.83 times as much in non-diabetic ones as compared to those using fistulas. The use of CVC also causes an increase in the frequency of hospitalization and thus in costs (Ishani et al., 2005; Inrig et al.,2006).

Central venous catheter infections are classified mainly in 3 groups.

1. **Infection in catheter exit-side:** A generally exudative lesion localized at the catheter exit-side (suspicion) and growth in the culture taken from this lesion (definite diagnosis)
2. **Infection in tunnels:** Signs of infection such as pain and swelling along the tunel of the catheter and purulent discharge from the exit-side (suspicion) and growth in the culture (definite diagnosis)
3. **Catheter-related bacteremia:** Growth in 2 or more blood cultures, but no infection signs exit-side the catheter (suspicion) and colonial unit growth 10 or more times as much in the catheter culture taken concurrently with the blood culture (Division of Nosocomial and Occupationl Infectious Diseases, Bureau of Infectious Diseases, Laboratory Centre for Disease Control, Health Canada. (CCDR) 1997; NKF KDOQI,2006).

The factors increasing the risk of a catheter infection include diabetes, peripheral atherosclerosis, previous history of bacteremia, being aged female gender, nasal carriage of Staphylococcus Aureus, long term use of a catheter, the catheter being used very frequently for infusion of various medications, and presence of local infections (NKF KDOQI,2006).

In order to reduce the risk of infection, the catheter exit-side should be checked by an experienced nurse or physician for infection symptoms in every dialysis session, the catheter outlet site should be dressed after every dialysis session and staff should observe the rules of asepsis and wear a mask when dealing with catheters (NKF KDOQI,2006). Catheter lock therapies involving antibiotics may be effective in preventing catheter infections. In the study made on the issue by Battistella et al in recent years, it was demonstrated that a tropical ointment containing polysporin triple ointment (500 U/g of bacitracin, 0.25 mg/g of gramicidin and 10000 U/g of polymixin B) (Lok et al., 2003; Battistella et al., 2011).

The treatment of infected hemodialysis catheters depends on the type and duration of the infection. All the catheter-related infections other than the infection in the exit-side should be treated with a parenteral antibiotherapy suitable for the suspected organisms. If there is growth in the culture taken from the exit-side, again a suitable antibiotherapy should be initiated. When the causative organism is isolated, the antibiotherapy should be adjusted accordingly. The catheters that are thought to have been infected should be replaced as soon as possible, often within 72 hours. A blood culture should be taken for checking a week after the completion of the antibiotics treatment (NKF KDOQI,2006).

2.4.1.2.3 Stenosis associated with the use of central venous stenosis

Prevalence of central venous stenosis (CVS) was reported to be as much as 30% in the literature (Lumsdenet al., 1997). The risk factors for developing a stenosis include a history of placing more than one catheter, the location of the placed catheter in the body and the catheter being with the patient for a long time. There is also a risk of stenosis when the catheter is placed in the subclavian vein (Agarwal al., 2007). While the prevalence of CVS after placing the catheter in the subclavian vein is 42%, it remains around 10% after placing it in the internal jugular vein (Schillinger et al.,1991).

Central venous stenosis is asymptomatic; it can be detected coincidentally or it may give signs depending on the site where it is placed. A subclavian vein stenosis usually causes a swelling in the arm of the same side and the breast tissue. The bilateral innominate vein stenosis in particular may lead to a vena cava superior syndrome. Insertion of an AVF on the side of stenosis and administration of hemodialysis cause an increase in the symptoms and signs. The stenosis restricts blood flow in the hemodialysis access in the clinic and results in an insufficient hemodialysis (Agarwal et al., 2007; Kundu, 2010). Occurrence of AVF complications particularly in patients with a subclavian vein stenosis is more common and the gold standard for its diagnosis is the digital subtraction venography (Lumsden et al., 1997).

A percutaneous transluminal angioplasty with or without a stent is recommended for treating the stenosis (NKF KDOQI,2006).

Nonetheless, the CVCs are important instruments as they enable urgent initiation of a treatment in some hemodialysis patients and maintain a long-term therapy in the others. Therefore, in order to prevent catheter withdrawal we mentioned earlier and the complications that result in morbidity or even mortality in patients, it is necessary that blood is easily aspirated from the catheter of a patient at the beginning of a hemodialysis session, sufficient blood flow is attained during the session and the patient's hemodialysis efficiency is monitored. When there is a deviation in the monitoring parameters it is important to check the catheter for any dysfunction and to employ an appropriate treatment approach. Moreover, the target should be that the percentage of CVC usage in the population of hemodialysis patients is less than 10%.

2.4.2 Use, complications and treatment of arteriovenous fistula/graft

2.4.2.1 Arteriovenous fistula

Use of AVF is recommended as it is superior in enabling sufficient blood flow in hemodialysis patient group and has fewer complications. NKF DOQI targets the percentage of AVF usage in hemodialysis units to be 65% (NKF KDOQI,2006). AVFs are more commonly preferred to AVGs. The reason for AVFs to be preferred more than grafts is that they have longer access life because there are fewer incidences of thrombosis or infection and fewer procedures requiring punctures, and the cost is less. It was shown in various studies that access-related complications were 3 to 7 times more in AVGs than in fistulae (Di Iorio et al., 2004; Enzler et al.,1996; Gibson et al., 2001a; Gibson et al., 2001b). The access potency was found in a study to be 85% in negative AVF while it was 40% in grafts (Hodges et al., 1997).

Besides its advantages, AVFs also involve some complications. While a maturation defect in AVFs lead to venous stenosis and thrombosis, low dialysis blood flow and inefficiency in dialysis, the high flow rate in fistulae may cause a high-output heart failure. Besides these, access-related infections, steal syndrome and aneurism are other complications associated with AVFs. Arteriovenous fistulae are required to mature in 6 weeks on the average. The factors influencing development of a maturation defect include age, DM, obesity and female gender (Allon et al., 2000; Enzler et al.,1996; Lin et al., 1998). A fistulography may be attempted in cases involving immature fistulae (NKF KDOQI,2006). A cause-oriented treatment may be employed.

AVF thrombosis is the major cause of access failure. An average of 0.5 to 0.8 fistula thrombosis is observed per patient in a year (Fan & Schwab, 1992). The cause in 85% of the cases is venous stenosis resulting from neointimal hyperplasia (Bent et al., 2011). The other reasons that create a tendency to fistula thrombosis are excessive compression on the fistula after dialysis, hypotension, hypovolemia, susceptibility to hypercoagulation, arterial stenosis and the fistula being made subject to a prolonged compression for some reason. The thromboses observed especially in the first month after the implantation of a fistula relate to the fistula implantation technique used and the use of fistula before its maturation (Fan & Schwab, 1992). When treating a fistula thrombosis, a thrombectomy should be employed as soon as possible. The thrombectomy may be conducted using surgical or percutaneous interventional techniques (Bent et al., 2011).

AVF stenosis is the most common cause of a fistula failure. Since a fistula-related stenosis may result in susceptibility to thrombosis, dialysis failure and consequently loss of the fistula, its early diagnosis and treatment is very important (Chandra et al.,2010, Tessitore et al.,2004). The Doppler USG is a noninvasive and reliable technique for its diagnosis (Chandra et al.,2010; Sands et al.,1999). Various studies have been done to determine at what stage of the stenosis the treatment should start. While some of these studies produced results evidencing that an angioplasty or a surgical intervention at the early stenosis stage prolonged fistula survival (Schwabet al.,2001;Tessitore et al.,2003,), other studies defended that an early intervention was not advantageous (Turmel-Rodrigues et al.,2000). The commonly accepted approach today is that the fistula should be treated via PTA or surgically if the stenosis is more than 50% and shows clinical signs (NKF KDOQI,2006).

The ischemia that develops as a result of diversion of the arterial flow to the access site is referred to as the steal syndrome. Although a steal syndrome is seen rarely, it produces significant clinical results. The risk factors are female gender, diabetes mellitus, old age, a history of an operation in the extremity which previously had an AVF and the use of a brachial artery rather than a radial artery in making a fistula (Maliket al., 2008). A short time after making the AVF, patients may experience chilling, pain, numbness and paleness in the fingers of their extremity where the fistula is located and after a few months, necrosis or permanent nerve damages may occur in the fingers (Akoh, 2009). Diagnosis of steal syndrome involves hearing the history and carrying out a physical examination followed by an arteriogram to support the diagnosis and viewing the extremity via duplex Doppler ultrasound (DDU). Surgical methods such as access banding, ligation, angioplasty, bypass and sympathectomy may be used in treating it (Berman et al.,1997; Jean-Baptiste et al., 2004; Schanzer et al., 1992).

Native AVF infections are seen less frequently than in CVCs and AVGs (Inrig et al., 2006; Hoen et al.,1998). In the case of an infection, an antibiotherapy should be administered in periods up to 6 weeks due to the risk of developing an infective endocarditis (NKF KDOQI,2006; Tordoir et al.,2007).

In preventing arteriovenous fistula complications, it is recommended to brief, patients with a GFR under 30 ml/min. / 1.73 m^2 about a permanent renal replacement therapy, to avoid any vascular puncture (for placing a catheter or taking blood) in the veins that are suitable for making an AVF and the large veins on that side in stage 4 and 5 patients, to make the AVF 6 months before the starting of hemodialysis when possible, to obtain patient histories and physically examine patients before making an AVF, to examine the upper extremity veins and arteries via a duplex USG and to view the central veins of those patients with a previous central vein catheterization history. The aseptic techniques should be adhered to in all vascular access cannulations. In order for an AVF to be ready, there must be a flow of more than 600 ml/min, and the fistula vein diameter must be at least 0.6 cm and its depth should not exceed 0.6 cm. It should be checked by an experienced physician or nurse at least once a month for any signs of dysfunction, which include any change in the characteristics of fistula trill and murmur during a physical examination, an increase in swelling, redness and heat in the arm carrying the fistula, and not being able to stop bleeding for a long time after pulling out the fistula needle. Direct flow measurement and dublex USG are preferred diagnostic methods in these cases. A fistulagraphy may also be carried out as an advanced diagnostic test (NKF KDOQI,2006; Tordoir et al.,2007).

2.4.2.2 AV graft

The use of grafts as vascular access in hemodialysis patient group varies from country to country. It is most common in the USA, but quite uncommon in the European countries (Hirth et al., 1996). Studies demonstrated that its primary and secondary potency is less as compared to native AVF and it involved more complications than native AVFs. Since it may involve more mortality and morbidity for this reason, the use of grafts as vascular access is only recommended for the patients who are problematic in making native AVFs (Coburn&Carney,1994; Di Iorio et al.,2004; Enzler et al.,1996; Gibson et al., 2001a; Gibson et al., 2001b). AVG may be used as an access in elderly patients, those with comorbid diseases, those whose vascular structures are impaired or those who require an early access. Grafts usually become ready for hemodialysis approximately in 3 weeks.

All the complications seen in native AVFs may also bee seen in AVGs. However, frequency of such complications is more in grafts (Coburn&Carney,1994; Di Iorio et al.,2004; Enzler et al.,1996; Gibson et al., 2001a; Gibson et al., 2001b).

There are some points to pay attention to in grafts that differ from the treatments of native AVF complications. These include spontaneous bleeding, suspecting graft rapture in the case of a fast increase in the diameter of pseudoaneurysm and a severe degenerative change in the graft material and considering an urgent surgery in this situation, the initial treatment of a graft infection needing to cover gram negatives and positives, then selection of a suitable antibiotherapy according to culture result, incision and drainage also possibly being useful, and replacing the graft material in prolonged infections. Furthermore, when an edema lasts more than 2 weeks in patients with AVGs, a fistulography should be made and if any stenosis is found, it should be treated via either surgery or PTA (NKF KDOQI,2006).

3. Cardiovascular complications of hemodialysis

Prevalence of cardiovascular diseases in dialysis patients increased as compared to the normal population. The most important reason of this increase is the increased number of incidences of diabetes mellitus (DM) and hypertension in this patient group. Cardiovascular diseases accounts for approximately 45% of the causes of mortality in dialysis patients (Shastri&Sarnak,2010). Besides the patient-related factors, the hemodialysis therapy itself brings about a number of cardiovascular complications.

3.1 Hypotension

The frequency of intradialytic hypotension (IDH) in patients receiving hemodialysis therapy has been assessed in various studies. For example, in a study made by Andrulli et al on 123 hemodialysis patients, IDH was considered to prevail if there was a decrease of 30 mmHg or more in Systolic blood pressure (SBP) or if IDH appeared symptomatically and the prevalence of IDH in the group that has a tendency to hypotension was found to be 44% (Andrulli et al., 2002). In another study made by Emily S et al, IDH was found in 608 (24%) of 2559 dialysis patients (Emili et al., 1999). Although the figures change in different studies, IDH is observed between 20 and 50% of the cases and continues to be an important problem (Cruz et al.,1997; Daugirdas, 2001). IDH is a significant clinical issue as it involves impairment in the quality of life, increased treatment costs and loss of time and effort on the part of the employees and leads to incidences of high mortality and morbidity such as cardiovascular, cerebrovascular and mesentery ischemia in the patients of the risk group (Emili et al., 1999; Daugirdas, 2001). There are two mechanisms suggested in the pathogenesis of IDH. First is failure to keep the plasma volume at an optimum level and the second is cardiovascular abnormalities. The first mechanism is related to excessive weight gain that requires low serum osmolarity and large volume ultrafiltration and the second to autonomic dysfunction, a shift of blood flow to the gastrointestinal area during eating, a decrease in vasoconstructive compounds and an increase in vasodilatatory compounds, vasodilatation associated with acetate-based dialysate, and impairment of compensatory response due to hypertrophy or ischemia (Emili et al., 1999). The causes of intradialytic hypotension are shown in the table 2. IDH may be accompanied by symptoms such as cramps, dizziness, nausea, vomiting, excessive fatigue and debility or it may show no symptoms at all (Perazella,2001). It becomes more symptomatic in the aged and women, and in the presence of a cardiac disease, autonomic neuropathy and DM (Perazella,2001, Davenport,2006). IDH-based extremity interactions may be seen in a chronic hypotensive patient when there is a drop in blood pressure < 30 mmHg and in a normotensive or hypertensive patient when the drop in blood pressure is > 30 mmHg (Schreiber, 2001).

Factor associated with the patient	
	Excessive interdialytic weight gain (more than 3% of body weight)
	Myocardial infarction
	Left ventricular hypertrophy
	Diastolic dysfunction
	Aritmia
	Pericardial tamponade
	Autonomic neuropathy
	Taking antihipertensive or other medications that lower blood pressure before dialysis
	İnterdialitic food consumption
Factros associated with the hemodialysis	
	High ultrafiltration rate
	Dialysis with acetate
	High dialysate temperature
	Electrolyte abnormalities
Factors associated with the doctor	
	Incorrect calculation of dry body weight

Table 2. Intradialytic hypotension causes

Prevention and treatment of intradialytic hypotension

Educating the patient should be the first consideration in preventing IDH. The patient should be educated to restrict his/her salt consumption so that the interdialytic weight gain is limited to 3% of his/her weight, to avoid taking any antihypertensive drugs before dialysis, and to avoid eating during dialysis (Schreiber, 2001). If the patient has anemia, it should be corrected. The patient's dry weight should be reassessed and the temperature of the dialisate should be optimized (Maggiore et al., 1982; Maggiore Q et al., 2002). A bicarbonate-based dialysate may be preferred (Sopngano et al.,1988; Velez et al.,1984), a dialysate with high calcium content may be used if the patient's calcium situation allows it (Maynard et al.,1986) and a sodium profiling may be carried out in the relevant patients (Emili et al.,1999; Schreiber, 2001). Nevertheless, conflicting results were obtained in the meta-analyses made for sodium profile applications. Therefore, it is recommended that it should be carried out in a way to avoid sodium overloading in selected patients (Stiller et al.,2001). Ultrafiltration profiles and relative blood volume measurements may relieve hemodialysis-related hypotension (Donauer et al.,2000; Andrulli et al.,2002).

In patients with sudden symptomatic hypotension, the patient's hemodynamic stability should be achieved first. To do this, the UF is closed, the patient is brought to a trendelenburg position and then a bolus of iv fluid is administered. These fluids may be normal saline, hypertonic saline, albumin, mannitol or hydroxyethylstarch (HES) (Schreiber, 2001). They may be given one by one or in incremental profiles (Emili et al.,1999). Additional dialysis sessions should be considered in patients gaining kilos more than 3% of their weight and those who are susceptible to hypotension. However, most of the patients do not agree with extra sessions. Therefore, a medical treatment may be considered for the patients with increased hypotension episodes in spite of all these measures. The treatment agents that were evidenced to have positive effects in pharmacologic therapy are carnitine, sertraline and midodrine (Perazella, 2001). L-carnitine is a naturally available amino acid and assumes the duty of carrying long-chain fatty acids to the mitochondria. It is either synthesized endogenously in the kidneys and liver or taken in by a diet. It may be insufficient in patients with chronic kidney failure. It was demonstrated in many studies that an iv administration of 20 mg/kg during each dialysis reduced the intradialytic hypotension (Perazella, 2001; Lynch et al.,2008). There are also studies showing that the use of sertraline, which is a reuptake inhibitor of the selective serotonin, in doses of 50 to 100 mg/day also reduced IDH (Perazella, 2001; Yalcin et al.,2003). Midodrine is an α1 agonist. Hypotension was shown to be reduced with its use 30 minutes before hemodialysis (the initial dose of 2.5 mg is increased to 30 mg by titration) in patients with IDH (Perazella, 2001; Cruz et al.,1997).

3.2 Hypertension

Hypertension (HT) is the most frequently observed complication in chronic hemodialysis patients. Over 80% of the patients have HT histories and the blood pressures of two thirds of these are not under control. The target values of blood pressure in hemodialysis patients are not clear today. While K-DOQI recommends a pre-dialysis blood pressure target of 140/90 mmHg and post-dialysis blood pressure target of 130/180 mmHg, such recommendation is not based on strong evidence (Hemodialysis Adequacy 2006 Work Group,2006). As a result of many observational studies, it was shown that low blood pressure (BP) increased mortality; the lowest mortality was in those with a pre-dialysis blood pressure between 140-160/70-90 mmHg and the highest mortality was in those patients with > 180/100 mmHg (Agarwal,2005; Lacson &Lazarus, 2007; Peixoto & Santos,2010). An intradialytic increase of >10 mmHg BP was observed in 12 to 13% of hemodialysis patients (Inrig et al.2007, Inrig et al., 2009). In another study made by the same researchers, it was shown that intradialytic hypertension caused mortality in patients with a pre-dialysis hypotension (<120/80 mmHg) (Inrig et al., 2009).

Most of them are hypertensions associated with high blood volume in the etiology of hemodialysis patients. Considering the prolonged patient survey among the hemodialysis

population in the Tassin dialysis center and the absence of any hypertension, lack of hypertension can be thought of as a synonym of normovolemia and presence of hypertension as a synonym of hypervolemia (Kooman, 2009). The volume balance in hemodialysis patients are adjusted by daily sodium intake, amount of urine, and removal of excess fluid through ultrafiltration. An imbalance of these factors leads to hypertension and a poor cardiovascular outcome (Hörl et al., 2002). A study showed that a weight gain of more than 4.8% between two dialysis sessions increased mortality (Foley et al.,1998). The patients need to be brought back to their dry weights to treat a HT associated with excess volume. The dry weight is clinically determined by measuring the BP and considering the presence of any signs of excess volume and the patient's tolerance to ultrafltration (Sherman, 2002). However, it should be noted here that there could be excessive volume in patients without any signs of hypervolemia (Mitch&Wilcox, 1982). Therefore, besides physical examination, chest radiography, vena cava echography and bioimpedance techniques can be employed in assessing the volume status and the changes in blood volume during dialysis can be monitored by observing the level of natriuretic peptide and the changes in hematocrit and proteins (Koomanet al., 2009).
Besides excessive volume, the other causes of hypertension in hemodialysis patients include arterial stiffness associated with atherosclerosis, salt-related decline in NO formation, overactivation of the sympathetic nervous system, activation of the rennin-angiotensin-aldosterone system, presence of other vasoconstructive agents, inadequacy of vasodilatatory compounds, erythropoietin therapy and genetic tendency (Hemodialysis Adequacy 2006 Work Group,2006).

Treatment

It is being argued in recent years that home measurements or ambulatory blood pressure measurements may be more realistic in diagnosing hypertension (Peixoto & Santos,2010). As no definite target BP values are provided to hemodialysis patients, it is suggested that the pre-hemodialysis BP is kept between 130-160 mmHg / 80-100 mmHg (140/90 mmHg) until more objective data is published (Hemodialysis Adequacy 2006 Work Group,2006; Peixoto & Santos,2010). In hypertensive HD patients, the first consideration should be whether the patient is in his/her dry weight. If not, intake of Na chloride should be restricted to 5 gm, weight gain between two dialyses to 1 kg during the week and to 1.5-2 kg at weekends; sodium profiling and use of dialisate with high amounts of sodium should be avoided; and the patients should not be made to lose more than 1-2 kg in a week when bringing them to their dry weight (Hemodialysis Adequacy 2006 Work Group,2006). Additional dialysis sessions and prolongation of dialysis time may also be helpful to attain the dry weight (Culleton et al.,2007). Some patients persist to remain hypertensive even though they are brought to their dry weight. In such cases, antihypertensive therapies are required. The rennin-angiotensin-aldosterone system (RAAS) blockers may be preferred as a first step. KDOQI recommends that they are to be preferred especially in patients with diabetics and/or heart failure (K/DOQI Workgroup, 2005). However, angiotensin converting enzyme inhibitors (ACE), which are RAAS blockers, are dialyzable with the exception of fosinopril. Therefore, a transition should be made to non-dialyzable fosinopril or angiotensin receptor blockers (ARB) in patients with intradialytic hypertension and patients taking RAS blockers should be monitored for any side-effects. There is not adequate number of studies made on aldosterone antagonists or Alliskrein. Beta blockers may be preferred in patients with coronary arterial disease and heart failure. Since water-soluble B blockers are dialyzable, additional doses should be given after dialysis. Calcium channel blockers are not dialyzable and can safely be used. In conclusion, RAS blockers may be used as the first line and alternative drugs such as combined alpha and beta blockers, calcium channel blockers and direct vazodilatators may be employed as the second line in patients with heart failure (Inrig,2010; Hörl MP& Hörl WH,2004).

3.3 Arrhythmias

Arrhythmias are complications that are frequently observed in patients attending to hemodialysis. They mostly occur during and after dialysis. Prevalence of arrhythmia varies between 17 to 76% (Buemi et al.,2009). Prevalence of arrhythmia was reported to be 5 to 75% in another study (Genovesi et al., 2008). ECG abnormalities were found in 65% of the patients in a study made by Abe S and associates (Abe et al.,1996). In a study made by Severi S et al, an increase in the heart rate was seen in 30% of the patients at the end of the hemodialysis (Severi et al.,2001). The differences in the figures of the studies are associated with patient characteristics and arrhythmia types.

Arrhythmia etiology of the hemodialysis patient group is multi-factorial. The dialysis therapy itself may lead to changes that can alter excitability of myocardium. Dialysis may be pro-arrhythmic as it changes the fluid composition in the body, the PH and the concentrations of heat and electrolytes. Patients with chronic kidney diseases who are undergoing a dialysis therapy are prone to arrhythmia since they usually have ischemic heart disease, left ventricle hypertrophy or autonomic neuropathy in high prevalence. Finally, the drugs used by some of the patients receiving anti-arrhythmic therapy may also be dialyzable. Such patients may, for this reason, be susceptible to arrhythmia during or after hemodialysis (Kimura et al.,1989; Weber et al., 1984). Prevalence of atrial fibrillation as one of the arrhythmia types was reported to be 27%, which is way above 0.5-1% seen in the general population (Genovesi et al.,2008). Another two types of arrhythmia, the complex ventricular arrhythmia and premature ventricular complexes, in particular increase the mortality and morbidity. Complex ventricular arrs (those defined as having a Lown score of 3 and more) prevail at a rate of 35% in the HD patient group (Burton et al.,2008).

Treatment

NKF-DOQI recommends that due to the susceptibility of hemodialysis patients to arrhythmia, every dialysis patient should undergo a 12-lead ECG regardless of his/her age and if an arrhythmia is found, he/she should be treated as in the normal population. In case of an atrial fibrillation, B blockers, calcium channel blockers and amiodarone may be used for controlling the rate (K/DOQI Workgroup, 2005). While the indications of using anticoagulants in preventing a stroke in patients with atrial fibrillation in the general population are distinct, this issue is controversial in the hemodialysis population because this patient group is prone to bleeding (Sood et al., 2009). In the trial made by Quinn RR et al, the cost of using either acetylsalicylic acid or warfarin in hemodialysis patients with atrial fibrillation was compared and no difference was found between the two costs (Quinn et al., 2007). At present, an anticoagulant therapy can be applied in a similar way as in the normal population, but the susceptibility of patients to bleeding and the reactions with other medication they use should be borne in mind and the patients should be closely monitored (Abbott et al.,2007). Doses should be adjusted depending on whether or not the drugs used in treatment are dialyzable and have potential side-effects or some drugs should be avoided altogether (K/DOQI Workgroup, 2005).

3.4 Pericarditis

We come across pericarditis in hemodialysis patients in two ways. The first is in the form of a uremic pericarditis. This type of pericarditis can be seen before starting the dialysis or in the first 8 weeks of dialysis. It is usually associated with uremia. The other type of pericarditis is a dialysis-related pericarditis that can be seen any time after the patient starts the dialysis. Although its definite cause is not known, insufficient dialysis and excess volume are the most blamed factors in pathogenesis (Rostand&Rutsky,1990; Rutsky& Rostand, 1987). Prevalence of pericarditis in dialysis patients is reported to be between 2 and 21% (Lange& Hillis,2004; Banerjee& Davenport,2006).

They can be clinically present as complaints such as a nonspecific chest pain, muscle weakness and coughing, but they can also come in as a hypotension and heart failure. A reduction of heart sounds and pericardial rubbing, and in serious cases, hypotension can be observed depending on the intensity of effusion during a physical examination. Classical ECG changes may not appear in uremic pericarditis. A final diagnosis is made using an ECHO (Shastri &Sarnak,2010).

Treatment

The treatment depends on the symptoms and the diameter of the effusion. A small scale asymptomatic effusion does not usually necessitate taking urgent measures. Those having a large amount of pericardial fluid may need to undergo an urgent drainage by way of pericardiotomy if it is hemodynamically unstable or an intensive hemodialysis therapy for 7 to 14 days and avoidance of heparinization during hemodialysis if it is hemodynamically stable. Glucocorticoid and non-steroidal anti-inflammatory drugs are usually ineffective (Banerjee& Davenport,2006; Shastri &Sarnak,2010). In uremic pericarditis, a response can be obtained from an intensive hemodialysis therapy in >85% (76-100%) of the patients and in dialysis-related pericarditis, in <60% (12.5-66%) of the patients (Alpert & Ravenscraft,2003).

3.5 Sudden cardiac death

Sudden cardiac death is held responsible for 62% of the cardiac-related deaths and is usually attributed to arrs (Herzog et al.,2008). The first year of hemodialysis is significant in terms of sudden cardiac deaths and a sudden death was reported in 93 of 1000 patients in the first year (Shastri &Sarnak,2010).

Ischemic heart diseases, cardiomyopathy, fast ion change and electrolyte during hemodialysis, changes in PH, microvascular diseases or endothelial dysfunction are blamed in its pathogenesis (Shastri &Sarnak,2010).

Treatment

It is the same as in the normal population. It is advisable that an external defibrillator is made available in hemodialysis units and the staff is trained in using it (K/DOQI Workgroup, 2005). There is not adequate data on the use of B blockers (Pun et al.,2007) and internal defibrillators (de Bie et al.,2009).

3.6 Myocardiac infarction

An increase is observed in the prevalence of coronary incidences in patients with end-stage renal failure and in mortality following a myocardial infarction (MI) (Herzog et al., 1998; Winkelmayer et al., 2006). A cardiac-related death is seen 10 to 20 times as much in this patient group as compared to the normal population (Foley et al., 1998).

Acute MI is diagnosed in the normal population at the presence of a high cardiac enzyme level, classical chest pain and ECG changes. However, there are some differences in MI presentation and laboratory findings of hemodialysis patient group. This situation causes a delay in diagnosing MI in this group and thus a less frequent use of the thrombolytic and early coronary angiography/coronary stent applications for treatment of MI as compared to the normal population.

For example, MI-associated classical chest pain is seen less in patients with renal failure in correlation with the intensity of such renal failure. The cause of this is thought to be the impairment of sensory and autonomic nerve functions seen in patients with renal failure. It was demonstrated in a study made by Komukai et al that as the renal function disorders increased, the prevalence of painless MI also increased (Komukai et al., 2007). In another study conducted by Pitsavos C et al, it was shown that MI patients with renal failure admitted to the hospital late and the possible reason for such late admission was thought to be the less occurence of alerting symptoms such as chest pain in this patient group (Pitsavos et al., 2007). Late admissions certainly mean that coronary interventions are less and mortality is more.

Cardiac troponin T (cTnT) and creatine kinase-MB, which are two of the enzymes used in the verification of a myocardial infarction diagnosis, were seen in high levels in the hemodialysis patient group without the presence of coronary ischemia. cTnT in particular was shown to be as high as 17 to 23.8% in this patient group (Chew, 2008). This situation leads to controversies in diagnosing MI in the hemodialysis patient group. Researches are still in progress to find an ideal marker that supports an MI diagnosis. For the time being, it is advisable to monitor the cardiac enzyme levels in patients clinically suspected of having an MI.

Another point to take into consideration is that 15 to 40% of the patients are seen to have ST depression during hemodialysis (Abe et al., 1996; Conlon et al., 1998). Dialysis therapy itself may cause subclinical myocardial ischemia in this patient group which is prone to atherosclerosis and left ventricular hypertrophy (Selby& McIntyre, 2007).

There is not sufficient data about the reliability of conducting a dialysis within 48 hours after a myocardial infarction (MI). In such a case, the volume status of the patient should be assessed together with its biochemical parameters and the hemodialysis therapy should be adjusted in a way to avoid hypotension (Coritsidis et al., 2009). The treatment of acute MI is recommended to be the same as in the normal population (K/DOQI Workgroup, 2005).

4. Neurologic complications

Neurologic complications may develop in the patients of end-stage renal failure due to a multiple metabolic disorder caused by a chronic kidney disease and due to the dialysis procedure. These complications may appear in the form of variations in consciousness, headache, nausea, vomiting, myoclonus, tremor, focal and generalized seizures, cerebrovascular events (infarct and bleeding) and disequilibrium syndrome.

4.1 Disequilibrium syndrome

Dialysis Disequilibrium syndrome (DDS) was first defined by Kennedy AC (Kennedy ,1970, Chen et al.,2007). Although the pathogenesis of DDS is controversial, the first theory blamed in etiology is the fast urea removal theory. According to this theory, the fast removal of urea from plasma in patients who newly started a hemodialysis therapy creates an osmotic gradient between the brain cells and plasma and the fluid enters the brain cells due to this osmotic gradient (Kennedy,1970; Attur et al.,2008; Chen et al.,2007; Trinh-Trang-Tanet al.,2005). Another theory is the idiogenic osmole effect. According to this theory, the diffusion of bicarbonate from the dialysate to plasma increases PH. Bicarbonate transforms into carbon dioxide (CO2) outside the cell. Blood with CO2 penetrates the brain barrier and enters the brain cells, causing an intracellular acidosis. This event then causes the cell proteins to break down to form idiogenic osmoles. An increase of idiogenic osmoles in the cell in turn results in an osmotic gradient and eventually causes the fluid to enter the cell (Arieff et al.,1976). DDS usually develops as a result of fast reduction of urea in patients with severe uremia. Risk factors include young age, a history of head trauma or cerebrovascular event, and an electrolyte imbalance such as a malign hypertension and hyponatremia (Trinh-Trang-Tanet al.,2005; Patel et al.,2008).

DDS is a diagnosis of exclusion, because its clinical signs resemble other neurologic complications. DDS is an acute neurologic complication of dialysis. It generally starts towards the end of dialysis or after it ends. Its symptoms and signs can be fatigue, slight headache, HT, nausea, vomiting, blurred vision, and muscle cramps, and it can cause arrhythmia, confusion, tremor, seizure, and coma. DDS may rarely result in death due to a brain edema (Patel et al.,2008).

To prevent a Dialysis Disequilibrium syndrome, the initial dialysis session may be performed using a slow flow and in a shorter time, sodium level may be raised in the dailysate and osmotic active compounds may be administrated. In a slow-flow shortened dialysis, it may be useful to limit the time to 2 hours and the blood flow rate to 200 ml/min and to use a dialyzer with a small surface area (Levin&Goldstein,1996; Sang et al.,1997). The target rate of urea reduction may be 0.4 to 0.45 for the first session. There are studies showing that adding urea to the dialysate is useful in preventing DDS (Hampl et al.,1983, Patel et al.,2008, Levin&Goldstein,1996; Sang et al.,1997). The aim in raising the level of Na in the dialysate is to reduce the osmolarity difference resulting from a fast urea removal by an increase in plasma Na. Na profile applications and use of fixed high-Na dialysate can be attempted in this respect, but they are not evidenced to be effective. Therefore, use of dialysate containing 143-146 mmmol/L is recommended in patients under DDS risk (Patel et al.,2008; Levin&Goldstein,1996, Sang et al.,1997). Administration of osmotic active compounds follows the same logic. Various studies showed that osmolarity change and DDS were reduced by administering a dialysate with high glucose content and 1 gr/kg mannitol (Rodrigo et al.,1977; Rosa et al.,1981).

4.2 Headache

The International Headache Society (ICHD, 2004) included the hemodialysis headache in the headache classification. To be able to mention a hemodialysis headache, the headache should prevail in at least half of the hemodialysis sessions, there should be 3 acute headache attacks meeting at least two criteria and the headache should be relieved within 72 hours after the hemodialysis (Gladstone& Dodick,2004,; Goksel et al.,2006). Although its prevalence is not certain, it was found to be 30% by Goksel et al and 48% by Göksan et al (Goksel et al.,2006; Göksan et al.,2004). Jesus AC et al, on the other hand, found a much lower prevalence of 6.7% in 2009 (Jesus et al.,2009).

Although its physiopathology is not fully clear, the factors triggering headache may be hypertension, hypotension, low level of sodium, decreased serum osmolarity, low level of plasma rennin, pre- and post-dialysis Bun values and low levels of magnesium (Bana et al.,1972; Bana& Graham,1976; Göksan et al.,2004; Goksel et al.,2006).

Treatment

After making sure that there is no migraine, cerebrovascular event or intracranial mass, the first step in treatment is to investigate if there is a hemodialysis headache. If a hemodialysis headache is suspected, the factors that are thought to trigger the headache should be reviewed and the necessary electrolyte replacements or a modification in the treatment modality should be made.

4.3 Cerebrovascular event

A cerebrovascular event constitutes the 3rd most common cause of death in the normal population. Patients with chronic kidney failure have an increased rate of cerebrovascular event risk as compared to the normal population (K/DOQI Workgroup, 2005). Although there is not any clear information on its prevalence, a study made in Japan revealed that cerebrovascular events were seen at a rate of 8% and cerebral hemorrhage was seen more frequently (Kawamura et al.,1998). According to the American data, the rates of hemorrhagic stroke and ischemic stroke were found equal, which were 5 to 10 times more than those seen in the normal population (Selinger et al.,2003). It was found in another study made in 2009 that ischemic stroke was seen more frequently (Sozio et al.,2009). There are just a few studies make on the etiologic risk factors of cerebrovascular event. Hypertension was defined as a risk factor in a study conducted in Japan (Iseki&Fukiyama,1996). In a study made by Selinger SL et al, the risk factors for cerebrovascular event were determined to be hypertension, low hemoglobin level and indicators of malnutrition (low weight, low level of albumin) (Selinger et al.,2003). The frequency of carotid artery atherosclerosis increased in patients with end-stage renal failure. This in turn may increase the rate of ischemic strokes. Hypertension, routine heparin use during dialysis therapy and tendency to bleeding diathesis in this patient group may result in an increase in hemorrhagic strokes (Selinger et al.,2003).

Screening and treatment

Since subclinical vascular disease is common in the dialysis population, ultrasonographic measurement of carotid artery elasticity during screening may be helpful (Pascazio et al.,1996). Likewise, since an increase in the thickness of carotid intima media is attributed to the increase in cardiovascular events, this can also be used during screening (Benedetto et al.,2001). Screening is not recommended in asymptomatic patients (K/DOQI Workgroup,2005). Screening of patients for cerebrovascular event is the same as recommended for the normal population. It only differs from the normal population in that it should be remembered to educate the patients who are planned to be given a heparinisation or thrombolytic therapy about the increased bleeding diathesis. Differentiation between the hemorrhagic and ischemic stroke should also be made before initiating the hemodialysis therapy (because heparinisation will be wrong in hemorrhagic stroke) (K/DOQI Workgroup).

5. Complications associated with use of anticoagulant therapy

5.1 Heparin-induced thrombocytopenia

Heparin is frequently used as an anticoagulant in hemodialysis therapy due to its low cost and short half life, but a heparin-induced thrombocytopenia (HIT) is a situation restricting the use of heparin and resulting in a significant amount of mortality. HIT is classified as Type-I and Type-II.

Type-I HIT is a commonly seen form. It develops as a result of a direct reaction between heparin and thrombocytes. It usually appears as a slight decline in the number of thrombocytes in the early stage of heparin administration and the number of thrombocytes goes back to normal despite the repeated heparin applications (Kapa& Qian, 2009). Type-II HIT is less common, its incidence being between 0.5 to 5% (Jang &Hursting,2005). It is an antibody immune response against platelet factor 4 and heparin complex (Visentin et al., 1994; Suranyi&Chow, 2010).

HIT generally appears with an acute systemic reaction, thrombocytopenia, thrombosis, skin necrosis and venous gangrene in the extremities 5 to 30 minutes after a bolus application of unfractioned heparin (Syed&Reilly, 2009).

In diagnosing a heparin-induced thrombocytopenia, the following criteria are used: thrombocytopenia appering 5-10 days after the initiation of heparin therapy, presence of any thrombotic event, having a normal number of thrombocytes before the heparin therapy, 50% decline in the number of thrombocytes from baseline, absence of any other reason to cause thrombocytopenia, thrombocytes returning to normal when heparin use is suspended and presence of HIT antibody seroconversion. A possible diagnosis of HIT is made after the scoring of these criteria (Warkentin, 2004).

The risk factors for developing a heparin-induced thrombocytopenia show racial differences and may vary according to the type and source of heparin used. For example, when a low molecule weight heparin (LMWH) is used, less HIT is observed as compared to the use of unfractioned heparin (UFH) (Prandoni et al., 2005). It was shown in a meta-analysis of 5 trials that unfractioned bovine heparin caused more HIT than the classical unfractioned porcine heparin (Syed&Reilly, 2009).

As the results of HIT antibodies can take time to be obtained, the treatments of high-risk patients in particular should not be delayed. When treating it, first all heparin therapies including flash and catheter lock therapies should be discontinued and then alternative non-heparin anticoagulant therapies should be initiated. However, a warfarin therapy should not be attempted until the number of thrombocytes returns to normal (Syed&Reilly, 2009). LMWH may be continued in the low-risk patients until the HIT antibody results are obtained (Warkentin et al., 2003).

Patients who developed HIT may be made subject to a non-heparin dialysis using flush or citrate anticoagulation in intervals or using the direct thrombin inhibitors lepirudin and argatroban or the Factor Xa inhibitor danaparoid (Matsuo&Wanaka, 2008, Syed&Reilly, 2009).

5.2 Bleeding diathesis

Bleeding is the most important factor restricting the use of heparin in hemodialysis treatment. Taking all methods of use into account, the level of bleeding is 10%-15%, while that of hemorrhage-associated morbidity is above 15% (Davenport et al.,1994, Martin et al.,1994; van de Wetering et al.,1996) Gastrointestinal (GIS) bleeding is observed in one-third of uremic patients. Upper GIS bleeding is more frequent in uremic patients undergoing hemodialysis in particular (Galbusera et al., 2009). Kutsumi et al. reported that 17% of patients presenting to the emergency department with GIS bleeding had received hemodialysis treatment (Kutsumi et al., 1998). Other reported hemorrhagic complications include hemorrhagic stroke, subdural hematoma, spontaneous retroperitoneal bleeding, spontaneous subcapsular hematoma of the liver, intraocular hemorrhage, and hemorrhagic pericarditis with cardiac tamponade (Remuzzi, 1989; Galbusera et al. 2009). Of these, hemorrhagic stroke and subdural hematoma are more prevalent in the hemodialysis population compared to the normal population. Hemorrhagic stroke incidence is 5-10 times greater than in the normal population (Seliger et al., 2003; Toyoda et al., 2005), while the incidence of subdural hematoma was 20 times greater in a study by Power et al. For these reasons, the mortality rate in this population group is 40% higher than in the normal population (Power et al., 2010). One study regarding the frequency of hemorrhagic complications and correlation with mortality determined 48 hemorrhagic complications in 37 patients undergoing 78 continuous renal replacements. Six of the 40 major hemorrhages were intra-abdominal, 18 involved bleeding around the catheter, 3 were GIS bleeding, 12 were oronasopharyngeal and 1 intracerebral. One intracerebral case, 1 intra-abdominal case and 1 with gastrointestinal bleeding died (van de Wetering et al., 1996).

In conclusion, the use of anticoagulant therapy in patients undergoing hemodialysis increases the tendency toward hemorrhage. The frequency of hemorrhage in vital organs in particular increases. The appropriate approach to preventing the progress of hemorrhagic complications in hemorrhagic patients during hemodialysis treatment is the restriction or avoidance of anticoagulants during hemodialysis. Systemic heparin as an alternative to anticoagulation in this patient group may be administered as regional anticoagulation with heparin and protamine, low-dose heparin, regional anticoagulation with citrate and hemodialysis without anticoagulation with intermittent saline flushes (Galbusera et al., 2009; Yixiong et al., 2010)

6. Electrolyte disorders

6.1 Impaired potassium balances

Chronic hemodialysis patients are usually predisposed to hyperkalemia at the beginning of dialysis sessions. The first reason for such tendency to hyperkalemia is this patient group does not have residual urine whose major duty is to remove potassium (K) from the body. Another reason is that K passes from inside the cells to outside to correct the acid-base balance and an increase being present in nitrogenous catabolites and inhibition of these Na / K ATPase (Weiner & Wingo, 1998). K is normally in balance inside and outside the cells. A small change in K in the extracellular area causes big changes in resting membrane potential (RMP). The myocardial tissue is affected the most from this situation. A decline in RMP may result in fetal arrhythmias. For this reason, if there is a change in ECG, hyperkalemia should be treated urgently (Browning & Channer, 1981). To prevent a cardiac interaction, iv calcium may be administered. It generally starts affecting in 1 to 3 minutes; if not, a second dose may be given (Schwarts, 1978). K starts dropping after dialysis therapy begins in the hemodialysis patient group, but if the interdialytic hyperkalemia persists, dietary compatibility should be questioned in these patients. Potassium binding resins may also be given to these patients (Acker et al., 1998).

During dialysis, potassium is removed 85% by diffusion and 15% by convection. Hypokalemia is seen more often in dialysis patients and especially in those whose pre-dialysis K levels are normal and who are administered a sodium profile technique (Buemi et al., 2009). Hypokalemia creates tendency to arrhythmia just like hyperkalemia. In order to avoid hypokalemia, the level of K in the dialysate should be arranged for each patient and the intracellular and extracellular shifts of K should be borne in mind. It is especially recommended in recent years to avoid using dialysates with very low levels of K during dialysis in order to prevent excessive decrease of K. For example, it is recommended to use a dialysate containing 2 mEq/L of K in patients whose serum K level is 4-6 mEq/L at the beginning of dialysis (Zehnder et al., 2001), and a dialysate containing 3 mEq/L of K in patients whose pre-dialysis K is in normal intervals (Weisberg& Rachoin, 2010).

6.2 Impaired calcium balances

Calcium plays an important role in the contraction of skeletal, smooth and cardiac muscle. The major factors causing increases and decreases in the Ca level in the hemodialysis patient group are secondary hyperparathyroidism and vitamin D used in treating it or its analogs, calcimimetics, and phosphorus binders containing calcium and magnesium. Since there is no urination in these patients, the excess calcium taken through diet may also cause increases in the serum calcium. In addition to these factors, the changes in Ca level are also associated with the concentration of calcium in the dialysate during hemodialysis therapy (Saha et al., 1996). Dialysates containing 3.5 mEq/L of Ca have been used for many years to help treat secondary hyperparathyroidism. However, this approach resulted in an increase both in hypercalcemia and adynamic bone disease. The relationship between a high serum calcium and mortality has been demonstrated in many studies conducted over years (Block et al., 2004; Kalantar-Zadeh et al., 2006). Due to the relationship between hypercalcemia and mortality, K-DOQI recommended that the target for serum Ca should be 8.4-9.5 mg/dl and for dialisate Ca to be 2.5 mEq/l (Hemodialysis Adequacy 2006 Work Group,2006). A tendency to hypocalcemia is seen in the hemodialysis patient group in recent years as a result of decreases in the use of calcimimetics, phosphorus binders with no Ca content and dialisates with low levels of Ca, and in the dietary intakes of Ca (Hemodialysis Adequacy 2006 Work Group,2006; Kalantar-Zadeh et al., 2006; Stevens et al.,2010). It was demonstrated in the study carried out recently by Miller JE and associates that the Ca values of < 9 mg/dl and >10 mg/dl were associated with increased mortality (Miller et al., 2010). Hypercalcemia causes mortality through tendency to arrhythmia, hypertension and vascular calcification, and hypocalcemia through tendency to arrhythmia. As a result, both hypercalcemia and hypocalcemia can cause an increase in mortality. The most important approach in the prevention and treatment of this electrolyte imbalance will be to assess each patient individually and prescribe hemodialysis accordingly.

6.3 Impaired sodium balances

The Na balance in the hemodialysis patient group is closely associated with the Na level in the dialysate and the volume situation. The Na balance in the HD patient group, on the other hand, is mainly maintained by the balance between the amount taken through the diet and the amount removed through dialysis. Various studies showed that HD patient group has been taking salt as much as taken by the normal population (Maduell& Navarro, 2000; Lambie et al., 2005). Intake of excessive salt in turn leads to an increase in thirstiness and interdialytic weight gain (Santos&Peixoto, 2010).

In a study made by Peixoto AJ and associates, 100 stable HD patients were observed for a period of 12 months and it was seen that the patients had lower pre-dialysis levels of salt, but they were stable in the 12-month period (Peixoto&Santos, 2010).

During hemodialysis, Na is removed mainly through diffusion and in fewer amounts through convection (Lambie et al., 2005). The level of Na being high or low in the dialysate directly affects the level of Na in patients. It is recommended, therefore, that the Na level in the dialysate is kept between 139 and 144 mEq/L to prevent development of hyponatremia or hypernatremia in patients (Henrich et al., 1982, Swartz et al., 1982). An Na modeling is made today in some patient groups (high level of Na at the beginning of dialysis and low levels in later hours). Such modeling is particularly made for patients with intradialytic hypotension, cramps or severe uremia or for those whose hemodynamics is not stable. However, modeling will not be appropriate for patients with hypernatremia or intradialytic hypertension (Palmer, 2001). Finally, preparation of individual HD prescriptions should be remembered in adjusting the Na balance.

7. Hematological complications

7.1 Hemolysis

Hemolysis was observed at a level of 2% in the initial years of the chronic dialysis program (Maher&Schreiner, 1965), and this has now declined considerably. Various factors lead to hemolysis. These include those arising through oxidizing agents and reducing agents, osmolar insults, thermal and mechanical injury or excessive uremia at initiation of dialysis (Abtahi et al., 2007; Sweet et al., 1996) Oxidizing agents result from contamination of the dialysate with copper, zinc, chloramine or nitrate. These agents lead to hemolysis by establishing oxidant damage in erythrocytes (Kjellstrand et al., 1974; Carlson&Shapiro 1970; Calderaro & Heller 2001; Blomfield et al., 1969). Reducing injury generally arises because of the formaldehyde used in the dialyzer sterilization process (Fonseca et al., 2004). Osmolar injury generally develops secondary to hypotonic dialysate use (Said et al., 1977). Thermal injury is observed when dialysate temperature reaches levels higher than body temperature (Berkes et al., 1975). Mechanical injury may develop in association with maloccluded blood pumps, arterial line collapse, kinked or obstructed hemodialysis tubing of the use of subclavian hemodialysis catheter (Abtahi et al., 2007; Sweet et al., 1996)

Acute hemolytic reaction symptoms include malaise, nausea, chest pain, shortness of breath, abdominal pain, back pain, emesis, cyanosis and headache. A positive pink test (pink-appearing serum) is seen in massive hemolysis. Pink test positivity is due to the almost total loss of haptoglobin, elevated levels of serum lactate dehydrogenase and the presence of free hemoglobin (Malinauskas, 2008; Murcutt, 2007). Acute hemolysis is a life-threatening condition that may lead to such complications as anemia, hyperkalemia, vasoconstriction in plasma hemoglobin and pancreatitis.

In treatment, dialysis must be brought to a conclusion and patients should not be given blood in sets. Emergency resuscitation should be performed depending on the patient's clinical condition, electrolyte imbalance and hemoglobin decrease evaluated, and appropriate treatments administered. The etiological factors leading to hemolysis must subsequently be investigated and eliminated.

7.2 Neutropenia

Neutropenia may be observed in correlation with membrane biocompatibility during hemodialysis. It generally begins within 2-3 min of the start of dialysis and reaches a maximum 10-15 min subsequently (Cheung et al., 1994; Deppisch et al.,1990; Twardowski, 2006). It generally reverts to normal levels after dialysis. Neutropenia observed during hemodialysis is associated with neutrophils accumulating on the hemodialysis membrane surfaces and with sequestration in the lungs in particular (Dodd et al., 1983). C5 and $C5a_{des\ Arg}$ binding to specific receptors and alterations to various receptors on the neutrophil surface are held responsible in the pathogenesis of dialysis-induced neutropenia. In addition, several studies have shown a correlation between complement activation and leukopenia. (Hakim et al., 1984; Huang et al., 2009; Lee et al., 1984; Takemoto et al., 2011) Temporary neutropenia does not generally lead to significant clinical problems. However, it is regarded as maybe one of the factors causing a predisposition to infection observed in hemodialysis patients.

8. Others

8.1 Nausea and vomiting

Nausea and vomiting is encountered in the hemodialysis patient group at rates up to 10% (Bregman H et al., 1994). While nausea and vomiting can be part of dialysis-related complications such as disequilibrium syndrome, hypotension, allergic reactions and electrolytic imbalance, they may also accompany acute coronary syndrome, cerebrovascular events and infections. Patients with nausea and vomiting should be examined for the causes of these events. One of the points to remember is that besides the factors enumerated above, prevalence of dyspeptic complaints and gastritis, duodenitis, peptic ulcer and colelithiasis has also increased in the dialysis patient group (Jain J & Thiele D, 2006). Therefore, hemodialysis-related complications should be set aside in the hemodialysis patients with nausea and vomiting, and the patients should be assessed in terms of any cerebrovascular and cardiovascular events, and infection. If these causes are absent, presence of other gastrointestinal symptoms should be assessed and a gastroscopy should be conducted. Nausea and vomiting not associated with hemodynamics may benefit from 5 to 10 mg of metoclopramide before dialysis (Bregman H et al., 1994).

8.2 Itching

Itching is one of the most frequently encountered symptoms in chronic kidney disease. Complaints of itching was found in 50 to 60% of the patients with end-stage renal failure who are undergoing a dialysis therapy (Narita et al., 2008). Although the etiology of uremic itching is not fully clarified, the factors held responsible include xerosis (Morton et al., 1996), peripheral neuropathy (Johansson et al.,1989), increases in divalent ions such as calcium, magnesium and phosphorus (Blachley et al., 1985), high level of parathyroid hormones (Morachiello et al., 1991) increases in the level of, and sensitivity to, histamine (Stockenhuber et al., 1987) and dialysis-related factors (Schwartz&Iaina 1999).

In diagnosing uremic itching, first the other causes of itching should be ruled out. Various tropical and systemic therapies have been tried in treating it for many years, but there have been patients who did not benefit from any of such therapies. For this reason, both the pathogenesis and the treatment of itching continue to be researched today. The recommended tropical therapy at present involves moisturizing creams and creams containing capsaicin (Breneman et al., 1992). Other treatment methods include phototherapy, acupuncture, a low-protein diet, long-chain fatty acids, lidocaine, orally activated charcoal, cholestramine, efficient dialysis, heparin, opioid antagonists, erythropoietin, parathyroidectomy, serotonin antagonists, thalidomide, antihistaminics and nicergoline (Schwartz&Iaina, 2000).

8.3 Cramps

Muscle cramps were being seen at a rate of 24 to 86% in the years when hemodialysis was first introduced (Kobrin&Berns,2007; Chou et al., 1985). Today, the intradialytic cramp rate fell down to 2% in a week owing to the improvements in the dialysis technology (Ahsan et al., 2004). Although cramps are mostly seen in the lower extremities, they can also occur in the abdomen, arms and hands.

Pathogenesis of muscle cramps is not fully clarified, but electromyographic research indicates that they more likely to originate from the neurons rather than the muscle itself (McGee, 1990). Subnormal muscle metabolism is considered as the most important factor in cramp etiology (Chang et al., 2002). For this reason, hypotension, changes in plasma osmolarity, hyponatremia, carnitine deficiency, hypomagnesemia and tissue hypoxia are thought to cause development of cramps (Ahsan et al., 2004; Chou et al., 1985; Khajehdehi et al., 2001). In these aforesaid situations, the muscle metabolism is impaired and cramps develop. Muscle cramps may lead to early finishing of dialysis sessions, failure to carry out sufficient ultrafiltration and finally dialysis inefficiency.

Hypertonic glucose, saline and mannitol may be administered in the acute treatment of cramps (Canzanello et al., 1991). Non-medical measures that can be taken to prevent cramps include avoidance of intradialytic hypotension and osmolarity changes, and regular exercise. There are studies showing that administration of 320 mg quinine sulfate 1 or 2 hours before hemodialysis therapy decreased muscle cramps (Kaji et al., 1976; Roca et al., 1992). However, use of quinine sulfate has side-effects such as cinchonism, optical atrophy, thrombocytopenia, arrhythmia, hemolytic uremic syndrome and interaction with drugs such as digoxin and warfarin (Wolf et al., 1992; Goldenberg&Wexler, 1988; Kojouri et al., 2001; Pedersen et al., 1985). There are also studies showing that muscle cramp development is reduced by administering 400 mg/day vitamin E, 250 mg/day vitamin C (Khajehdehi et al., 2001), 12 gm of creatinin monohydrate before dialysis (Chang et al.,2002), prozosin (0.25-1 mg) (Sidhom et al., 1994) and L-carnitine (Bellinghieri et al., 1983). However, the safety of using vitamin C above 200 mg for a long time is not proven (Kobrin et al., 2007).

9. References

Abbott, K.C., Neff, R.T., Bohen, E.M. & Narayan, R. (2007). Anticoagulation for chronic atrial fibrillation in hemodialysis patients: which fruit from the decision tree? *Am J Kidney Dis,* 50,3, 345-8.

Abe, S., Yoshizawa, M., Nakanishi, N., Yazawa, T., Yokota, K., Honda, M. & Sloman, G. (1996). Electrocardiographic abnormalities in patients receiving hemodialysis. Am Heart J, 131,6,1137-44

Abtahi, M., Uzan, M. & Souid, M. (2007). Hemolysis-induced acute pancreatitis secondary to kinked hemodialysis blood lines. *Hemodial Int,* 11, 1, 38-41

Acker, C.G., Johnson, J.P., Palevsky, P.M. & Greenberg, A. (1998). Hyperkalemia in hospitalized patients: causes, adequacy of treatment, and results of an attempt to improve physician compliance with published therapy guidelines. *Arch Intern Med,* 27,158,917-24.

Agarwal, R. (2005). Hypertension and survival in chronic hemodialysis patients--past lessons and future opportunities. *Kidney Int,* 67, 1, 1-13

Agarwal, A.K., Patel, B.M. & Haddad NJ. (2007). Central vein stenosis: a nephrologist's perspective. *Semin Dial,*. 20,1,53-62.

Ahmed, J., Besarab, A., Lubkowski, T. & Frinak, S. (2004). Effect of differing blood lines on delivered blood flow during hemodialysis. *Am J Kidney Dis,* 44,3,498-508

Ahsan, M., Gupta, M., Omar, I., Frinak, S., Gendjar, S., Osman-Malik, Y.& Yee, J. (2004).Prevention of hemodialysis-related muscle cramps by intradialytic use of sequential compression devices: a report of four cases. *Hemodial Int,* 1,8,283-6.

Akoh, J.A. (2009). Prosthetic arteriovenous grafts for hemodialysis. *J Vasc Access,* 10,3,137-47

Allon, M., Ornt, D.B., Schwab, S.J., Rasmussen, C., Delmez, J.A., Grene, T., Kusek, J.W., Martin, A.A. & Minda, S. (2000). Factors associated with the prevalence of arteriovenous fistulas in hemodialysis patients in the HEMO study. Hemodialysis (HEMO) Study Group. *Kidney Int,* 58, 5, 2178-85

Alomari, A.I. & Falk, A. (2007). The natural history of tunneled hemodialysis catheters removed or exchanged: a single-institution experience. *J Vasc Interv Radiol,* 18,2, 227-35

Alpert, M.A., & Ravenscraft, M.D. (2003). Pericardial involvement in end-stage renal disease. *Am J Med Sci,* 325, 4, 228-36

Alter, M.J., Tokars, J.I., Arduino M.J. & Favero M.S.(2004). Nosocomial infections associated with hemodialysis, *In: Hospital Epidemiology and Infection Control, Mayhall, C.G.*1139-1160 Lippincott Williams& Wilkins, ISBN: 0781742587, Philadelphia

Andrulli, S., Colzani, S., Mascia, F., Lucchi, L., Stipo, L., Bigi, M.C., Crepaldi, M., Redaelli, B., Albertazzi, A. & Locatelli, F. (2002). The role of blood volume reduction in the genesis of intradialytic hypotension. *Am J Kidney Dis,* 40, 6, 1244-54

Arieff, A.I., Guisado, R., Massry, S.G. & Lazarowitz, V.C. (1976). Central nervous system pH in uremia and the effects of hemodialysis. *J Clin Invest,* 58,2,306-11

Attur, R.P., Kandavar, R., Kadavigere, R. & Baig, W.W. (2008). Dialysis disequilibrium syndrome presenting as a focal neurological deficit. *Hemodial Int,* 12,3,313-5

Azar, A.T. (2009). The influence of maintenance quality of hemodialysis machines on hemodialysis efficiency. *Saudi J Kidney Dis Transpl,* 20, 1, 49-5

Bana, D.S., Yap, A.U.& Graham, J.R.(1972). Headache during hemodialyis. *Headache,* 12:1-14

Bana, D.S. & Graham, J.R.(1976). Renin response during hemodialysis headache. *Headache,* 16,168-172

Barak, M., Nakhoul, F. & Katz, Y. (2008). Pathophysiology and clinical implications of microbubbles during hemodialysis. *Semin Dial,* 21,3,232-8

Battistella, M., Bhola, C. & Lok, C.E. (2011). Long-term Follow-up of the Hemodialysis Infection Prevention With Polysporin Ointment (HIPPO) Study: A Quality Improvement Report. *Am J Kidney Dis,* 57, 3, 432-41

Banerjee, A. & Davenport, A.(2006). Changing patterns of pericardial disease in patients with end-stage renal disease. *Hemodial Int,* 10, 249-55.

Benedetto, F.A., Mallamaci, F., Tripepi, G.&Zoccali, C. (2001). Prognostic value of ultrasonographic measurement of carotid intima media thickness in dialysis patients. *J Am Soc Nephrol,* 12, 11, 2458-64

Breneman, D.L., Cardone, J.S., Blumsack, R.F., Lather, R.M., Searle, E.A. & Pollack V.E. (1992). Topical capsaicin for treatment of hemodialysis-related pruritus. *J Am Acad Dermatol,* 26,1,91-4

Bellinghieri, G., Savica, V., Mallamace, A., Di Stefano, C., Consolo, F., Spagnoli, L.G., Villaschi, S., Palmieri, G., Corsi, M.&Maccari, F. (1983). Correlation between increased serum and tissue L-carnitine levels and improved muscle symptoms in hemodialyzed patients. *Am J Clin Nutr,* 38, 4, 523-31.

Bent, C.L., Sahni, V.A. & Matson, M.B. (2011). The radiological management of the thrombosed arteriovenous dialysis fistula. *Clin Radiol,* 66, 1,1-12.

Berman, S.S., Gentile, A.T., Glickman, M.H., Mills, J.L., Hurwitz, R.L., Westerband, A., Marek, J.M., Hunter, G.C., McEnroe, C.S., Fogle, M.A. & Stokes, G.K. (1997). Distal revascularization-interval ligation for limb salvage and maintenance of dialysis access in ischemic steal syndrome. *J Vasc Surg,* 26, 3, 393-402

Berkes, S.L., Kahn, S.I., Chazan, J.A. & Garella, S. (1975). Prolonged hemolysis from overheated dialysate. *Ann Intern Med,* 83,3, 363-4

Blachley, J.D., Blankenship, D.M., Menter, A., Parker, T.F. 3rd. & Knochel, J.P. (1985). Uremic pruritus: skin divalent ion content and response to ultraviolet phototherapy. *Am J Kidney Dis,* 5:237-41.

Block, G.A., Klassen, P.S., Lazarus, J.M., Ofsthun, N., Lowrie, E.G. & Chertow, G.M. (2004). Mineral metabolism, mortality, and morbidity in maintenance hemodialysis. *J Am Soc Nephrol,* 15, 8, 2208-18.

Blomfield, J., McPherson, J. & George, C.R. (1969). Active uptake of copper and zinc during haemodialysis. *Br Med J,* 19,2,141-5

Bour, E.S. & Weaver, A.S. (1990). Experience with the double lumen silastic catheter for hemoaccess. Surg Gynecol Obstet, 171, 33-39.

Bregman, H., Daugirdas, J.T.& Ing, T.S. (Daugirdas, JT, Ing, TS (Eds)), (1994). Complications during hemodialysis. In: Handbook of Dialysis, Little, Brown, ISBN 0-190852954-6, New York

Browning, J.J. & Channer, K.S. (1981). Hyperkalaemic cardiac arrhythmia caused by potassium citrate mixture. *Br Med J,* 283,1366

Brunet, P. & Water, Y.B. (2000). quality and complications of haemodialysis. *Nephrol Dial Transplant,* 15, 578-580

Buemi, M., Coppolino. G., Bolignano. D., Sturiale. A., Campo. S., Buemi, A., Crascì, E. & Romeo, A. (2009). Arrhythmias and hemodialysis: role of potassium and new diagnostic tools. *Ren Fail,* 31,1,75-80.

Burton, J.O., Korsheed, S., Grundy, B.J. & McIntyre, C.W. (2008). Hemodialysis-induced left ventricular dysfunction is associated with an increase in ventricular arrhythmias. *Ren Fail,* 30, 7, 701-9

Buturović, J., Ponikvar, R., Kandus, A., Boh, M., Klinkmann, J. & Ivanovich, P. (1998). Filling hemodialysis catheters in the interdialytic period: heparin versus citrate versus polygeline: a prospective randomized study. *Artif Organs,* 22,11, 945-7.

Canzanello, V.J., Hylander-Rossner, B., Sands, R.E., Morgan, T.M., Jordan, J.&Burkart, J.M. (1991).Comparison of 50% dextrose water, 25% mannitol, and 23.5% saline for the treatment of hemodialysis-associated muscle cramps. *ASAIO Trans,*37, 4, 649-52

Calderaro, R.V. & Heller, L. (2001). Outbreak of hemolytic reactions associated with chlorine and chloramine residuals in hemodialysis water. *Rev Saude Publica,* 35,5,481-6.

Carlson DJ& Shapiro FL. (1970). Methemoglobinemia from well water nitrates: a complication of home dialysis. *Ann Intern Med,* 73,5,757-9.

Can, M.R. (2008).Hemodialysis central venous catheter dysfunction. *Sem Dial,*21, 516-521.

Chandra, A.P., Dimascio, D., Gruenewald, S., Nankivell., B, Allen, R.D. & Swinnen, J. (2010). Colour duplex ultrasound accurately identifies focal stenoses in dysfunctional autogenous arteriovenous fistulae. *Nephrology (Carlton),* 15,3,300-6.

Chang, C.T., Wu, C.H., Yang, C.W., Huang, J.Y. & Wu, M.S. (2002). Creatine monohydrate treatment alleviates muscle cramps associated with haemodialysis. *Nephrol Dial Transplant,* 17,11,1978-81

Chen, C.L., Lai, P.H., Chou. K.J., Lee, P.T., Chung, H.M. & Fang, H.C. (2007). A preliminary report of brain edema in patients with uremia at first hemodialysis: evaluation by diffusion-weighted MR imaging. *AJNR Am J Neuroradiol,*28,1,68-71

Cheung, A.K., Faezi-Jenkin, B. & Leypoldt, J.K. (1994). Effect of thrombosis on complement activation and neutrophil degranulation during in vitro hemodialysis. *J Am Soc Nephrol,* 5,1,110-5.

Chew, H.C. (2008). Cardiac troponin T in acute coronary syndrome with renal insufficiency. *Asian Cardiovasc Thorac Ann,* 16, 4, 284-7.

Chou, C.T., Wasserstein, A., Schumacher, H.R. Jr. & Fernandez, P. (1985). Musculoskeletal manifestations in hemodialysis patients. *J Rheumatol,* 12,1149-53.

Coburn, M.C. &Carney, W.I. Jr. (1994). Comparison of basilic vein and polytetrafluoroethylene for brachial arteriovenous fistula. *J Vasc Surg,* 20,6,896-902

Conlon, P.J., Krucoff, M.W., Minda, S., Schumm, D. & Schwab, S.J. (1998). Incidence and long-term significance of transient ST segment deviation in hemodialysis patients. *Clin Nephrol,* 49, 4,236-9.

Coritsidis, G., Sutariya, D., Stern, A., Gupta, G., Carvounis, C., Arora, R., Balmir, S. &Acharya, A. (2009). Does timing of dialysis in patients with ESRD and acute myocardial infarcts affect morbidity or mortality? *Clin J Am Soc Nephrol,* 4,8,1324-30

Cruz, D.N., Mahnensmith, R.L. & Perazella, M.A. (1997). Intradialytic hypotension: is midodrine beneficial in symptomatic hemodialysis patients? *Am J Kidney Dis,* 30,6,772-9.

Culleton, B.F., Walsh, M., Klarenbach, S.W., Mortis, G., Scott-Douglas, N., Quinn, R.R., Tonelli, M., Donnelly, S., Friedrich, M.G, Kumar, A., Mahallati, H., Hemmelgarn, B.R. & Manns, B.J. (2007). Effect of frequent nocturnal hemodialysis vs conventional hemodialysis on left ventricular mass and quality of life: a randomized controlled trial. *JAMA,* 298,1291-9.

Daugirdas, J.T.,&Ing, T.S. (1988). First-use reactions during hemodialysis: a definition of subtypes. *Kidney Int,* 24, 37–S43

Daugirdas, J.T. (2001). Pathophysiology of dialysis hypotension: an update. *Am J Kidney Dis,* 38,11-7

Davenport, A., Will, E.J. & Davison, A.M. (1994). Comparison of the use of standard heparin and prostacyclin anticoagulation in spontaneous and pump-driven extracorporeal circuits in patients with combined acute renal and hepatic failure. *Nephron,*66, 4, 431-7

Davenport, A. (2006). Intradialytic complications during hemodialysis. *Hemodial Int,* 10,2,162-7.

De Backer, W.A., Verpooten, G.A., Borgonjon, D.J., Vermeire, P.A., Lins, R.R. &De Broe, M.E. (1983). Hypoxemia during hemodialysis: effects of different membranes and dialysate compositions. *Kidney Int,* 23,5,738-43.

De Broe, M.E. &De Backer, W.A. (1989).Pathophysiology of hemodialysis-associated hypoxemia. *Adv Nephrol Necker Hosp,* 18, 297-315 de Bie, M.K., van Dam, B., Gaasbeek, A., van Buren, M., van Erven, L., Bax, J.J., Schalij, M.J., Rabelink, T.J. & Jukema, J.W. (2009). The current status of interventions aiming at reducing sudden cardiac death in dialysis patients. *Eur Heart J*, 30,13,1559-64

Depner, T.A., Rizwan, S. & Stasi, T.A. (1990). Pressure effects on roller pump blood flow during hemodialysis. *ASAIO Trans*, 36,3,456-9

Deppisch, R., Schmitt, V., Bommer, J., Hänsch, G.M., Ritz, E. & Rauterberg, E.W. (1990). Fluid phase generation of terminal complement complex as a novel index of bioincompatibility. *Kidney Int*, 37, 2, 696-706

Di Iorio, B.R., Bellizzi, V., Cillo, N., Cirillo, M., Avella, F., Andreucci, V.E. & De Santo, N.G. (2004). Vascular access for hemodialysis: the impact on morbidity and mortality. *J Nephrol*, 17, 1,19-25

Dinarello, C.A., Lonnemann, G., Maxwell, R. & Shaldon, S. (1987). Ultrafiltration to reject human interleukin-1-inducing substances derived from bacterial cultures. *J Clin Microbiol*, 25,7,1233-8.

Dinwiddie, L.C. (2004). Managing catheter dysfunction for better patient outcomes: a team approach. *Nephrol Nurs J*, 31,6, 653-60

Division of Nosocomial and Occupationl Infectious Diseases, Bureau of Infectious Diseases, Laboratory Centre for Disease Control, Health Canada. (1997). Preventing infections associated with indwelling intravascular access devices. *Can Commun DisRep*, 23, 1-32

Dodd, N.J., Gordge, M.P., Tarrant, J., Parsons, V. & Weston, M.J. (1983). A demonstration of neutrophil accumulation in the pulmonary vasculature during haemodialysis. *Proc Eur Dial Transplant Assoc*, 20, 186-9.

Dolan, M.J., Whipp, B.J., Davidson, W.D., Weitzman, R.E. & Wasserman, K. (1981). Hypopnea associated with acetate hemodialysis: carbon dioxide-flow-dependent ventilation. *N Engl J Med*, 305,2,72-5

Donauer, J., Kölblin, D., Bek, M., Krause, A. & Böhler, J. (2000). Ultrafiltration profiling and measurement of relative blood volume as strategies to reduce hemodialysis-related side effects. *Am J Kidney Dis*,36,115-23.

Dumler, F., Zasuwa, G. & Levin, N.W. (1987). Effect of dialyzer reprocessing methods on complement activation and hemodialyzer-related symptoms. *Artif Organs*, 11,128-31

Ebo, D.G., Bosmans, J.L., Couttenye, M.M. & Stevens, W.J. (2006). Haemodialysis-associated anaphylactic and anaphylactoid reactions. *Allergy*, 61, 211-20.

Emili, S., Black, N.A., Paul, R.V., Rexing, C.J. & Ullian, M.E. (1999). A protocol-based treatment for intradialytic hypotension in hospitalized hemodialysis patients. *Am J Kidney Dis*, 33, 1107-14.

Enzler, M.A., Rajmon, T., Lachat, M. & Largiadèr, F. (1996). Long-term function of vascular access for hemodialysis. *Clin Transplant*, 10,511-5.

Faintuch, S. & Salazar, G.M. (2008). Malfunction of dialysis catheters: management of fibrin sheath and related problems. *Tech Vasc Interv Radiol*, 11,3,195-200.

Fan, P.Y.&Schwab, S.J. (1992).Vascular access: concepts for the 1990s. *J Am Soc Nephrol*, 3, 1, 1-11.

Farrell, J., Walshe, J., Gellens, M. & Martin, K.J. (1997). Complications associated with insertion of jugular venous catheters for hemodialysis: the value of postprocedural radiograph. *Am J Kidney Dis*, 30, 5, 690-2

Feldman, H.I., Kobrin, S. & Wasserstein, A. (1996). Hemodialysis vascular access morbidity. *J Am Soc Nephrol*,7,4, 523-35.

Fiaccadori, E., Gonzi, G., Zambrelli, P. &Tortorella, G. (1996). Cardiac arrhythmias during central venous catheter procedures in acute renal failure: a prospective study. *J Am Soc Nephrol*, 7,7,1079-84.

Filiopoulos, V., Hadjiyannakos, D., Koutis, I., Trompouki, S., Micha, T., Lazarou, D. & Vlassopoulos, D. (2011). Approaches to prolong the use of uncuffed hemodialysis catheters: results of a randomized trial. *Am J Nephrol*, 33, 3, 260-8.

Foley, R.N., Herzog, C.A. &Collins, A.J. (2002). United States Renal Data System Blood pressure and long-term mortality in United States hemodialysis patients: USRDS Waves 3 and 4 Study. *Kidney Int*, 62,5,1784-90

Foley, R.N, Parfrey, P.S. & Sarnak, M.J. (1998). Epidemiology of cardiovascular disease in chronic renal disease. *J Am Soc Nephrol*, 9, 16-23.

Floege, J., Lonnemann, G. (2000).Complications Related to Water Treatment, Substitution Fluids, and Dialysate Composition. *In: Complications of Dialysis*, (Lameire N, Mehta R.L.(29-40)), Markel Dekker,(0-8247-8871-0) New York

Fonseca, H.E., Chiba, A.K., Junior, A.F., Draibe, S.A. &Bordin, J.O. (2004). Anti-N-like and anti-Form red cell antibodies in chronic hemodialysis patients. *Ren Fail*, 26, 5, 553-6

Galbusera, M., Remuzzi, G. &Boccardo, P. (2009). Treatment of bleeding in dialysis patients. *Semin Dial*, 22,3,279-86

Genovesi, S., Vincenti, A., Rossi, E., Pogliani, D., Acquistapace, I., Stella, A. & Valsecchi, M.G. (2008). Atrial fibrillation and morbidity and mortality in a cohort of long-term hemodialysis patients. *Am J Kidney Dis*, 51, 2, 255-62.

Gibson, K.D., Caps, M.T., Kohler, T.R., Hatsukami, T.S., Gillen, D.L., Aldassy, M., Sherrard, D.J. & Stehman-Breen, C.O. (2001). Assessment of a policy to reduce placement of prosthetic hemodialysis access. *Kidney Int*, 59, 6, 2335-45.

Gibson, K.D., Gillen, D.L., Caps, M.T., Kohler, T.R., Sherrard, D.J. & Stehman-Breen, C.O. (2001). Vascular access survival and incidence of revisions: a comparison of prosthetic grafts, simple autogenous fistulas, and venous transposition fistulas from the United States Renal Data System Dialysis Morbidity and Mortality Study. *J Vasc Surg*, 34, 4, 694-700.

Gladstone, J.P. & Dodick, D.W. (2004). Revised 2004 International Classification of Headache Disorders: new headache types.*Can J Neurol Sci*, 31,3,304-14

Glorieux, G., Schepers, E., Schindler, R., Lemke, H.D., Verbeke, F., Dhondt, A. Lameire, N. &Vanholder, R. (2009). A novel bio-assay increases the detection yield of microbiological impurity of dialysis fluid, in comparison to the LAL-test. *Nephrol Dial Transplant*, 24, 2,548-54

Goksel, B.K., Torun, D., Karaca, S., Karatas, M., Tan, M., Sezgin, N., Benli, S., Sezer, S. & Ozdemir, N. (2006). Is low blood magnesium level associated with hemodialysis headache? *Headache*, 46,1, 40-5.

Goldenberg, A.M. & Wexler, L.F. (1988). Quinine overdose: review of toxicity and treatment. *Clin Cardiol*, 11,10,716-8.

Göksan, B., Karaali-Savrun, F., Ertan, S. &Savrun, M. (2004).Haemodialysis-related headache. *Cephalalgia*, 24,4, 284-7.

Graf, H., Stummvoll, H.K., Haber, P. & Kovarik, J. (1980). Pathophysiology of dialysis related hypoxaemia. *Proc Eur Dial Transplant Assoc*, 17,155-61.

Hakim, R.M.,& Lowrie, E.G. (1982).Hemodialysis-associated neutropenia and hypoxemia: the effect of dialyzer membrane materials. *Nephron,* 32,1,32-9

Hakim, R.M., Fearon, D.T. & Lazarus, J.M. (1984). Biocompatibility of dialysis membranes: effects of chronic complement activation. *Kidney Int,* 26, 2, 194-200

Hampl, H., Klopp, H.W., Michels, N., Mahiout, A., Schilling, H., Wolfgruber, M., Schiller, R., Hanefeld, F. & Kessel, M. (1983). Electroencephalogram investigations of the disequilibrium syndrome during bicarbonate and acetate dialysis. *Proc Eur Dial Transplant Assoc,* 19, 351-9

Hanly, P.J. & Pierratos, A. (2001). Improvement of sleep apnea in patients with chronic renal failure who undergo nocturnal hemodialysis. *N Engl J Med,* 344,2,102-7.

Heckmann, J.G., Lang, C.J., Kindler, K., Huk, W., Erbguth, F.J. & Neundörfer, B. (2000). Neurologic manifestations of cerebral air embolism as a complication of central venous catheterization. *Crit Care Med,* 28,5,1621-5.

Hemmelgarn, B.R., Moist, L.M., Lok, C.E., Tonelli, M., Manns, B.J., Holden, R.M., LeBlanc, M., Faris, P., Barre, P., Zhang, J. & Scott-Douglas, N. (2011). Prevention of Dialysis Catheter Lumen Occlusion with rt-PA versus Heparin Study Group. Prevention of dialysis catheter malfunction with recombinant tissue plasminogen activator. *N Engl J Med* 364, 4, 303-12

Hemodialysis Adequacy 2006 Work Group. (2006). Clinical practice guidelines for hemodialysis adequacy, update 2006. *Am J Kidney Dis,* 48, 2-90

Henrich, W.L., Woodard, T.D. & McPhaul, J.J. Jr. (1982). The chronic efficacy and safety of high sodium dialysate: double-blind, crossover study. *Am J Kidney Dis,* 2,3,349-53

Herzog, C.A., Mangrum, J.M., & Passman, R. (2008). Sudden cardiac death and dialysis patients. *Semin Dial,* 21, 300-7

Herzog, C.A., Ma, J.Z. &Collins, A.J. (1998). Poor long-term survival after acute myocardial infarction among patients on long-term dialysis. *N Engl J Med,* 339,12, 799-805

Hirth, R.A., Turenne, M.N., Woods, J.D., Young, E.W., Port, F.K., Pauly, M.V. & Held, P.J. (1996). Predictors of type of vascular access in hemodialysis patients. *JAMA,* 276,16,1303-8

Hodges,T.C., Fillinger, M.F., Zwolak, R.M., Walsh, D.B., Bech, F. & Cronenwett, J.L. (1997). Longitudinal comparison of dialysis access methods: risk factors for failure. *J Vasc Surg,* 26, 6, 1009-19.

Hoen, B., Paul-Dauphin, A., Hestin, D. & Kessler, M. (1998). EPIBACDIAL: a multicenter prospective study of risk factors for bacteremia in chronic hemodialysis patients. *J Am Soc Nephrol,* 9, 5, 869-76.

Hoenich, N.A.&Levin, R. (2003). The implications of water quality in hemodialysis. *Semin Dial,* 16, 6, 492-7

Hörl, M.P. & Hörl, W.H. (2002). Hemodialysis-associated hypertension: pathophysiology and therapy. *Am J Kidney Dis,*39, 2, 227-44.

Hörl, M.P.& Hörl W.H. (2003). Hypertension and dialysis. *Kidney Blood Press Res,* 26, 2, 76-81

Hörl, M.P. & Hörl, W.H. (2004). Drug therapy for hypertension in hemodialysis patients. Semin Dial,17,4, 288-94.

Huang, Z., Gao, D., Letteri, J.J. & Clark, W.R. (2009). Blood-membrane interactions during dialysis. *Semin Dial,* 22, 6, 623-8

Inrig, J.K., Reed, S.D., Szczech, L.A., Engemann, J.J., Friedman, J.Y., Corey, G.R., Schulman, K.A., Reller, L.B. & Fowler, V.G. Jr. (2006). Relationship between clinical outcomes and vascular access type among hemodialysis patients with Staphylococcus aureus bacteremia. *Clin J Am Soc Nephrol,* 1,3,518-24

Inrig, J.K., Oddone, E.Z., Hasselblad, V., Gillespie, B., Patel, U.D., Reddan, D., Toto, R., Himmelfarb, J., Winchester, J.F., Stivelman, J., Lindsay, R.M. & Szczech, L.A. (2007). Association of intradialytic blood pressure changes with hospitalization and mortality rates in prevalent ESRD patients. *Kidney Int,* 71, 5, 454-61

Inrig, J.K., Patel, U.D., Toto, R.D. & Szczech, L.A. (2009). Association of blood pressure increases during hemodialysis with 2-year mortality in incident hemodialysis patients: a secondary analysis of the Dialysis Morbidity and Mortality Wave 2 Study. *Am J Kidney Dis,* 54, 5, 881-90

Inrig, J.K. (2010). Antihypertensive agents in hemodialysis patients: a current perspective. *Semin Dial,* 23, 3, 290-7.

Iseki, K. & Fukiyama, K. (1996). Predictors of stroke in patients receiving chronic hemodialysis. *Kidney Int,* 50, 5, 1672-5

Ishani, A., Collins, A.J., Herzog, C.A. & Foley, R.N. (2005). Septicemia, access and cardiovascular disease in dialysis patients: the USRDS Wave 2 study. *Kidney Int,* 68, 1, 311-8.

Jaber, B.L. & Pereira, B.J.G. (1997). Dialysis reactions. *Semin Dial,* 10, 158-165

Jain, J. &Thiele, D., (2006) Gastrointestinal and hepatic manifestations of systemic diseases. (In Feldman. M. & Friedman, L, Brandt LJ. (Eds)). *Sleisenger and Fordtran's Gastrointestinal and Liver Disease.8th ed. vol 1.* Philadelphia, PA: Saunders Elsevier

Jang, I.K. & Hursting, M.J. (2005). When heparins promote thrombosis: review of heparin-induced thrombocytopenia. *Circulation,* 111, 20, 2671-83.

Jean-Baptiste, R.S. & Gahtan, V. (2004). Distal revascularization-interval ligation (DRIL) procedure for ischemic steal syndrome (ISS) after arteriovenous fistula placement. *Surg Technol Int,* 12, 201-5.

Jenson, B.M., Dobbe, S.A., Squillace, D.P. & McCarthy, J.T. (1994). Clinical benefits of high and variable sodium concentration dialysate in hemodialysis patients. *ANNA J,* 21:115-20

Jesus, A.C., Oliveira, H.A., Paixão, M.O., Fraga, T.P., Barreto, F.J. &Valença, M.M. (2009). Clinical description of hemodialysis headache in end-stage renal disease patients. *Arq Neuropsiquiatr,* 67, 4, 978-81

Johansson, O., Hilliges, M. & Ståhle-Bäckdahl, M. (1989). Intraepidermal neuron-specific enolase (NSE)-immunoreactive nerve fibres: evidence for sprouting in uremic patients on maintenance hemodialysis. *Neurosci Lett,* 8, 99:281-6

Kaji, D.M., Ackad, A., Nottage, W.G. & Stein, R.M. (1976). Prevention of muscle cramps in haemodialysis patients by quinine sulphate. *Lancet,* 10, 2, 66-7

Kalantar-Zadeh, K., Kuwae, N., Regidor, D.L., Kovesdy, C.P., Kilpatrick, R.D., Shinaberger, C.S., McAllister, C.J., Budoff, M.J., Salusky, I.B. & Kopple, J.D. (2006). Survival predictability of time-varying indicators of bone disease in maintenance hemodialysis patients. *Kidney Int,* 70, 4, 771-80

Kapa, S. & Qian, Q. (2009). 84-year-old woman with hemodialysis-associated shortness of breath. *Mayo Clin Proc,* 84, 2, 187-90

Kawamura, M., Fijimoto, S., Hisanaga, S., Yamamoto, Y. & Eto, T. (1998). Incidence, outcome, and risk factors of cerebrovascular events in patients undergoing maintenance hemodialysis. *Am J Kidney Dis,* 31, 6, 991-6.

K/DOQI, Workgroup. (2005).K/DOQI clinical practice guidelines for cardiovascular disease in dialysis patients. *Am J Kidney Dis.* 2005, 45, 1-153

Ken-ichi, Kimura., Kaoru, Tabie., Yasushi, Asano. & Saichi, Hosoda. (1989). Cardiac Arrhythmias in Hemodialysis Patients A Study of Incidence and Contributory Factors *Nephron,* 53:201–207

Kennedy, A.C. (1970). Dialysis disequilibrium syndrome. *Electroencephalogr Clin Neurophysiol,* 29, 2, 213

Khajehdehi, P., Mojerlou, M., Behzadi, S. & Rais-Jalali, G.A. (2001). A randomized, double-blind, placebo-controlled trial of supplementary vitamins E, C and their combination for treatment of haemodialysis cramps. *Nephrol Dial Transplant,* 16,7, 1448-51

Kjellstrand, C.M., Eaton, J.W., Yawata, Y., Swofford, H., Kolpin, C.F., Buselmeier, T.J., von Hartitzsch, B. & Jacob, H.S. (1974). Hemolysis in dialized patients caused by chloramines. *Nephron,* 13, 6, 427-33

Kobrin, S.M. & Berns, J.S. (2007). Quinine--a tonic too bitter for hemodialysis-associated muscle cramps? *Semin Dial,* 20, 396-401

Kojouri, K., Vesely, S.K. & George, J.N. (2001). Quinine-associated thrombotic thrombocytopenic purpura-hemolytic uremic syndrome: frequency, clinical features, and long-term outcomes. *Ann Intern Med,* 135, 12, 1047-51

Komukai, K., Ogawa, T., Yagi, H., Date, T., Suzuki, K., Sakamoto, H., Miyazaki, H., Takatsuka, H., Shibayama, K., Ogawa, K., Kanzaki, Y., Kosuga, T., Kawai, M., Hongo, K., Yoshida, S., Taniguchi, I. & Mochizuki, S. (2007). Renal insufficiency is related to painless myocardial infarction. *Circ J,* 71, 9, 1366-9

Koman, J.P., van der Sande, F.M. & Leunissen, K.M. (2009). Wet or dry in dialysis--can new technologies help? *Semin Dial,* 22,1, 9-12

Kundu, S. (2010). Central venous disease in hemodialysis patients: prevalence, etiology and treatment. *J Vasc Access,*11,1,1-7

Kutsumi, H, Fujimoto, S & Rokutan, K. (1998). Risk factors for gastrointestinal bleeding]. *Nippon Rinsho,* 56 , 9, 2309-13

Lacson, E. Jr. & Lazarus, J.M. (2007). The association between blood pressure and mortality in ESRD-not different from the general population? *Semin Dial,* 20,510-7

Lambie, S.H., Taal, M.W., Fluck, R.J. & McIntyre, C.W. (2005). Online conductivity monitoring: validation and usefulness in a clinical trial of reduced dialysate conductivity. *ASAIO J,* 51, 1, 70-6

Lange, R.A. & Hillis, L.D. (2004). Clinical practice. Acute pericarditis. *N Engl J Med,* 351,21, 2195-202

Lee, J., Hakim, R.M. & Fearon, D.T. (1984). Increased expression of the C3b receptor by neutrophils and complement activation during haemodialysis. *Clin Exp Immunol,* 56, 1, 205-14

Levin, A. & Goldstein, M.B. (1996). The benefits and side effects of ramped hypertonic sodium dialysis. *J Am Soc Nephrol,* 7, 2, 242-6

Lin, S.L., Huang, C.H., Chen, H.S., Hsu, W.A., Yen, C.J. &Yen, T.S. (1998). Effects of age and diabetes on blood flow rate and primary outcome of newly created hemodialysis arteriovenous fistulas. *Am J Nephrol,* 18, 2, 96-100

Lindley, E. & Canaud, B. (2002). New European guidelines for microbiological quality of dialysis fluid: a review. *Nephrol News Issues,* 16, 7, 46-8

Lok, C.E., Stanley, K.E, Hux, J.E., Richardson, R., Tobe, S.W. & Conly, J. (2003). Hemodialysis infection prevention with polysporin ointment. *J Am Soc Nephrol,* 14, 1,169-79

Lumsden, A,B., MacDonald, M.J., Isiklar, H., Martin, L.G., Kikeri, D., Harker, L.A. & Allen R.C. Central venous stenosis in the hemodialysis patient: incidence and efficacy of endovascular treatment. *Cardiovasc Surg.* 1997, 5, 5, 504-9

Lynch, K.E., Feldman, H.I., Berlin, J.A., Flory, J., Rowan, C.G. & Brunelli, S.M. (2008). Effects of L-carnitine on dialysis-related hypotension and muscle cramps: a meta-analysis. *Am J Kidney Dis,* 52, 5, 962-71

Maduell, F. &Navarro, V. (2000). Dietary salt intake and blood pressure control in haemodialysis patients. *Nephrol Dial Transplant,* 15, 12, 2063

Maggiore, Q., Pizzarelli, F., Sisca, S., Zoccali, C., Parlongo, S., Nicolò, F. & Creazzo, G. (1982). Blood temperature and vascular stability during hemodialysis and hemofiltration. *Trans Am Soc Artif Intern Organs,* 28, 523-7

Maggiore, Q., Pizzarelli, F., Santoro, A., Panzetta, G., Bonforte, G., Hannedouche, T., Alvarez de Lara, M.A., Tsouras, I., Loureiro, A., Ponce, P., Sulkovà, S., Van Roost, G., Brink, H. & Kwan, J.T. (2002). Study Group of Thermal Balance and Vascular Stability. The effects of control of thermal balance on vascular stability in hemodialysis patients: results of the European randomized clinical trial. *Am J Kidney Dis,* 40, 2, 280-90

Maher, J.F. & Schreiner, G.E. (1965). Hazards and complications of dialysis. N Engl J Med, 273, 7, 370-7

Maki, D.G., Ash,S.R., Winger, R.K. & Lavin, P. for the AZEPTIC Trial Investigators. (2010). A novel antimicrobial and antithrombotic lock solution for hemodialysis catheters: A multi-center, controlled, randomized trial. *Crit Care Med*

Malinauskas, R.A. (2008). Decreased hemodialysis circuit pressures indicating postpump tubing kinks: a retrospective investigation of hemolysis in five patients. *Hemodial Int,* 12, 3, 383-93

Malik, J., Tuka, V., Kasalova, Z., Chytilova, E., Slavikova, M., Clagett, P., Davidson, I., Dolmatch, B., Nichols, D. & Gallieni, M. (2008). Understanding the dialysis access steal syndrome. A review of the etiologies, diagnosis, prevention and treatment strategies. *J Vasc Access.* 9, 3, 155-66

Malinauskas, R.A. (2008). Decreased hemodialysis circuit pressures indicating postpump tubing kinks: a retrospective investigation of hemolysis in five patients. *Hemodial Int,* 12, 3, 383-93

Mandolfo, S., Piazza, W. & Galli, F. (2002). Central venous catheter and the hemodialysis patient: a difficult symbiosis. *J Vasc Access,* 3, 2, 64-73

Mandolfo, S. & Gallieni, M. (2010). Use of oral anticoagulants to prevent central venous catheter-related thrombosis in hemodialysis. *G Ital Nefrol,* 27, 5, 490-7

Martin, P.Y., Chevrolet, J.C., Suter, P. & Favre, H. (1994). Anticoagulation in patients treated by continuous venovenous hemofiltration: a retrospective study. *Am J Kidney Dis,* 24, 5, 806-12

Matsuo, T. & Wanaka, K. (2008). Management of uremic patients with heparin-induced thrombocytopenia requiring hemodialysis. *Clin Appl Thromb Hemost,* 14, 4, 459-64

Maynard, J.C., Cruz, C., Kleerekoper, M. & Levin, N.W. (1986). Blood pressure response to changes in serum ionized calcium during hemodialysis. *Ann Intern Med,* 104,3,358-61

McGee, S.R. (1990). Muscle cramps. *Arch Intern Med,* 150, 511-8

Miller, J.E., Kovesdy, C.P, Norris, K.C., Mehrotra, R., Nissenson, A.R., Kopple, J.D. & Kalantar-Zadeh, K. (2010) Association of cumulatively low or high serum calcium levels with mortality in long-term hemodialysis patients. *Am J Nephro,* 32,5,403-13

Mitch, W.E. & Wilcox, C.S. (1982) Disorders of body fluids, sodium and potassium in chronic renal failure. *Am J Med,* 72,3,536-50

Moini, M., Rasouli, M.R., Kenari, M.M. & Mahmoodi, H.R.(2009) Non-cuffed dual lumen catheters in the external jugular veins versus other central veins for hemodialysis patients. *Saudi J Kidney Dis Transp,.* 20,1,44-8

Montanari, L.B., Sartori, F.G., Cardoso, M.J., Varo, S.D., Pires, R.H., Leite, C.Q., Prince, K. & Martins, C.H.(2009) Microbiological contamination of a hemodialysis center water distribution system. *Rev Inst Med Trop Sao Paulo,* 51,1,37-43

Morachiello, P., Landini, S., Fracasso, A., Righetto, F., Scanferla, F., Toffoletto, P., Genchi, R. & Bazzato, G.(1991) Combined hemodialysis-hemoperfusion in the treatment of secondary hyperparathyroidism of uremic patients. *Blood Purif,* 9,3,148-52

Morton, C.A., Lafferty, M., Hau, C., Henderson, I., Jones, M. & Lowe, J.G.(1996) Pruritus and skin hydration during dialysis. *Nephrol Dial Transplant,* 11,2031-6

Murcutt, G. (2007) Guarding against hidden haemolysis during dialysis: an overview. Summary of the EDTNA/ERCA Journal Club discussion Spring. *J Ren Care.* 334,191-5

Narita, I., Iguchi, S., Omori, K. &Gejyo, F. (2008)Uremic pruritus in chronic hemodialysis patients. *J Nephrol.* 21,161-5

National Kidney Foundation: K/DOQI (2006). Clinical Practice Guidlines for Vascular Access *Am J Kidney Dis,* 48,5248-5257

National Kidney Foundation. K/DOQI (2005). Clinical practice guidelines for cardiovascular disease in dialysis patients. *Am J Kidney Dis,* 45:1-153

[No authors listed*] Nephrol Dial Transplant.* (2002)17 :45-62. Section IV. Dialysis fluid purity.

Oguzkurt, L., Tercan, F., Kara, G., Torun, D., Kizilkilic, O. & Yildirim, T.(2005) US-guided placement of temporary internal jugular vein catheters: immediate technical success and complications in normal and high-risk patients. *Eur J Radiol,* 55,1,125-9

Oh, M.S., Uribarri, J., Del Monte, M.L., Heneghan, W.F., Kee, C.S., Friedman, E.A. & Carroll, H.J.(1985) A mechanism of hypoxemia during hemodialysis. Consumption of CO2 in metabolism of acetate. *Am J Nephrol,* 5,5,366-71

Orebaugh, S.L.(1992) Venous air embolism: Clinical and experimental considerations. *Crit Care Med* 20,1169-1177

Palanchon, P., Bouakaz, A., van Blankenstein, J.H., Klein, J., Bom, N. & de Jong, N.(2001) New technique for emboli detection and discrimination based on nonlinear characteristics of gas bubbles. *Ultrasound Med Biol,* 27,6,801-8

Pascazio, L., Bianco, F., Giorgini, A., Galli, G., Curri, G. & Panzetta, G.(1996) Echo color Doppler imaging of carotid vessels in hemodialysis patients: evidence of high levels of atherosclerotic lesions. *Am J Kidney Dis,* 28,5,713-20

Patel, N., Dalal, P. & Panesar, M.(2008) Dialysis disequilibrium syndrome: a narrative review. *Semin Dial,* 21,5,493-8

Palmer, B.F.(2001) Individualizing the dialysate in the hemodialysis patient. *Semin Dial,* 1,41-9

Pedersen, K.E., Lysgaard Madsen, J., Klitgaard, N.A., Kjaer, K. & Hvidt, S.(1985) Effect of quinine on plasma digoxin concentration and renal digoxin clearance. *Acta Med Scand,* 218,2,229-32

Peixoto, A.J. & Santos, S.F.(2010) Blood pressure management in hemodialysis: what have we learned? Curr *Opin Nephrol Hypertens,* 19,561-6

Peixoto, A.J., Gowda, N., Parikh, C.R. & Santos, S.F.(2010) Long-term stability of serum sodium in hemodialysis patients. *Blood Purif,* 29,3,264-7

Perazella, M.A.(2001) Pharmacologic options available to treat symptomatic intradialytic hypotension. *Am J Kidney Dis,* 38,S26-36

Pisoni, R.L., Young, E.W., Dykstra, D.M., Greenwold, R.N., Hecking, E., Gillespie, B., Wolfe, R.A., Goodkin & D.A., Held, P.J.(2002) Vascular access use in Europe and the United States: results from the DOPPS. *Kidney Int,* 61,305-316

Pitsavos, C., Kourlaba, G., Panagiotakos, D.B., Kogias, Y., Mantas, Y., Chrysohoou, C. & Stefanadis, C. (2007) Association of creatinine clearance and in-hospital mortality in patients with acute coronary syndromes: the GREECS study. *Circ J,* 71,1,9-14

Polaschegg , H.D.(2007) Hemodialysis machine air detectors need not detect microbubbles. *Artif Organs,* 31,12,911-2

Power ,A., Hamady, M., Singh, S., Ashby, D., Taube, D. & Duncan, N.(2010) High but stable incidence of subdural haematoma in haemodialysis--a single-centre study. *Nephrol Dial Transplant,* 25,7, 2272-5

Prandoni, P., Siragusa, S., Girolami, B. & Fabris, F. (2005) BELZONI Investigators Group. The incidence of heparin-induced thrombocytopenia in medical patients treated with low-molecular-weight heparin: a prospective cohort study. *Blood,* 1,106,9, 3049-54

Pun, P.H., Lehrich, R.W., Smith, S.R. & Middleton, J.P.(2007) Predictors of survival after cardiac arrest in outpatient hemodialysis clinics. *Clin J Am Soc Nephrol,* 2,3,491-500

Quinn, R.R., Naimark, D.M., Oliver, M.J. & Bayoumi, A.M.(2007) Should hemodialysis patients with atrial fibrillation undergo systemic anticoagulation? A cost-utility analysis. *Am J Kidney Dis,* 50,3,421-32

Remuzzi, G. (1989) Bleeding disorders in uremia: pathophysiology and treatment. *Adv Nephrol Necker Hosp,* 18,171-86

Roca, A.O, Jarjoura, D., Blend, D., Cugino, A., Rutecki, G.W., Nuchikat, P.S. & Whittier, F.C.(1992) Dialysis leg cramps. Efficacy of quinine versus vitamin E. *ASAIO J,* 38,3,481-5

Rodrigo, F., Shideman, J., McHugh, R., Buselmeier, T. & Kjellstrand, C.(1977)Osmolality changes during hemodialysis. Natural history, clinical correlations, and influence of dialysate glucose and intravenous mannitol. *Ann Intern Med,* 86,5,554-61

Rosa, A.A., Shideman, J., McHugh, R., Duncan, D. & Kjellstrand, C.M.(1981) The importance of osmolality fall and ultrafiltration rate on hemodialysis side effects. Influence of intravenous mannitol. *Nephron,* 27,3,134-41

Rostand, S.G. & Rutsky, E.A.(1990) Pericarditis in end-stage renal disease. *Cardiol Clin,* 8,4,701-7

Rutsky, E.A &Rostand, S.G.(1987)Treatment of uremic pericarditis and pericardial effusion. *Am J Kidney Dis.* 10,1,2-8

Saha , H., Harmoinen, A., Pietilä, K., Mörsky, P. & Pasternack, A.(1996) Measurement of serum ionized versus total levels of magnesium and calcium in hemodialysis patients. *Clin Nephrol,* 46,5,326-31

Said, R., Quintanilla, A., Levin, N. & Ivanovich, P.(1997) Acute hemolysis due to profound hypo-osmolality. A complication of hemodialysis. *J Dial,* 1,5,447-52

Sands, J.J., Jabyac, P.A., Miranda, C.L. & Kapsick, B.J.(1999) Intervention based on monthly monitoring decreases hemodialysis access thrombosis. *ASAIO J,* 45,3,147-50

Sang, G.L, Kovithavongs, C., Ulan, R. & Kjellstrand, C.M.(1997) Sodium ramping in hemodialysis: a study of beneficial and adverse effects. *Am J Kidney Dis,* 29,5,669-77

Santos, S.F. & Peixoto, A.J.(2010) Sodium balance in maintenance hemodialysis. *Semin Dial,* 23,6,549-55

Schanzer, H., Skladany, M. & Haimov, M .(1992) Treatment of angioaccess-induced ischemia by revascularization. *J Vasc Surg,* 16,6,861-4

Schillinger, F., Schillinger, D., Montagnac, R. & Milcent, T.(1991) Post catheterisation vein stenosis in haemodialysis: comparative angiographic study of 50 subclavian and 50 internal jugular accesses. *Nephrol Dial Transplant,* 10,722-4

Schreiber, M.J. Jr.(2001) Clinical case-based approach to understanding intradialytic hypotension. *Am J Kidney Dis,* 38,37-47

Schwab, S.J., Oliver, M.J., Suhocki, P. & McCann, R.(2001) Hemodialysis arteriovenous access: detection of stenosis and response to treatment by vascular access blood flow. *Kidney Int.* 59,1,358-62

Schwartz, A.B. (1978) Potassium-related cardiac arrhythmias and their treatment. *Angiology,* 29,3,194-205

Schwartz, I.F. & Iaina, A .(1999) Uraemic pruritus. *Nephrol Dial Transplant,* 14,4,834-9

Schwartz, I.F. & Iaina, A.(2000) Management of uremic pruritus. *Semin Dial,* 13,177-80

Seliger, S.L., Gillen, D.L., Longstreth, W.T. Jr., Kestenbaum, B. & Stehman-Breen, C.O. (2003) Elevated risk of stroke among patients with end-stage renal disease. *Kidney Int,* 64,2,603-9

Seliger, S.L., Gillen, D.L., Tirschwell, D., Wasse, H., Kestenbaum, B.R. & Stehman-Breen, C.O.(2003) Risk factors for incident stroke among patients with end-stage renal disease. *J Am Soc Nephrol,* 14,10,2623-31

Seliger, S.L., Gillen, D.L., Longstreth, W.T. Jr., Kestenbaum, B. & Stehman-Breen, C.O.(2003) Elevated risk of stroke among patients with end-stage renal disease. *Kidney Int,* 64,2,603-9

Selby, N.M. & McIntyre, C.W.(2007) The acute cardiac effects of dialysis. *Semin Dial,* 20,3,220-8

Severi, S., Cavalcanti, S., Mancini, E. & Santoro, A.(2001) Heart rate response to hemodialysis-induced changes in potassium and calcium levels. *J Nephrol.*14,488-96

Shaldon, S. & Koch, K.M.(1995) Biocompatibility in hemodialysis: clinical relevance in 1995. *Artif Organs,* 19,5,395-7

Shastri, S. & Sarnak, M.J.(2010) Cardiovascular disease and CKD: core curriculum 2010. *Am J Kidney Dis,* 56,2,399-417

Sherman, R.A.(2002) Intradialytic hypotension: an overview of recent, unresolved and overlooked issues. *Semin Dial,* 15,3,141-3

Sidhom, O.A., Odeh, Y.K., Krumlovsky, F.A., Budris, W.A., Wang, Z., Pospisil, P.A., Atkinson, & A.J. Jr. (1994) Low-dose prazosin in patients with muscle cramps during hemodialysis. *Clin Pharmacol Ther,* 56,4,445-51

Sood, M.M., Komenda, P., Sood, A.R., Rigatto, C. & Bueti, J.(2009) The intersection of risk and benefit: is warfarin anticoagulation suitable for atrial fibrillation in patients on hemodialysis? *Chest,*136,4,1128-33

Sozio, S.M., Armstrong, P.A., Coresh, J., Jaar, B.G., Fink, N.E., Plantinga, L.C., Powe, N.R. & Parekh, R.S.(2009) Cerebrovascular disease incidence, characteristics, and outcomes in patients initiating dialysis: the choices for healthy outcomes in caring for ESRD (CHOICE) study. *Am J Kidney Dis,* 54,3,468-77

Spongano, M., Santoro, A., Ferrari, G., Badiali, F., Rossi, M., Parrino, A., Lamberti, C., Sarti, E. & Zucchelli, P.(1988) Continuous computerized monitoring of hemodynamic parameters during acetate dialysis, bicarbonate dialysis, and acetate-free biofiltration. *Artif Organs,* 12,6,476-81

Stevens, L.A., Li, S., Wang, C., Huang, C., Becker, B.N., Bomback, A.S., Brown, W.W., Burrows, N.R., Jurkovitz, C.T., McFarlane, S.I., Norris, K.C., Shlipak, M., Whaley-Connell, AT., Chen, S.C., Bakris, G.L. & McCullough, P.A.(2010) Prevalence of CKD and comorbid illness in elderly patients in the United States: results from the Kidney Early Evaluation Program (KEEP). *Am J Kidney Dis,* 55,3,Suppl 2,S23-33

Stiller, S., Bonnie-Schorn, E., Grassmann, A., Uhlenbusch-Körwer, I. & Mann, H.(2001). A critical review of sodium profiling for hemodialysis. *Semin Dial,* 14,337-47

Stockenhuber, F., Sunder-Plassmann, G. & Balcke, P. (1987) Increased plasma histamine levels in chronic renal failure. *N Engl J Med,* 317,386

Stuart, R.K., Shikora, S.A., Akerman, P., Lowell, J.A., Baxter, J.K., Apovian, C., Champagne, C., Jennings, A., Keane-Ellison, M. & Bistrian, B.R.(1990) Incidence of arrhythmia with central venous catheter insertion and exchange. *JPEN J Parenter Enteral Nutr,* 14,2,152-5

Suranyi , M. & Chow, J.S.(2010). Review: anticoagulation for haemodialysis. *Nephrology (Carlton),* 15,4,386-92

Swartz, R.D., Somermeyer, M.G. & Hsu, C.H.(1982) Preservation of plasma volume during hemodialysis depends on dialysate osmolality. *Am J Nephrol,* 2,4,189-94

Sweet, S.J., McCarthy, S., Steingart, R. & Callahan, T.(1996) Hemolytic reactions mechanically induced by kinked hemodialysis lines. *Am J Kidney Dis,* 27,2,262-6

Syed, S. & Reilly, R.F.(2009) Heparin-induced thrombocytopenia: a renal perspective. *Nat Rev Nephrol,* 5,9,501-11

Takemoto, Y., Naganuma, T. & Yoshimura, R.(2011) Biocompatibility of the dialysis membrane. *Contrib Nephrol,* 68,139-45

Tessitore, N., Mansueto, G., Bedogna, V., Lipari, G., Poli, A., Gammaro, L., Baggio, E., Morana, G., Loschiavo, C., Laudon, A., Oldrizzi, L. & Maschio, G.(2003) A prospective controlled trial on effect of percutaneous transluminal angioplasty on functioning arteriovenous fistulae survival. *J Am Soc Nephrol,*14,6,1623-7

Tessitore, N., Lipari, G., Poli, A., Bedogna, V., Baggio, E., Loschiavo, C., Mansueto, G. & Lupo, A.(2004) Can blood flow surveillance and pre-emptive repair of subclinical stenosis prolong the useful life of arteriovenous fistulae? A randomized controlled study. *Nephrol Dial Transplant,*19,9,2325-33

Tordoir, J., Canaud, B., Haage, P., Konner, K., Basci, A., Fouque, D., Koman, J., Martin-Malo, A., Pedrini, L., Pizzarelli, F., Tattersall, J., Vennegoor, M., Wanner, C., ter Wee, P. & Vanholder, R.(2007) EBPG on Vascular Access. *Nephrol Dial Transplant*

Toyoda, K., Fujii, K., Fujimi, S., Kumai, Y., Tsuchimochi, H., Ibayashi, S. & Iida, M. (2005) Stroke in patients on maintenance hemodialysis: a 22-year single-center study. *Am J Kidney Dis,* 45,6,1058-66

Trerotola, S.O., Johnson, M.S., Haris, V.J., Shah, H., Ambrosius, W.T., McKusky, M.A. & Kraus, M.A.(1997) Outcome of tunneled hemodialysis catheters placed via the right internal jugular vein by interventional radiologists. *Radiology,* 203,489-495

Trinh-Trang-Tan, M.M., Cartron, J.P. & Bankir, L.(2005) Molecular basis for the dialysis disequilibrium syndrome: altered aquaporin and urea transporter expression in the brain. *Nephrol Dial Transplant,* 20,9,1984-8

Turmel-Rodrigues, L., Pengloan, J., Baudin, S., Testou, D., Abaza, M., Dahdah, G., Mouton & A., Blanchard, D.(2000) Treatment of stenosis and thrombosis in haemodialysis fistulas and grafts by interventional radiology. *Nephrol Dial Transplant,*15,12,2029-36

Twardowski, Z.J.(2008) History of hemodialyzers' designs. *Hemodial Int,*12,173-210

Twardowski, Z.J.(2006) Dialyzer reuse--part II: advantages and disadvantages. *Semin Dial,* 19,3,217-26

van de Wetering, J., Westendorp, R.G., van der Hoeven, J.G., Stolk, B., Feuth, J.D. & Chang, P.C.(1996) Heparin use in continuous renal replacement procedures: the struggle between filter coagulation and patient hemorrhage. *J Am Soc Nephrol* 7,1,145-50

Vanholder, R.C., Pauwels, R.A., Vandenbogaerde, J.F., Lamont, H.H., Van der Straeten, M,E, & Ringoir, S,M.(1987) Cuprophan reuse and intradialytic changes of lung diffusion capacity and blood gases. *Kidney Int,* 32,1,117-22

Velez, R.L., Woodard, T.D. & Henrich, W.L.(1984) Acetate and bicarbonate hemodialysis in patients with and without autonomic dysfunction. *Kidney Int,* 26,1, 59-65.

Versluis, M., Goertz, D.E., Palanchon, P., Heitman, I.L., van der Meer, S.M., Dollet, B., de Jong, N. & Lohse, D.(2010) Microbubble shape oscillations excited through ultrasonic parametric driving. *Phys Rev E Stat Nonlin Soft Matter Phys,* 82,2 Pt 2,026321.

Visentin, G.P., Ford, S.E., Scott, J.P. & Aster, R.H.(1994) Antibodies from patients with heparin-induced thrombocytopenia/thrombosis are specific for platelet factor 4 complexed with heparin or bound to endothelial cells. *J Clin Invest,* 93,1,81-8

Wadełek, J.(2010)Haemodialysis catheters.*Anestezjol Intens Ter,*42,4,213-7

Walter, J. & Taraba, I.(1991) Dialysis hypersensitivity. *Nephrol Dial Transplant,* 3,47-9

Ward, R.A. & Ronco, C.(2006) Dialyzer and machine technologies: application of recent advances to clinical practice. *Blood Purif,* 24,1,6-10

Ward, R.A. (2004) Ultrapure dialysate. *Semin Dial,* 17,6,489-97

Warkentin, T.E.(2004) Heparin-induced thrombocytopenia: diagnosis and management. *Circulation,* 2,110,18

Warkentin, T.E., Aird, W.C. & Rand, J.H.(2003) Platelet-endothelial interactions: sepsis, HIT, and antiphospholipid syndrome. *Hematology Am Soc Hematol Educ Program,* 497-519

Weber, H., Schwarzer, C., Stummvoll, H.K., Joskowics, G., Wolf, A., Steinbach, K. & Kaindl, F.(1984) Chronic Hemodialysis: High Risk Patients for Arrhythmias? *Nephron,* 37,180–185

Weiner, I.D. & Wingo, C.S.(1998) Hyperkalemia: a potential silent killer. *J Am Soc Nephrol,* 9,8,1535-43

Weisberg, L.S. & Rachoin, J.S.(2010) The safety of low-potassium dialysis. *Semin Dial,* 23,6,556-60

Whittier, W.L. (2009) Surveillance of hemodialysis vascular access. *Semin Intervent Radiol,* 26,2,130-8

Winkelmayer, W.C., Charytan, D.M., Levin, R. & Avorn, J.(2006) Poor short-term survival and low use of cardiovascular medications in elderly dialysis patients after acute myocardial infarction.*Am J Kidney Dis,* 47,2,301-8

Wolf, L.R., Otten, E.J. & Spadafora, M.P.(1992) Cinchonism: two case reports and review of acute quinine toxicity and treatment. *J Emerg Med,* 10,3,295-301

Yalcin, A.U., Kudaiberdieva, G., Sahin, G., Gorenek, B., Akcar, N., Kuskus, S., Bayrak, F. & Timuralp, B.(2003) Effect of sertraline hydrochloride on cardiac autonomic dysfunction in patients with hemodialysis-induced hypotension. *Nephron Physiol,* 93,21-8

Yavascan, O., Mir, S. & Tekguc, H.(2009) Supraventricular tachycardia following insertion of a central venous catheter. *Saudi J Kidney Dis Transpl,* 20,6,1061-4

Yu, A.S. & Levy, E.(1997) Paradoxical cerebral air embolism from a hemodialysis catheter. *Am J Kidney Dis,* 29,3,453-5

Yixiong, Z., Jianping, N., Yanchao, L. & Siyuan, D. (2010) Low dose of argatroban saline flushes anticoagulation in hemodialysis patients with high risk of bleeding. *Clin Appl Thromb Hemost,* 16,4,440-5

Zehnder, C., Gutzwiller, J.P., Huber, A., Schindler, C. & Schneditz, D.(2001) Low-potassium and glucose-free dialysis maintains urea but enhances potassium removal. *Nephrol Dial Transplant,* 16,1,78-84

17

Review of the Effectiveness of Cellulose- and Polysulfone-Based Vitamin E-Bonded Dialysis Membranes

Masaharu Aritomi[1] and Francesco Galli[2]
[1]*Asahi Kasei Kuraray Medical Co., Ltd. Tokyo*
[2]*Dept of Internal Medicine, University of Perugia*
[1]*Japan*
[2]*Italy*

1. Introduction

Reduction of the stressful effects of extracorporeal circulation is a major target in hemodialysis (HD) therapy. These effects can be attributed to the HD-associated uremic comorbidity and the oxidative and non-oxidative events that occur because of the extracorporeal treatment. Anemia, cardiovascular disease, chronic inflammation, immunosuppression and intradialytic hypotension are among the most common complications in patients receiving HD, which show a causal relationship with oxidative stress (Galli, 2002 and Del Vecchio et al., 2011). During HD, the patient's blood is repeatedly exposed to components of the extracorporeal circulation, a key component of which is the hollow-fiber dialyzer membrane. This phenomenon may lead to leukocyte and platelet activation, thereby causing oxidative stress. Moreover, bioactive contaminants, e.g., bacterial endotoxins in the dialysis fluids, to which the patient's blood is eventually exposed through the dialyzer membrane, may further sustain leukocyte activation. These variables, which are usually included under the definition of "bio-incompatibility," should be carefully monitored by dialysis centers because these variables are responsible for causing pro-inflammatory events, oxidative stress, and pro-thrombotic effects. Leukocyte activation and oxidative stress are also reported to cause erythrocyte damage that is further aggravated by shear stress and other mechanical injuries. Plasma proteins and lipids show signs of oxidative damage (Piroddi et al., 2007 and Galli, 2007), and this may influence the burden of uremic toxicity by inducing cell and tissue reactions, abnormal metabolism of these oxidation products, vascular and immune reactions, etc. To reduce the risk of oxidative stress and other adverse reactions that can be caused by poor biocompatibility of HD treatment, highly purified dialysis fluids and dialyzer membranes with greater biocompatibility have been developed, and are currently under investigation for further improvement.

The bio-incompatibility of prototypical dialyzer membranes made of regenerated cellulose has been associated with the contact of blood components with the hydroxyl groups of beta-D-glucose. These groups trigger intradialytic activation of the complement system and cause leucopenia (Rousseau et al., 1999). Biocompatibility of regenerated cellulose dialyzer membranes was tentatively improved by the chemical modification of the hydroxyl groups, e.g., by acetylation to obtain tri-acetate cellulose, or by adding polyethylene glycol (PEG) chains to obtain PEG-grafted cellulose. Another and more successful approach was the de novo development of synthetic polymer membranes such as polysulfone or polyether sulfone membranes with no bio-incompatible groups in their chemical structures (Bowry, 2002). At present, high-flux synthetic membranes are more frequently used, and represent a cost-effective solution with proven clinical superiority over cellulosic membranes (Krane et al., 2007).

Antioxidants such as vitamin C, vitamin E, and glutathione have been used as oral supplements to alleviate HD-induced oxidative stress (Galli and Azzi, 2010). The clinical course of chronic kidney disease (CKD) includes a progressive decrease in the levels of blood antioxidants such as vitamins C, vitamin E, and glutathione. As a result, CKD patients who undergo regular HD treatment show severe deficiencies, particularly of water-soluble antioxidants (such as vitamin C). Few studies, however, provided clear evidence of the clinical advantage of oral antioxidants. The most convincing evidence was obtained from the randomized clinical trial on vitamin E supplementation in HD patients. This trial, known as SPACE study (Boaz et al., 2000), showed a significant reduction (54%) of the primary endpoint variable (a composite variable including myocardial infarction, ischemic stroke, peripheral vascular disease, and unstable angina) and 70% reduction in myocardial infarction.

One of the most original approaches for antioxidant therapy in HD involved the use of vitamin E as a lipophilic modifier of the surface of the dialysis membrane. The bonded vitamin E on the surface of the dialyzer membrane is expected to reduce the production of reactive oxygen species (ROS) at the site where blood cells are exposed to the dialyzer membrane, thereby providing the blood cells with antioxidant protection in a timely and targeted manner. Two generations of vitamin E-bonded dialyzers based on this concept, namely, cellulosic- and polysulfone-based membrane dialyzers, have been successfully developed and launched in the market over the last 2 decades. This chapter provides a review of the literature and a critical examination of the available clinical data on vitamin E-bonded dialyzer membranes.

2. Cellulose-based vitamin E-bonded dialyzer membranes

2.1 Development

In 1990, cellulose-based vitamin E-bonded dialyzer membranes (Excebrane) were developed and introduced into the market by Terumo Corporation. The base membrane was made of regenerated cellulose hollow fiber, and the surface of the hollow fiber was covalently modified by hydrophilic polymers as well as by oleic alcohol. Vitamin E (α-tocopherol) was then bonded to oleic alcohol via hydrophobic interaction. Sasaki et al., 2000, reported the outline of the production process as well as the results of *in vitro* and *in vivo* studies on Excebrane, which showed much better biocompatibility than the original regenerated cellulose membrane.

2.2 Clinical outcomes

Early trials using Excebrane indicated that its use would have positive clinical effects (Galli, 2002). The potential therapeutic effects of using this membrane in HD were reduction of oxidative stress and inflammation. Cardiovascular endpoints were investigated in several small clinical trials and in a meta-analysis of 14 peer-reviewed articles by Sosa et al., 2006; these studies concluded that Excebrane treatment was associated with a significant decrease in the plasma levels of lipid-peroxidation biomarkers, thereby suggesting the potential benefit of these membranes in clinical usage. Actually, these biomarkers have a cause-effect relationship with low density lipoprotein (LDL) damage and endothelial dysfunction in CKD. Preliminary evidence of better management of uremic anemia by these dialyzer membranes was obtained in the pioneering studies by Usberti et al., 2002; Nakatani et al., 2003; and Kobayashi et al., 2003. These authors found improved erythrocyte life span and rheology in patients receiving HD with Excebrane. A larger multicenter study (172 patients) reported by Cruz et al., 2008, confirmed that the impact of Excebrane dialyzers on anemia parameters was better than that of other high-flux biocompatible dialyzer membranes, including cellulose acetate, polysulfone, and polymethylmethacrylate.

Other reports demonstrated positive effects such as (1) decreased oxidative stress (Tarng et al., 2000; Miyazaki et al., 2000; Clermont et al., 2001; Westhuyzen et al., 2003; Bufano et al., 2004; Mydlik et al., 2004; Calò et al., 2004; Yang et al., 2006; and Odetti et al., 2006), (2) suppression of leukocyte activation (Omata et al., 2000; Zaluska et al., 2001;Pertosa et al., 2002; Tsuruoka et al., 2002; Libetta et al., 2004; and Kojima et al., 2005), (3) dosage reduction of anticoagulants (Huraib et al., 2000), (4) improved biocompatibility (Yoshida et al., 2002), and (5) decreased levels of advanced glycation end products (AGEs) (Baragetti et al., 2006). Moreover, a recent study reported by Kirmizis D et al., 2010, showed that the levels of inflammatory markers such as C-reactive protein (CRP), interleukin (IL)-6, and soluble intercellular adhesion molecule (sICAM)-1 in 35 patients treated with Excebrane were lower than those in the baseline evaluation carried out with conventional low- or middle-flux dialyzers. Whereas, no change was observed throughout the experimental period in a matched control group of 25 patients who underwent treatment with the unmodified dialyzers.

3. Polysulfone-based vitamin E-bonded dialyzer membranes

3.1 Development

Synthetic membrane dialyzers have been developed by many manufacturers in the past decades to achieve higher depurative and biocompatibility standards. Polysulfone has shown better performance among these synthetic biomaterials; as a result, it has become popular in clinical practice (Bowry, 2002). In order to achieve the synergistic effect of the biocompatibility of synthetic membranes and the antioxidant activity of vitamin E, polysulfone-based vitamin E-coated membranes were developed and introduced in the market in 1998. These dialyzers were initially developed by Terumo Corporation; subsequently, they were produced using a new technique and are now manufactured by Asahi Kasei Kuraray Medical Co. Ltd., with the membrane name of VitabranE. Preliminary *in vitro* analyses on these membranes were reported by Sasaki, 2006; the antioxidant capacity of VitabranE was recently confirmed and quantified by Floridi A, et al., 2009, by means of *in vitro* re-circulation tests carried out on mini-module dialyzers. These tests, which used an unbiased procedure, showed that at least one-third of the vitamin E present on the membrane participates in the one-electron transfer reaction with transition metals. This reaction, together with scavenging of peroxyl radicals, characterizes the antioxidant mechanism of vitamin E and is of putative relevance in its biological function.

3.2 Improvement of anemia

On the basis of the early evidence obtained in the Excebrane studies described in section 2.2, VitabranE was proposed as a more biocompatible dialyzer membrane to achieve a better control of anemia in HD patients. This aspect was investigated in clinical trials that compared VitabranE with polysulfone membranes. A pilot study by Andrulli et al., 2010, carried out with a 2-arm randomized controlled design showed that 8-month treatment with VitabranE decreased the erythropoiesis-stimulating agent (ESA)-resistance index (ERI); ERI is calculated as the ratio between ESA dosage (IU/kg/w) and hemoglobin levels (g/dL). In the primary analysis, ERI showed no significant deference between the groups treated with VitabranE and the control polysulfone membrane. However, in the secondary analysis where the baseline parathyroid hormone (PTH) and serum vitamin E levels were included as covariates, the ERI was significantly decreased in the group treated with VitabranE than in the group treated with the control polysulfone membrane. Therefore, the authors concluded that VitabranE membranes have potentially beneficial effects on ERI of HD patients. This conclusion was confirmed in another and more recent multicenter study by Panichi et al., 2011. In this report, a crossover design was employed and 62 HD patients from 13 dialysis units were randomized to receive treatments with VitabranE or polysulfone dialyzer controls. The patients were studied for 2 steps of 6 months in each treatment. In this study, hemoglobin levels significantly increased after 6 months of VitabranE treatment, whereas these remained unchanged in the control group. Moreover, at the same ESA dose, the ERI was significantly lower during the VitabranE treatment period.

Further support for the findings of these randomized trials came from a pilot cross-over study by Mandolfo et al. (in press), which was conducted on patients using central venous catheters for blood access. Sixteen patients were enrolled and divided into 2 treatment groups (VitabranE dialyzer versus synthetic membrane dialyzers) and were followed for 2 periods of 6 months each. The results showed that the ERI decreased significantly in the group that received treatment with VitabranE, whereas it did not change in the control group. Hemoglobin levels were not affected; thus, the authors concluded that VitabranE membranes might help reducing the ESA dose required in anti-anemic therapy.

3.3 Improvement of inflammatory markers

In the report by Panichi et al., 2011, the authors observed that beside of ERI reduction, CRP and IL-6 levels decreased during VitabranE treatment, whereas no significant changes were found during the control polysulfone treatment. The study by Mandolfo et al. (in press) on catheterized patients with a high inflammatory burden also reported a better control of CRP levels during the VitabranE treatment. In these studies, a lower inflammatory response was associated with improved ERI, which is consistent with the role of chronic inflammation and oxidative stress as pathogenic factors of uremic anemia (Del Vecchio et al., 2011).

Calò et al., 2011, conducted a 1-year study on 25 HD patients to evaluate the effects of VitabranE on the biochemical markers of inflammation. The authors employed a molecular approach by using immunoblot (western blot) analysis to assess the expression of $p22^{phox}$, plasminogen activator inhibitor (PAI)-1, phosphorylated extracellular signal-regulated kinase (pERK)1/2 and heme oxygenase (HO)-1 in circulating mononuclear leukocytes at the beginning of the study and after 6 and 12 months of treatment with VitabranE. The treatment with VitabranE significantly decreased the expression of inflammatory markers of $p22^{phox}$, PAI-1, and pERK1/2, while the treatment increased the expression of anti-inflammatory marker of HO-1.

3.4 Reduction in the levels of oxidative stress makers

Preliminary investigations of blood levels of advanced protein oxidation products (AOPP) and fluorescent AGEs were performed in the randomized controlled pilot trial reported by

Andrulli et al., 2010. In this study, these protein-damaged markers were investigated as oxidative and carbonyl stress indices associated with the correction of ERI. Although IL-6 and CRP levels were not affected, the 2 indices showed better control in the patients receiving with VitabranE than in those receiving treatment with polysulfone dialyzer (Galli et al., manuscript in preparation).

Vitamin E-bonded dialyzer membranes were originally developed with the aim of reducing oxidative stress. As shown in the section 2.2, lowered lipid peroxidation was observed in clinical trials with Excebrane, a cellulose-based vitamin E-bonded membrane. In the case of VitabranE, 2 studies were conducted, considering LDL oxidation as an end point. Morimoto et al., 2005, reported that the 15 patients who received 6 months of treatment with VitabranE showed significant reduction in the levels of asymmetric dimethylarginine (ADMA), malondialdehyde low density lipoprotein (MDA-LDL), and oxidized low density lipoprotein (Ox-LDL). The levels returned to baseline when the membrane was changed to a polysulfone dialyzer membrane. In a matched control group, patients treated with polysulfone dialyzers showed no change in ADMA, Ox-LDL, and MDA-LDL levels during the entire treatment period of 18 months. The other report from Calò et al., 2011, showed that VitabranE improved the levels of inflammation markers and also reduced plasma levels of Ox-LDL, which was evaluated by enzyme-linked immunosorbent assay.

3.5 Improvement of intradialytic hypotension

Intradialytic hypotension (IDH) is a common clinical trait in HD patients. Matsumura et al., 2010, conducted a pilot study to assess the effectiveness of VitabranE in improving IDH. Eight IDH patients who had been receiving HD with conventional dialyzers were switched to VitabranE dialyzers, and intradialytic blood pressure (BP) was monitored regularly for 10 months. The results showed that hypotension, monitored during the session by measuring systolic BP (SBP), diastolic BP (DBP), and pulse pressure (PP), improved after changing the dialyzer membrane. Moreover, after 8 to 10 months, SBP recorded before dialysis was significantly lower than that at baseline, which suggests a stable improvement in the vascular compliance to intra- and inter-dialysis control of BP.

3.6 Anticoagulation management

In a recent report, Aoun et al., 2010, described the potential clinical advantages of VitabranE in anticoagulant management. In an observational trial, these authors evaluated the minimum requirement of low molecular weight heparin (LMWH) in pediatric dialysis patients. Seven children and adolescent patients received HD with VitabranE dialyzer and their LMWH dose was decreased every week without any other change in the clinical management; the findings of this study consistently indicated a lower requirement of anticoagulants, which may help reducing bleeding problems and simplifying post-dialysis hemostasis.

4. Conclusion

The available literature suggests that vitamin E bonding on the cellulosic membrane Excebrane can reduce oxidative stress, as assessed by the levels of lipid peroxidation markers, and improve laboratory indices of inflammation and uremic anemia. The newly developed synthetic polysulfone-based dialysis membrane VitabranE appears to produce even more relevant clinical advantages as it is a homologue of most widely used synthetic membrane dialyzers. Randomized studies carried out in the past few years, which have reported positive effects on ERI and anemia management, provide convincing and clinically relevant evidence. Early findings also suggest a better control of inflammatory and oxidative stress parameters. Anticoagulation and IDH are other potentially relevant aspects in the clinical application of VitabranE. These results suggest that VitabranE has superior performance than other synthetic membranes. Further and more comprehensive trials are needed for detailed verification of these clinical outcomes.

5. References

Andrulli, S.; Di Filippo, S.; Manzoni, C.; Stefanelli, L.; Floridi, A.; Galli, F. & Locatelli, F. (2010). Effect of Synthetic Vitamin E-Bonded Membrane on Responsiveness to Erythropoiesis-Stimulating Agents in Hemodialysis Patients: A Pilot Study. *Nephron Clin Pract.* 115(1):c82–c89.

Aoun, B.; Janssen-Lozinska, Y. & Ulinski, T. (2010). Effect of vitamin E coated dialyzers on anticoagulation requirement in hemodialyzed children. *Saudi J Kidney Dis Transpl.* 21(3):466–70.

Baragetti, I.; Furiani, S.; Vettoretti, S.; Raselli, S.; Maggi, FM.; Galli, F.; Catapano, AL. & Buccianti, G. (2006). Role of vitamin E-coated membrane in reducing advanced glycation end products in hemodialysis patients: a pilot study. *Blood Purif.* 24(4):369–76.

Boaz, M.; Smetana, S.; Weinstein, T.; Matas, Z.; Gafter, U.; Iaina, A.; Knecht, A.; Weissgarten, Y.; Brunner, D.; Fainaru, M. & Green, MS. (2000). Secondary prevention with antioxidants of cardiovascular disease in endstage renal disease (SPACE): randomised placebo-controlled trial. *Lancet.* 356(9237):1213-8.

Bowry, SK. (2002). Dialysis membranes today. *Int J Artif Organs.* 25(5):447-60.

Bufano, G.; Usberti, M.; Mandolfo, S.; Malberti, F.; Piroddi, M. & Galli, F. (2004). Von Willebrand factor and autoantibodies against oxidized LDL in hemodialysis patients treated with vitamin E-modified dialyzers. *Int J Artif Organs.* 27(3):214–21.

Calò, LA.; Naso, A.; Pagnin, E.; Davis, PA.; Castoro, M.; Corradin, R.; Riegler, P.; Cascone, C.; Huber, W. & Piccoli, A. (2004). Vitamin E-coated dialyzers reduce oxidative stress related proteins and markers in hemodialysis--a molecular biological approach. *Clin Nephrol.* 62(5):355–61.

Calò, LA; Naso, A; D'Angelo, A.; Pagnin, E.; Zanardo, M. & Puato, M. (2011). Rebeschini M, Landini S, Feriani M, Perego A, Malagoli A, Zagatti R, Calzavara P, Cascone C, Davis PA. Molecular biology-based assessment of vitamin E-coated dialyzer effects on oxidative stress, inflammation, and vascular remodeling. *Artif Organs.* 35(2):E33–9.

Clermont, G.; Lecour, S.; Cabanne, JF.; Motte, G.; Guilland, JC.; Chevet, D. & Rochette, L. (2001). Vitamin E-coated dialyzer reduces oxidative stress in hemodialysis patients. *Free Radic Biol Med.* 31(2):233–41.

Cruz, DN.; De Cal, M.; Garzotto, F.; Brendolan, A.; Nalesso, D.; Corradi, V. & Ronco, C. (2008). Effect of vitamin E-coated dialysis membranes on anemia in patients with chronic kidney disease: an Italian multicenter study. *Int J Artif Organs.* 31(6):545–52.

Del Vecchio, L.; Locatelli, F. & Carini, M. (2011). What we know about oxidative stress in patients with chronic kidney disease on dialysis-clinical effects, potential treatment, and prevention. *Semin Dial.* 24(1):56–64.

Floridi, A.; Piroddi, M.; Pilolli, F.; Matsumoto, Y.; Aritomi, M. & Galli F. (2009). Analysis method and characterization of the antioxidant capacity of vitamin E-interactive polysulfone hemodialyzers. *Acta Biomater.* 5(8):2974–82.

Galli, F. (2002). Vitamin E-modified dialyzers. *Contrib Nephrol.* 137:95–105.

Galli, F.; Floridi, A. & Buoncristiani U. (2002). Oxidant stress in hemodialysis patients. *Contrib Nephrol.* 137:371–8.

Galli, F. (2007). Protein damage and inflammation in uraemia and dialysis patients. *Nephrol Dial Transplant.* 22 Suppl 5:v20–36.

Galli, F. & Azzi, A. (2010). Present trends in vitamin E research. *Biofactors* 36(1):33-42.

Huraib, S.; Tanimu, D.; Shaheen, F.; Hejaili, F.; Giles, C. & Pagayon, V. (2000). Effect of vitamin-E-modified dialysers on dialyser clotting, erythropoietin and heparin dosage: a comparative crossover study. *Am J Nephrol.* 20(5):364–8.

Kirmizis, D.; Papagianni, A.; Belechri, AM. & Memmos, D. (2010). Effects of vitamin E-coated membrane dialyser on markers of oxidative stress and inflammation in patients on chronic haemodialysis. *Nephrol Dial Transplant.* [Epub ahead of print].

Kobayashi, S.; Moriya, H.; Aso, K. & Ohtake, T. (2003) Vitamin E-bonded hemodialyzer improves atherosclerosis associated with a rheological improvement of circulating red blood cells. *Kidney Int.* 63(5):1881–7.

Kojima, K.; Oda, K.; Homma, H.; Takahashi, K.; Kanda, Y.; Inokami, T. & Uchida, S. (2005). Effect of vitamin E-bonded dialyzer on eosinophilia in haemodialysis patients. *Nephrol Dial Transplant.* 20(9):1932–5.

Krane, V.; Krieter, DH.; Olschewski, M.; Marz, W.; Mann, JF.; Ritz, E. & Wanner, C. (2007). Dialyzer membrane characteristics and outcome of patients with type 2 diabetes on maintenance hemodialysis. *Am J Kidney Dis.* 49(2):267–75.

Libetta, C.; Zucchi, M.; Gori, E.; Sepe, V.; Galli, F.; Meloni, F.; Milanesi, F. & Dal Canton, A. (2004). Vitamin E-loaded dialyzer resets PBMC-operated cytokine network in dialysis patients. *Kidney Int.* 65(4):1473–81.

Mandolfo, S.; Corradi, B.; Bucci, R.; Barbisoni, F.; Farina, M; Pilolli F. & Galli, F. (in press) Evaluation of the impact of a new synthetic Vitamin E-bonded membrane on anemia and rHuEPO requirement in ESRD patients with central venous catheter: a pilot study. *Int J Nephrol.*

Matsumura, M.; Sasaki, H.; Sekizuka, K.; Sano, H.; Ogawa, K.; Shimizu, C.; Yoshida, H.; Kobayashi, S.; Koremoto, M.; Aritomi, M. & Ueki, K. (2010). Improved management of intradialytic hypotension (IDH) using vitamin E-bonded polysulfone membrane dialyzer. *Int J Artif Organs.* 33(3):147–153.

Miyazaki, H.; Matsuoka, H.; Itabe, H.; Usui, M.; Ueda, S. & Okuda, S. (2000). Imaizumi T. Hemodialysis impairs endothelial function via oxidative stress: effects of vitamin E-coated dialyzer. *Circulation.* 101(9):1002–6.

Morimoto, H.; Nakao, K.; Fukuoka, K.; Sarai, A.; Yano, A.; Kihara, T.; Fukuda, S.; Wada, J. & Makino, H. (2005). Long-term use of vitamin E-coated polysulfone membrane reduces oxidative stress markers in hemodialysis patients. *Nephrol Dial Transplant.* 20(12):2775–82.

Mydlik, M.; Derzsiova, K.; Racz, O.; Sipulova, A.; Lovasova, E.; Molcanyiova, A. & Petrovicova, J. (2004). Vitamin E-coated dialyzer and antioxidant defense parameters: three-month study. *Semin Nephrol.* 24(5):525–31.

Nakatani, T.; Takemoto, Y. & Tsuchida, AK. (2003). The effect of vitamin E-bonded dialyzer membrane on red blood cell survival in hemodialyzed patients. *Artif Organs.* 27(3):214–7.

Odetti, P.; Traverso, N.; Monacelli, F.; Menini, S.; Vazzana, J.; Tasso, B.; Pronzato, MA.; Robaudo, C. & Deferrari, G. (2006). Vitamin E-coated filter decreases levels of free 4-hydroxyl-2-nonenal during haemodialysis sessions. *Free Radic Res.* 40(2):207–12.

Omata, M.; Higuchi, C.; Demura, R.; Sanaka, T. & Nihei, H. (2000). Reduction of neutrophil activation by vitamin E modified dialyzer membranes. *Nephron.* 85(3):221–31.

Panichi, V.; Rosati, A.; Paoletti, S.; Ferrandello, P.; Migliori, M.; Beati, S.; Bernabini, G.; Daini, R.; Casani, A.; Angelini, D.; Parrini, M.; Rossi, A.; Petrone, I.; Barsotti, G.; Donadio, C.; Donati, G.; Grazi, G.; Manca Rizza, G.; Garosi, G.; Sansoni, E.; Braccagni, B.; Sidoti, A.; Boracelli, D.; Biagioli, M.; Moriconi, L.; Finato, V.; Mannarino, A.; Grimaldi, C.; Pansa, F.; Imperiali, P.; Mura, C.; Bianchi, S. & Bigazzi, R. (2011). A Vitamin E-Coated Polysulfone Membrane Reduces Serum Levels of Inflammatory Markers and Resistance to Erythropoietin-Stimulating Agents in Hemodialysis Patients: Results of a Randomized Cross-Over Multicenter Trial. *Blood Purif.* 32(1):7–14.

Pertosa, G.; Grandaliano, G.; Soccio, M.; Martino, C.; Gesualdo, L. & Schena, FP. (2002). Vitamin E-modified filters modulate Jun N-terminal kinase activation in peripheral blood mononuclear cells. *Kidney Int.* 62(2):602–10.

Piroddi, M.; Depunzio, I.; Calabrese, V.; Mancuso, C.; Aisa, CM.; Binaglia, L.; Minelli, A.; Butterfield, AD. & Galli, F. (2007). Oxidatively-modified and glycated proteins as candidate pro-inflammatory toxins in uremia and dialysis patients. *Amino Acids.* 32(4):573–92.

Rousseau, Y.; Carreno, MP.; Poignet, JL.; Kazatchkine, MD. & Haeffner-Cavaillon, N. (1999). Dissociation between complement activation, integrin expression, and neutropenia during hemodialysis. *Biomaterials.* 20(20):1959–67.

Sasaki, M.; Hosoya, N. & Saruhashi, M. (2000). Vitamin E modified cellulose membrane. *Artif Organs.* 24(10):779–89.

Sasaki, M. (2006). Development of vitamin E-modified polysulfone membrane dialyzers. *J Artif Organs.* 9(1):50–60.

Sosa, MA.; Balk, EM.; Lau, J.; Liangos, O.; Balakrishnan, VS.; Madias, NE.; Pereira, BJ. & Jaber, BL. (2006). A systematic review of the effect of the Excebrane dialyser on biomarkers of lipid peroxidation. *Nephrol Dial Transplant.* 21(10):2825–33.

Tarng, DC.; Huang, TP.; Liu, TY.; Chen, HW.; Sung, YJ. & Wei, YH. (2000). Effect of vitamin E-bonded membrane on the 8-hydroxy 2'-deoxyguanosine level in leukocyte DNA of hemodialysis patients. *Kidney Int.* 58(2):790–9.

Tsuruoka, S.; Kawaguchi, A.; Nishiki, K.; Hayasaka, T.; Fukushima, C.; Sugimoto, K.; Saito, T. & Fujimura, A. (2002). Vitamin E-bonded hemodialyzer improves neutrophil function and oxidative stress in patients with end-stage renal failure. *Am J Kidney Dis.* 39(1):127–33.

Usberti, M.; Gerardi, G.; Bufano, G.; Tira, P.; Micheli, A.; Albertini, A.; Floridi, A.; Di Lorenzo, D. & Galli, F. (2002). Effects of erythropoietin and vitamin E-modified membrane on plasma oxidative stress markers and anemia of hemodialyzed patients. *Am J Kidney Dis.* 40(3):590–9.

Westhuyzen, J.; Saltissi, D. & Stanbury, V. (2003). Oxidative stress and erythrocyte integrity in end-stage renal failure patients hemodialysed using a vitamin E-modified membrane. *Ann Clin Lab Sci.* 33(1):3–10.

Yang, CC.; Hsu, SP.; Wu, MS.; Hsu, SM. & Chien, CT. (2006). Effects of vitamin C infusion and vitamin E-coated membrane on hemodialysis-induced oxidative stress. *Kidney Int.* 69(4):706–14.

Yoshida, K.; Kitauchi, T.; Kimura, S.; Yoneda, T.; Uemura, H.; Ozono, S. & Hirao, Y. (2002). Serum neopterin monitoring and vitamin E-modified, regenerated hemodialyzer membrane influence on biocompatibility. *Artif Organs.* 26(1):54–7.

Zaluska, WT.; Ksiazek, A. & Roliski, J. (2001). Effect of vitamin E modified cellulose membrane on human lymphocyte, monocyte, and granulocyte CD11b/CD18 adhesion molecule expression during hemodialysis. *ASAIO J.* 47(6):619–22.